The Interphalangeal Joints

Editorial Advisory Board

Douglas W. Lamb FRCS Chairman
Princess Margaret Rose Orthopaedic Hospital,
Fairmilehead, Edinburgh, UK

Nicholas Barton FRCS
Department of Hand Surgery, University Hospital,
Queen's Medical Centre, Nottingham, UK

W. Bruce Conolly FRCS FRACS FACS
Hand Unit, Sydney Hospital, Macquarie Street,
Sydney, New South Wales, Australia

Lee W. Milford Jr BS MS MD
The Campbell Clinic, Madison Avenue,
Memphis, Tennessee, USA

Volumes in preparation

The Paralysed Hand
Douglas W. Lamb

Unsatisfactory Results in Hand Surgery
R. M. McFarlane

Fractures of the Hand and Wrist
Nicholas Barton

The Thumb
James W. Strickland

Microsurgical Procedures
Viktor E. Meyer and Michael J. M. Black

Joint Replacement in the Upper Limb
William A. Souter

Congenital Malformations of the Hand and Forearm
Dieter Buck-Gramcko

Skin Cover in the Injured Hand
David M. Evans

Dupuytren's Disease
D. A. McGrouther, R. M. McFarlane and M. L. Flint

THE HAND AND UPPER LIMB   Volume 1

The Interphalangeal Joints

EDITED BY
William H. Bowers MS MD
Attending Hand Surgeon,
Memorial Mission Hospital and St. Joseph's Hospital,
Asheville, North Carolina, USA

FOREWORD BY
Lee W. Milford Jr BS MS MD
The Campbell Clinic, Madison Avenue,
Memphis, Tennessee, USA

CHURCHILL LIVINGSTONE
EDINBURGH LONDON MELBOURNE AND NEW YORK 1987

CHURCHILL LIVINGSTONE
Medical Division of Longman Group UK Limited

Distributed in the United States of America by Churchill Livingstone Inc., 1560 Broadway, New York, N.Y. 10036, and by associated companies, branches and representatives throughout the world.

© Longman Group UK Limited 1987

All rights reserved. No part of this publication may be reproduced, stored in a retrieval system, or transmitted in any form or by any means, electronic, mechanical, photocopying, recording or otherwise, without the prior permission of the publishers (Churchill Livingstone, Robert Stevenson House, 1–3 Baxter's Place, Leith Walk, Edinburgh EH1 3AF).

First published 1987

ISBN 0 443 03216 5
ISSN 0269-4743

British Library Cataloguing in Publication Data
The Interphalangeal joints.—(The Hand and
   upper limb, ISSN 0269-4743; v. 1)
   1. Joints—Diseases   2. Hand—Diseases
   3. Wrist—Diseases
   I. Bowers, William H.   II. Series
   617'.575   RC932

Library of Congress Cataloging in Publication Data
The Interphalangeal joints.
   (The Hand and upper limb, ISSN 0269-4743; vol. 1)
   Includes index.
   1. Finger joint—Surgery. 2. Finger joint—Wounds and injuries. 3. Finger joint—Diseases. I. Bowers, William H. II. Series. [DNLM: 1. Finger Joint. WE 835 161]
   RD559.I58   1987   617'.575   86-20701

Typeset by CCC, printed and bound in Great Britain by William Clowes Limited, Beccles and London

Foreword

It may be inconceivable even to most surgeons that the nine interphalangeal joints of the hand justify an entire treatise dedicated to their anatomy and pathology. Yet, the timeliness of this work is obvious when one analyses the uniqueness of this small hand joint.

These comparatively small joints may be compared to the retina of the eye, in that they reflect symptoms of systemic disease and many times are seen as the site of the first symptom of various pathological processes. All major functions of movement of the hand are dependent on these joints.

The movement of the PIP joint is almost entirely in one plane. It is quite tight compared to its more proximal neighbour, the MP joint, with very little lateral tilt or rotation. There is a greater arch of motion ($\pm 125°$) than with any other joint of the hand. It is surrounded almost entirely by the extensor mechanism and, on the flexor surface, it is covered by the flexor tendon and its supporting ligaments. With this arrangement, there is little wonder why it may become stiff from just a little oedema or with a slight irregularity of the articular surface. Its strength is almost a marvel, for with the help of musculotendinous structures it may lift well beyond the person's total body weight without coming apart.

Even if all of the joints of the hand, with the exception of the PIP joint, become quite stiff, it is still capable of creating useful function by pinch against a stable thumb.

The DIP joint is the final regulator of movement of the tip of the fingers. It adjusts the amount of surface of the touch pad of the digit, whether it be to pick up a pen, a pencil, or the handle of a hammer. In concert with this movement is the most sensitive part of the hand, the terminal finger pad.

William H. Bowers has brought together some of the world's greatest authorities to present their knowledge of the intricacies and pathology of these joints. I am not aware of any other place in the literature where all of this information can be found so concentrated.

Memphis, 1987   L.W.M.

Preface

'Trifles make perfection and perfection is no trifle'. This statement by Michaelangelo infers the need and goals for a volume focused on the interphalangeal joints. As Urist has noted, 'nowhere else in the human frame are anatomy and function so interrelated as in these small joints'. Still, to present readers with this concentrated information package, several presumptions have been made. These, in no particular order, are:

1. The interphalangeal joints are of interest to a significant number of hand specialty teams.
2. Problems involving these joints are difficult to manage.
3. These problems are frequent.
4. The morbidity of disorders involving the joints is significant.
5. There is too little known regarding the anatomy and disorders of these joints.
6. A focus for new ideas would be useful.
7. The chapter authors have something to contribute.

I make no apologies for these presumptions; for me, they are perhaps facts. It is my belief that those who reflect on their experience with disorders of these articulations have continual problems with:

1. Over treatment vs. under treatment.
2. Stability (with perhaps stiffness) or motion (with perhaps instability?).
3. Surgery or no surgery.
4. Repair? Reconstruct? Salvage?
5. Primum non nocere!
6. Is there a better way?

Ray Curtis considered the proximal interphalangeal joint to be the 'epicenter' of hand surgery. It is no less. As editor, I had hoped to make this effort all inclusive but, as work progressed, I have found that it has simply expanded the questions beyond our abilities to answer them. At best, this book will be a brick in the wall of experience, being built over many years by many individuals.

Asheville, 1987   W.H.B.

Acknowledgements

I would like to thank Ray Curtis for his stimulus to learn more about these joints. I thank Hans Landsmeer and Cas Kuzinski for the time each has spent teaching me about anatomy. I appreciate the thoughtfulness of Lee Milford and Douglas Lamb, who gave me the chance to undertake this work. I want especially to thank Jim Thompson and Gary Kuzma, my partners, for their encouragement.

The contributors to this volume are a diverse group both in experience and location. Each has demonstrated real concern for the questions to be asked. They have enormous expertise and have given more than I envisioned toward the answers. My appreciation and congratulations go to each of them.

In this book are several unique contributions. Paul Brand has produced a monumental work on the biomechanics of these articulations particularly in regard to their movement in health and disease. It is the most intriguing presentation of finger motion that I have read. Peggy Carter's contribution is a therapist's dream—excellent writing covers the field and the illustrations are outstanding. Shellye Bittinger discusses joint mobilization—a manual art that has had no exposure to date in the field of joint rehabilitation. Spring Harkins Torkelson adds her expertise in the care of the 'splinted finger'. Nicholas Barton, Erik Rosenthal and Rick Honner present trauma in a lucid and stimulating fashion. Joe Imbriglia and Dean Louis have outdone themselves in the area of arthritis. Jim Thompson and Geoff Hooper discuss reconstruction in a detailed and methodical fashion that presents new techniques along with the old. Although often left to other texts, John Varian and Dieter Buck-Gramcko enhance the book with their compilation of congenital and developmental conditions. J. William Littler adds the spice with some new artwork and sage commentary.

The staff of Churchill Livingstone have been very helpful and encouraging over a long distance and a long time.

The office staff of the Asheville Hand Center—particularly Joyce Rice—have responded 'above and beyond' when presented with the myriad challenges of producing this book. My thanks go to each of them.

Finally, Bob Carroll and Shellye Bittinger share my gratitude for their continual inspiration to do more and do it better.

> Good—Better—Best,
> Never let them rest,
> Until your good is better
> And your better best.

W.H.B.

Contributors

Nicholas Barton FRCS
Consultant Hand Surgeon, Nottingham University Hospital and Harlow Wood Orthopaedic Hospital, Nottinghamshire, UK; Civilian Consultant in Hand Surgery to the Royal Air Force, UK

Shellye Bittinger CTR/L BS
Director, Hand Rehabilitation Unit, Memorial Mission Hospital, Asheville, North Carolina, USA

William Hampton Bowers MS MD
Attending Hand Surgeon, Memorial Mission Hospital and St. Joseph's Hospital, Asheville, North Carolina, USA

Paul W. Brand MD MRCS LRCP MB BS FRCS
Chief, Rehabilitation Branch, Gillis W. Long Hansen's Disease Center, Carville, Louisiana; Clinical Professor of Orthopaedics and Surgery, Louisiana State University Medical School, Louisiana, USA

Dieter Buck-Gramcko MD FRCPS
Chief, Department of Hand Surgery and Plastic Surgery, Berufsgenossenschaftliches Unfallkrankenhaus, Hamburg; Associate Professor of Hand Surgery and Plastic Surgery, University of Hamburg Medical School, Hamburg, Federal Republic of Germany

Margaret S. Carter OTR BS
Director, Hand Rehabilitation Unit, Phoenix, Arizona, USA

Richard Honner FRCS FRACS
Hand Surgeon, Royal Prince Alfred Hospital, Sydney, New South Wales, Australia

Geoffrey Hooper MSc FRCS
Senior Lecturer in Orthopaedic Surgery, University of Edinburgh, Edinburgh, UK

Joseph E. Imbriglia MD FACS
Assistant Clinical Professor of Orthopaedic Surgery, University of Pittsburgh, Pittsburgh, Philadelphia, USA

J. W. Littler MD
Attending Surgeon, The St. Luke's-Roosevelt Hospital Center, New York City, New York, USA

Dean S. Louis MD
Professor of Surgery and Chief, Orthopaedic Hand Service, University of Michigan Hospitals, Ann Arbor, Michigan, USA

John Micks MD AAOS ASSH
Assistant Clinical Professor (Retired), University of California at Los Angeles and University of Southern California, California, USA

Erik A. Rosenthal MD
Director, Hand Surgery Service, Baystate Medical Center, Springfield, Massachusetts; Associate Clinical Professor of Orthopaedic Surgery, Tufts University School of Medicine, Boston, Massachusetts; Assistant Clinical Professor of Orthopaedic Surgery, University of Connecticut School of Medicine, Farmington, Connecticut, USA

David E. Thompson BSME MSME PhD
Professor of Mechanical Engineering, Louisiana State University, Baton Rouge, Louisiana; Professor of Orthopaedic Surgery, Louisiana State University School of Medicine, New Orleans, Louisiana, USA

James S. Thompson MD
Assistant Professor of Orthopaedic Surgery, The Johns Hopkins University School of Medicine, Baltimore, Maryland; Director, Hand Clinic, Department of Orthopaedic Surgery, Francis Scott Key Medical Center, Baltimore, Maryland, USA

Spring Harkins Torkelson OTR/L BS
Hand Therapist, Asheville Hand Center, Asheville, North Carolina, USA

John P. W. Varian MA FRCS FRACS
Consultant Hand Surgeon, Blackrock Clinic, Dublin, Eire

Contents

SECTION 1. Anatomy 1

1. The anatomy of the interphalangeal joints 2
   W. H. Bowers
2. Surgical and functional anatomy 14
   J. W. Littler and J. S. Thompson
3. The biomechanics of the interphalangeal joints 21
   P. W. Brand, D. E. Thompson and J. E. Micks

SECTION 2. Repair and Reconstruction of Injury 55

4. Injuries and complications of injuries to the capsular structure of the interphalangeal joints 56
   W. H. Bowers
5. Intra-articular fractures and fracture-dislocations 77
   N. J. Barton
6. Extensor surface injuries at the proximal interphalangeal joint 94
   E. A. Rosenthal
7. Acute and chronic flexor and extensor mechanism injuries at the distal joint 111
   R. Honner

SECTION 3. Arthritis and Arthrosis: Reconstruction 119

8. Rheumatoid and related arthritides of the interphalangeal joints 120
   J. E. Imbriglia

9. Degenerative arthritis and allied conditions involving the interphalangeal joints 142
   Dean S. Louis
10. Interphalangeal joint arthroplasties 156
    J. S. Thompson
11. Techniques of interphalangeal arthrodesis 174
    G. Hooper

SECTION 4. Congenital and Developmental Conditions 187

12. Congenital and developmental conditions 188
    D. Buck-Gramcko
13. Developmental conditions 203
    J. P. W. Varian

SECTION 5. Rehabilitation 211

14. Therapeutic management of the proximal interphalangeal joint 212
    M. S. Carter
15. Splinting the interphalangeal joints 252
    S. Harkins Torkelson
16. The art of joint mobilization: the restoration of joint play 262
    S. Bittinger

Index 269

SECTION 1

Anatomy

W. H. Bowers

1

The anatomy of the interphalangeal joints

INTRODUCTION

The proximal interphalangeal joint has been termed by Ray Curtis as the 'epicentre' of hand surgery. Nowhere in the human frame are anatomy and function so interrelated as in these small joints. These statements correctly emphasize the importance of the interphalangeal joints and their anatomy. The following discussion is from the viewpoint of a functional anatomist and hand surgeon.

OSSEOUS ANATOMY

The interphalangeal joints have been referred to as 'hinge joints'. While generally descriptive, this concept implies a stationary axis with motion perpendicular to the shaft of the phalanges. Another analogy is that of a pulley—with the distalward phalanx sliding around the head of the proximalward phalanx as part of a loop completed by the flexor and extensor tendons (Santos 1968) (Fig. 1.1). This concept allows visualization of the relative motion of the articulating phalanges. The comparison can be furthered in this illustration by considering how lateral stability might be achieved within the mechanical articulating system. The human interphalangeal articulation bears some resemblance to this illustration. The condyles of the proximalward phalanx when viewed end-on do resemble a grooved pulley (trochlea); however, they are, in fact, asymmetric in shape and contour. The distalward articular surface mirrors the bicondylar configuration in its intercondylar ridge and condylar depressions, but the fit is far from fully congruous (Fig. 1.2). Nevertheless, when the two surfaces are held firmly opposed by tension within the musculotendinous system, the articulation possesses good resistance to lateral force, even in the complete absence of capsular support. The *lack of complete congruity* allows movement in planes other than flexion–extension. These movements or displacements of the articulating surfaces are not generated by muscular action, but occur in response to passive stresses generated by power grip (Barnett et al 1961). They may be termed rotation and translation. The asymmetry of the articulation

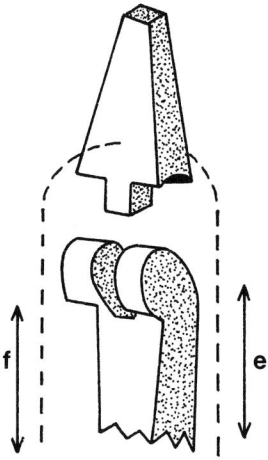

Fig. 1.1 A mechanical representation of interphalangeal joint motion as part of a pulley system. The distalward phalanx is part of a loop completed by flexor (f) and extensor (e) tendons. Lateral stability is obtained by a perfect fit of the tongue and groove plus tension within the loop system. (Redrawn by permission from Kuczynski 1975.)

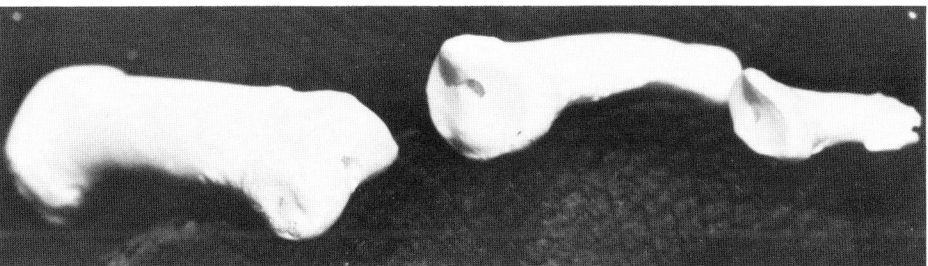

Fig. 1.2 The disarticulated digit shows the condylar depression in the proximal phalanx from which the proper collateral accessing collateral system originates. The various articular facets of the distal face of the proximal interphalangeal joint are clearly seen. The phalangeal perspective dramatizes the size difference between the two joints. (Reproduced by permission from Bowers 1983.)

is apparent when joint motion is analysed. The axis of rotation shifts palmarly (Landsmeer 1955) and is not perpendicular to the longitudinal phalangeal shaft axis. The resulting motion is helicoid. The assembled digits describe convergent arcs in flexion, the tips approaching a common target at the base of the thumb. The non-parallel motion of each articulation coupled with potential translation and rotational displacements allow the digits to adapt to irregular shapes when power grip is applied.

The bicondylar configuration present in each of the eight joints under discussion (four proximal interphalangeal and four distal interphalangeal joints) is unique for each joint. The characteristics have been studied by Kuczynski (1975) and Gigis & Kuczynski (1982) (Fig. 1.3). The general shape of the proximal interphalangeal (PIP) joint condyles viewed end-on is that of a trapezoid with the palmar margin twice that of the dorsal margin. The articular surface extends much further palmarly than dorsally when viewed from the lateral side. This favours flexion. The average contact surface area is 100 mm^2.

At the distal interphalangeal (DIP) joint, the end-on view is less trapezoidal and the articular

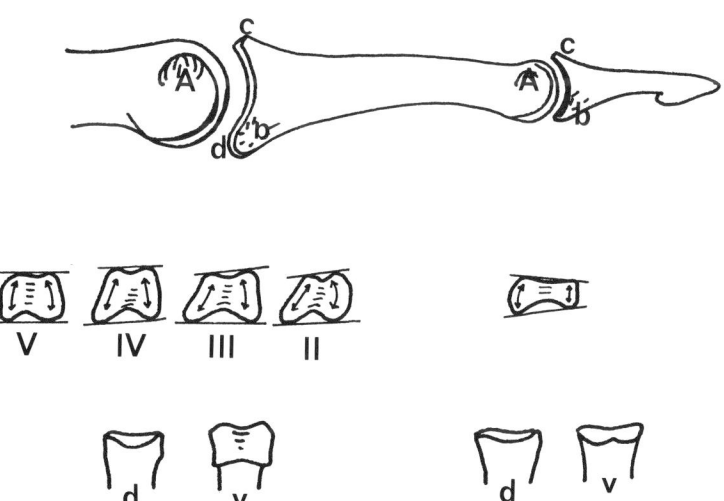

Fig. 1.3 Comparison lateral, end-on, dorsal, and volar drawings of the joint configurations at the proximal and distal interphalangeal joints. The different configurations of the proximal phalangeal condyles II–V are emphasized.
(**a**) Eccentric concavity on lateral condylar face for proximal attachment of collateral system (see also Figs. 1.2 and 1.5). (**b**) Volar lateral tubercles.
(**c**) Insertional areas for extensor apparatus. (**d**) Volar articular facet of distal articular face proximal joint only (see Figs. 1.2 and 1.16). (Portions redrawn with permission from Kuczynski 1968, 1975 and Gigis & Kuczynski 1982.)

4 THE INTERPHALANGEAL JOINTS

surface favours flexion little more than extension. The average articular contact surface area is 40 mm^2, less than half that of the proximal interphalangeal joint. The lateral face of the condyle falls sharply away from the articular margin. On this face is a slightly eccentric concavity from which comes the collateral ligament (Fig. 1.3**a**). On the lateral volar corner of the distalward phalanx of both joints there are prominent tubercles for the attachment of the collateral ligaments (Fig. 1.3**b**). Dorsally, there are distinct lips for insertion of the central slip and the extensor digitorum communis (Fig. 1.3**c**). The attachment area for the central slip is thick and centrally located, while that of the extensor digitorum communis is thin and wide (see Fig. 1.2). Palmarly, there are tubercles on each side of a roughened area where the volar plate (at the PIP joint) and the volar plate and flexor digitorum profundus (at the DIP joint) attach. The distal articular surface of the PIP joint has an articular facet volarly (Fig. 1.3**d**). This surface opposes the meniscal leaf of the volar plate (see below). Its cartilage occasionally wraps completely around onto the palmar surface. At the distal joint, this articular facet is less well developed and there is no significant meniscus of the volar plate.

CAPSULE

Dorsal capsular elements

There is no formal capsular structure dorsal to the collateral ligament system. The extensor mechanism directly covers this area (Fig. 1.4). The deeper layers of the synovial membrane merge with the central slip and its expansion into the lateral bands (see pertinent anatomy in Ch. 6). The large dorsal pouch of synovium blends proximally with the retrocondylar periosteum and the subtendinous areolar tissue proximally and laterally. The synovium then folds over the dorsal margin of the collateral ligament system to cover its deep surfaces (Fig. 1.5).

Lateral capsule

The major element of the lateral capsule is the collateral ligament system. This ligament system

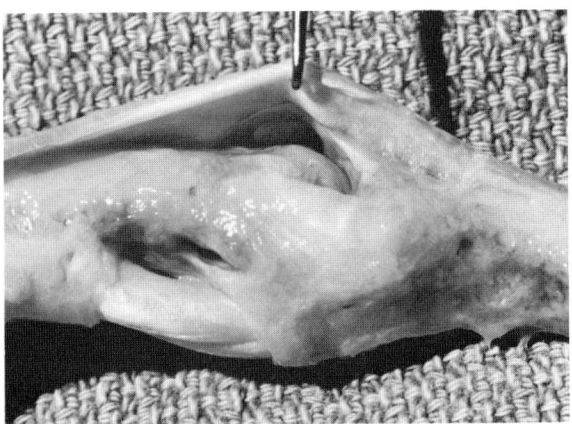

Fig. 1.4 The skin hook lifts the lateral band to show the dorsal capsular space between the central slip insertion and dorsal border of the proper collateral ligament. The proper and accessory collateral systems are shown together. The volar capsular space (retrocondylar recess) can be seen proximal to the accessory collateral ligament and dorsal to the proximal attachment of the volar plate (compare to Figs. 1.5, 1.6 and 1.16).

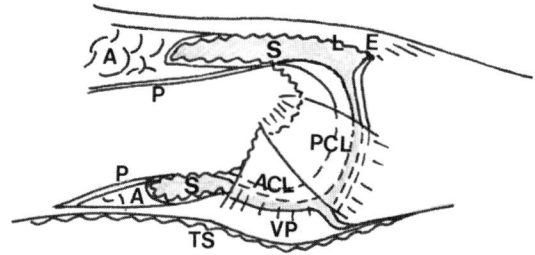

Fig. 1.5 The synovial space at the proximal interphalangeal joint. PCL: proper collateral ligament; ACL: accessory collateral ligament; VP: volar plate; A: areolar tissue; S: synovial space; P: periosteum; L: synovial lining; TS: parietal tenosynovium; E: extensor control slip.

has been considered to have two major components: the thick component which is the major restraint to lateral deviating force is called the proper collateral ligament (PCL), the lateral collateral ligament, or the cord ligament; the remaining element is called the accessory collateral ligament (ACL) or the suspensory ligament. This is volar to the proper collateral ligament. Both ligaments may be seen in their undissected state in Figure 1.4 and illustrated together in Figures 1.5 and 1.16. The proximal attachment of the proper collateral ligament is eccentrically located in the concave area on the lateral face of the proximal condyle (Figs. 1.3**a**, 1.6 and 1.7). The ligament proceeds distally in fan fashion to attach on the entire volar three-quarters of the distalward phalanx—not just on the volar lateral tubercles. Its volarmost fibres share some attachment with the most lateral fibres of the volar plate. This has been termed the 'critical corner', emphasizing its importance as an anatomical area in the stability of the joint.

The distal attachment of the proper collateral ligament is longitudinally extensive. It begins in the epiphyseal area just at the margin of the articular cartilage, but extends well beyond the epiphyseal plate area onto the metaphysis (Bogumil 1983). Some fibres wind around the phalanx volarly and can be traced into the area of the flexor sheath A-4 pulley. The proper collateral ligaments are thick, measuring up to 35% of the total width of the joint (see Fig. 1.9). The volar edge of the proper collateral ligaments blends with the accessory collateral ligament (suspensory ligament of the volar plate). This capsular element is thin and flexible; its fibres continue the volarward fan of the lateral capsule. The origin of the accessory collateral ligament is co-extensive with the proper collateral ligament, but its destination is the lateral margin of the volar plate cupping the wide volar surface of the condylar trapezoid as its fibres tighten in full extension and ballooning as the volar plate slides proximally in flexion. Its intra-articular surface is covered by the synovial membrane of the volar recess (see Fig. 1.5).

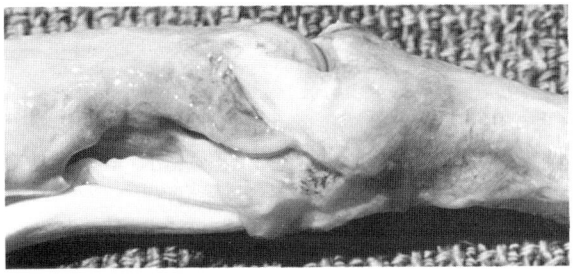

Fig. 1.6 The proper collateral ligament is shown with the joint extended. The extensor apparatus and accessory collateral ligament have been removed. Note the eccentric location of its proximal attachment and the extensive dorso-volar and longitudinal attachment distally. The thickness of the volar plate and its relationship to the A-3 pulley is well shown. (Compare with Figs. 1.4, 1.5 and 1.16.)

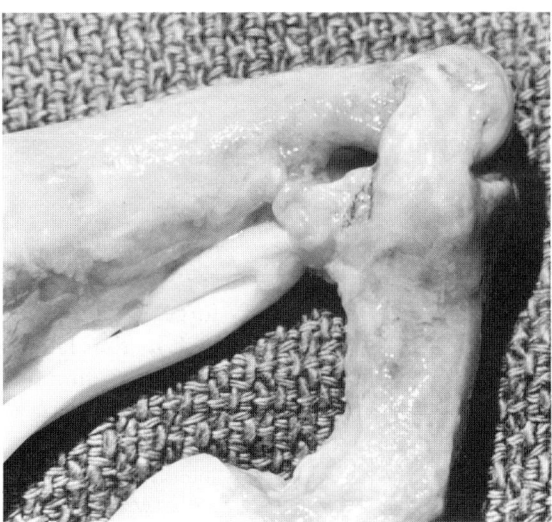

Fig. 1.7 The specimen in Figure 1.6 is now fully flexed to dramatize the eccentric proximal attachment of the proper collateral ligament. Note the torsion developed in its dorsal proximal fibres. Compare the location of the dorsal tubercle with that in Figure 1.6 to appreciate the excursion of the extensor control slip.

Lateral stability and the collateral ligament system

The lateral stability of the interphalangeal joint depends on several factors. These may be considered under the general headings of dynamic and passive stability. Compression of the bicondylar articulation occurs when muscular forces are generated in the digits. The articulation, under these circumstances, possesses a degree of lateral stability even in the total absence of supporting capsular structures. When these muscular forces are resisted, as in grip or pinch, the compressive forces are greatly increased, the joint nearing 'physiological fusion'. Lateral stability increases as long as the compressive forces remain perpendicular to the axis of motion. This element of dynamic stability may be used to advantage when the collateral ligaments must be released or excised in circumstances of capsular contracture (Eaton 1971). This 'dynamic stability' depends on the integrity of the osseous configuration of the joint. If the condylar configuration is violated (displaced condylar fracture, arthritic or tumour disruption of a condyle), the compressive forces are no longer perpendicular to the normal axis of motion. These forces then contribute to *instability*.

Lateral stability conferred on the articulation by the passive capsular system is dependent on the osseous structure as well. The oblique course of the PCL from proximal to distal and the trapezoidal shape of the condyle viewed end-on create an anatomical circumstance such that the joint is extremely stable in flexion (Fig. 1.8). The tension of the PCL increases rapidly as it proceeds volarly over the condylar bulge creating a very tight fit of the joint. In the range from 60° to full flexion, the PCL is thus the major factor in lateral stability—a range in which joint compressive force by longitudinal muscular tension is much less a factor. In terminal extension (as opposed to the 0° position), most of the PCL is somewhat lax and, left to itself, would allow several degrees of instability in response to lateral stress (Fig. 1.9 and see Fig. 1.11). In this position, however, the accessory collateral ligament and volar plate become the major stabilizing elements. The accessory collateral ligament fibres are tightened over the bulges of the condylar flare as the joint becomes fully extended. The suspensory ligament fibres hold the volar plate firmly to the under surface of the joint. When longitudinal tension in the volar plate is fully developed, the combined system provides a capsular cup around the volar hemi-circumference of the joint that has significant resistance to deviating

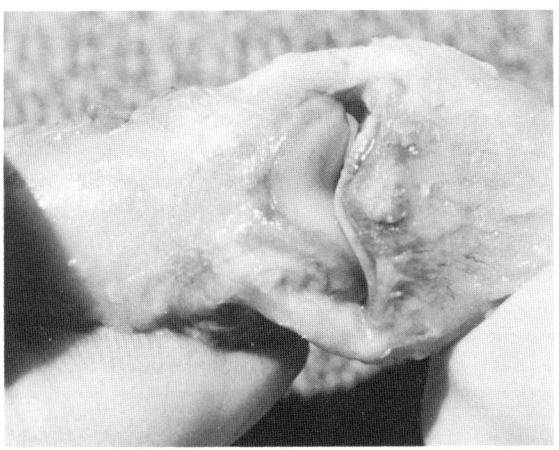

Fig. 1.9 Lateral tilt of the joint permitted by the proper collateral ligament at the zero degree position. In this specimen, the accessory collateral ligament (ACL) and volar plate (VP) have been excised. The same tilt is permitted as the joint is hyperextended, unless the ACL and VP are present. If the VP and ACL are present, the joint becomes fully stable at the position of terminal extension—usually 10–15° of hyperextension. (See Figs. 1.10 and 1.11.)

forces (Fig. 1.10). In addition, the leading fibres of the accessory collateral ligament assume a functional bone-to-bone attachment through the volar plate attachment at the critical corner. This justifies its designation as a ligament. It should be noted that the lower fibres of the proper collateral ligament are also tight in this position and help to stabilize the joint in both the zero position of extension (Stern et al 1985) and in the terminal position of extension.

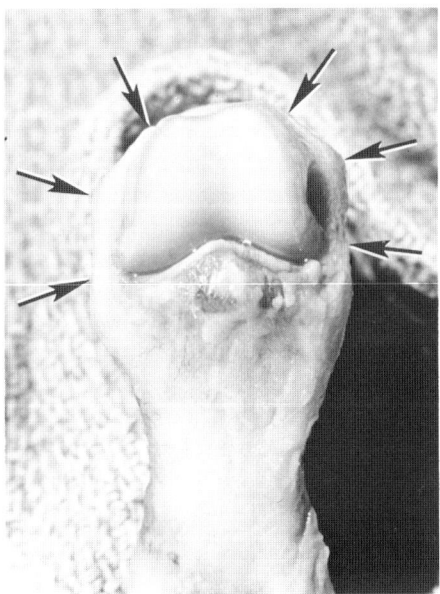

Fig. 1.8 End-on view of the proximal joint flexed to 90°. Note the trapezoidal shape of the condylar cross sections and the tight fit of the joint.

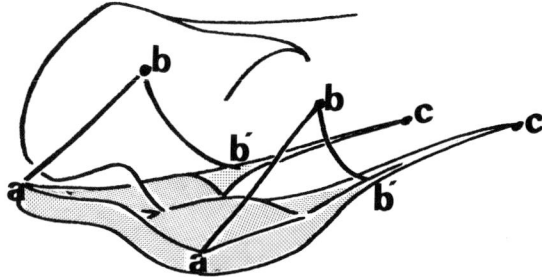

Fig. 1.10 In terminal extension, tension developed along AB, AC and perhaps B, B′, C confers a significant degree of lateral stability at the proximal joint. **a** Volar lateral attachment points of the volar plate to middle phalanx. **b** Attachment of accessory collateral ligament to proximal phalanx. **a–b′** Attachment of accessory collateral ligament to volar plate. **c** Proximal attachment of volar plate via proximal reins (swallow's tails, check reins) to proximal phalanx.

The joint, therefore, is fully stabilized by the proper collateral ligament in flexion greater than 60° and in terminal extension by the accessory collateral ligament–volar plate system. Between these ranges, the joint may have up to 7–8° of lateral tilt before the proper collateral ligament develops enough tension to resist the applied force (Stern et al 1985) (see Fig. 1.11). This arc of relative laxity allows translational and rotational movements to occur (see above). The capsular system, when influenced by oedema or the collagen rearrangement associated with immobilization, will tighten further, creating the tight 'cam-home' condition several degrees short of full extension and well short of full flexion. This reduces the arc of normally allowed motion to the arc of relative capsular laxity, generally from 10° to 60°.

The data in Figure 1.11 were gained by sequential cutting of the capsular elements felt to be important in the lateral stability of the joint. Several points can be made:

1. With all elements intact, the joint was stable (no lateral tilt) in terminal extension. This quickly progressed to a maximum of 7–10° of lateral tilt, then again became fully stable at approximately 75° of flexion
2. When the PCL was completely excised, the joint remained stable in terminal extension. It possessed a reasonable degree of stability up to 15° of flexion (15° lateral tilt). This stability is attributed to the accessory collateral ligament–volar plate system
3. If the volar plate–accessory collateral ligament (ACL) system is excised, leaving the proper collateral ligament intact, the joint did not possess full stability even at 30° of extension, nor did it achieve the same stability as the fully intact system until after 30° of flexion had occurred
4. When the PCL and ACL were excised, leaving only the volar plate, the system was stable at 15° of extension (terminal extension), but rapidly lost this stability as flexion began
5. The area represented by the arrow on the graph may reflect the contribution of the ACL to lateral stability of the joint

Stern et al (1985) studied the failure of the capsular mechanism to lateral stress at the *zero* position of flexion (they did not study the joint in the terminal

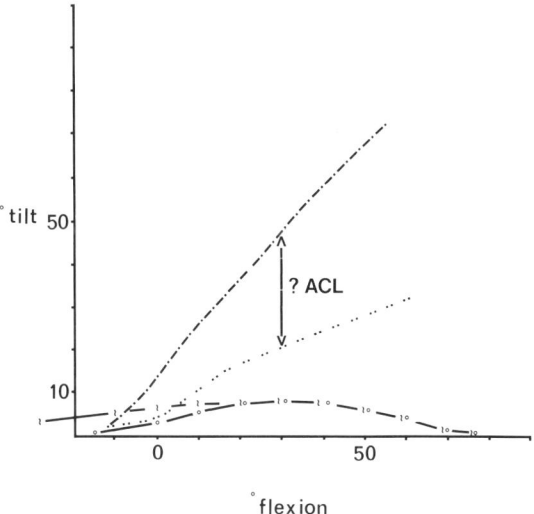

Fig. 1.11 This graph represents the average data obtained from 12 joints. The experiment was designed to estimate the contribution of lateral and volar capsular elements to lateral stability in varying degrees of flexion. The average position of terminal extension was 15°. ʃ–ʃ–ʃ Volar plate (VP), accessory collateral ligament (ACL) excised, proper collateral ligament (PCL) intact; ○–○– all capsular elements intact; · · · · PCL excised, ACL, VP intact; –·–·– PCL, ACL excised, VP intact (see text).

position of extension nor other degrees of flexion). They noted that the major stabilizing element at this position is the PCL. At the zero position, a variable normal laxity of up to 15° (total arc) was observed. As lateral stress is applied and the angulation exceeds its normal laxity, this distal-ward phalanx supinates, such that the oblique course of the PCL becomes straight. This places the PCL in a more effective position to resist the bending moment, and also brings the lateral fibres of the volar plate under tension. Failure of the lateral capsular support is sequential, beginning with rupture of the volar fibres of the PCL and progressing to the more dorsal fibres. Almost always, the failure is from the *proximal* phalanx without fracture. The tear then disrupts the PCL–ACL junction and the volar plate is last to fail at its *distal* margin. The data led Stern et al to conclude that stress testing of the PIP joint at zero degrees could be correlated with degree of injury. At greater than 20°, the PCL was consistently disrupted and the greater the angulation, the greater the likelihood that a displaced PCL would not return to its normal position with reduction of the joint. At less than 20° there was a 47% chance that the PCL was completely disrupted. However, there was also an excellent chance that it would have been found in its proper anatomical position. They concluded that joints demonstrating greater than 20° of angulation on a stress X-ray have a high probability of being improved by exploration, whereas under 20°, the potential for improvement with exploration is less.

Volar capsule

The volar capsule is a complex capsular structure which acts as a static volar restraint limiting interphalangeal extension. It provides a movable floor for the flexor sheath volar to the joint and provides a protected subsheath midline access for vascular feeders to the vincular system. In addition, it may participate in the lateral stability of the joint in terminal extension (see above). The structure is seen in gross dissection (Figs. 1.12**a**, 1.13 and 1.14), histological section (Fig. 1.15) and drawings (Figs. 1.12**b** and 1.16). In the undissected state, these features are blended with other connective tissue elements to provide a smooth, movable transitional floor across the phalangeal condyles and the joint cavity. The intrasheath surface of the volar capsule is covered by parietal tenosynovium while its intra-articular surface is covered by synovial reflections of the volar recess, except immediately subjacent to the condyles themselves, where articular fibrocartilage presents to the volar condylar surface.

The proximal attachment of the volar plates of the proximal interphalangeal joint resembles a swallow's tail, each tail (proximal rein, check ligament) coming firmly from bone just inside the walls of the second annular pulley (A-2) at its distal margin (Figs. 1.12 and 1.14). This proximal volar plate attachment is co-extensive with the proximal attachment of the first cruciate pulley, which straddles the sharp margin of the A-2 pulley (Bowers et al 1980). The limbs of the proximal attachment (swallow's tail) bridge the retrocondylar recess. Through the resulting hiatus, the transverse arterial feeders proceed medially, join, and form the major vincular vessel which then passes volarly through the arch of the swallow's tail to the flexor tendons (Fig. 1.12**a**). Distally, the volar plate is attached strongly, only at its lateral margin on the volar lateral surface of the critical corner (Figs. 1.13 and 1.14). The central 80% is meniscoid and the meniscal leaf faces the articular facet at the base of the distalward phalanx (Figs. 1.15 and 1.16). The attachment of this central portion is by thin extension onto the roughened area of the volar metaphysis under the flexor digitorum superficialis insertion. The meniscal recess, or space adjacent to the articular facet and facing the meniscal portion of the central plate, is well seen in these two figures. The subcondylar portion of the volar plate averages 1.5 mm in thickness and increases the moment arm of the flexors up to 35% over that offered by the condylar radius alone. This may be appreciated by a review of Figures 1.6 and 1.14. Its absence by retraction or excision would affect the joint posture, not only by loss of a static restraint, but also by decreasing the flexion turning moment of the tendons (Bowers et al 1980).

The distal interphalangeal joint volar plate differs from the proximal interphalangeal joint volar plate in several respects. Its proximal portion resembles the swallow's tail structure of the proximal interphalangeal joint, but when these tails are followed serially, in a proximal direction as by Landsmeer (1976), they can be seen to blend into the distalmost fibres of the flexor superficialis and the A-4 pulley walls with no clear insertion into bone (Fig. 1.17). It appears that the flexor superficialis absorbs the swallow's tail-like volar plate anchors. This confluence occurs in the wall and floor of the A-4 pulley area (Fig. 1.18). The volar plate at the distal joint thus has *no* clear attachment to bone (as is present at the PIP joint). Therefore, proximal detachment of the plate is much more likely in response to hyperextension stress (Landsmeer 1976, Gigis & Kuczynski 1982). The boundary of the distal vascular porthole (retrocondylar recess for the distal transverse digital artery) is the A-4 pulley margin, whereas at the proximal interphalangeal joint, the proximal boundary is the swallow's tail insertion into bone. The capsular recess between the meniscal leaf of the volar plate and the volar articular facet is much less distinct at the distal interphalangeal joint than at the proximal one. The flexor superficialis has no attachment whatsoever to the volar plate at the proximal joint, whereas the flexor profundus

THE ANATOMY OF THE INTERPHALANGEAL JOINTS 9

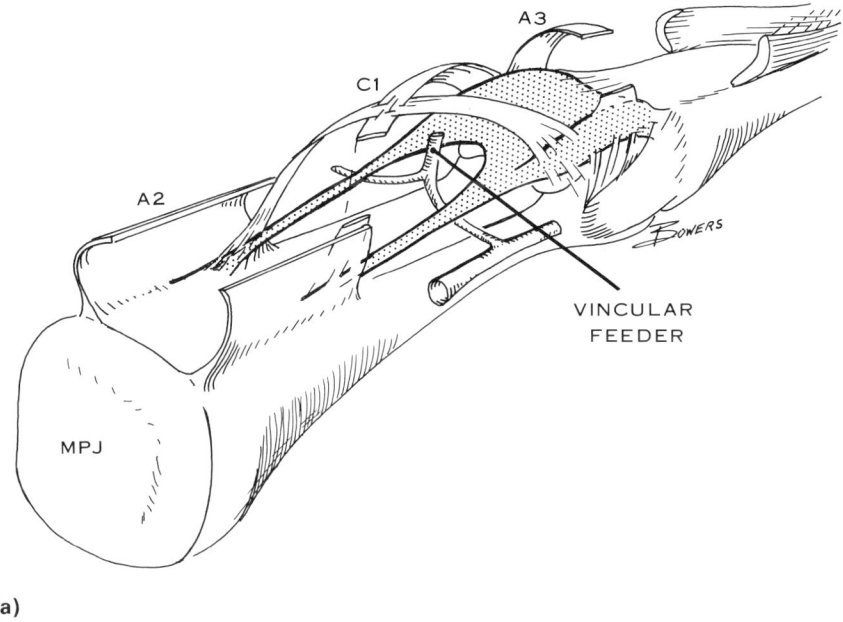

(a)

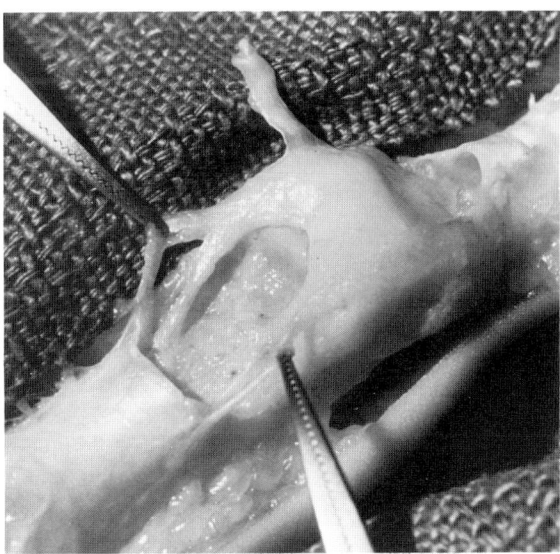

(b)

Fig. 1.12 The proximal interphalangeal joint: oblique volar view of volar plate, collateral ligament, and sheath relationships in (**a**) drawing and (**b**) photograph. Note especially the relationship of the first cruciate pulley (C-1) to the volar plate.

10 THE INTERPHALANGEAL JOINTS

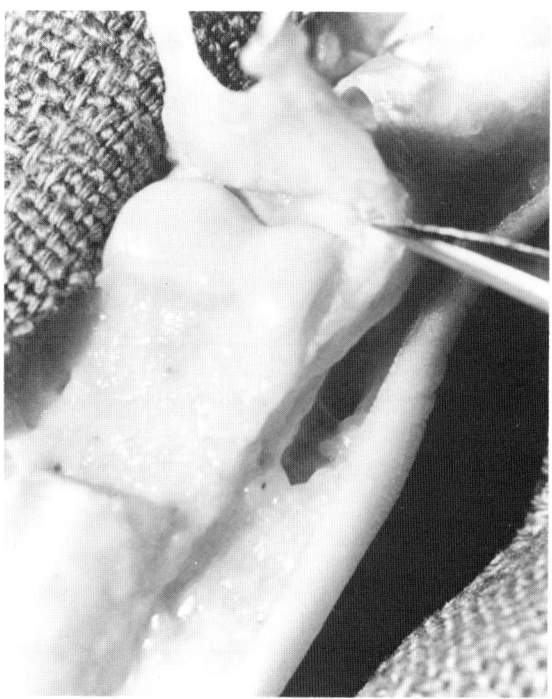

Fig. 1.13 The volar plate has been turned distally and the scissors point at the area where the lateral volar plate and volar fibres of the collateral ligament share attachment. This is termed the 'critical corner'—a reference to its importance in joint stability.

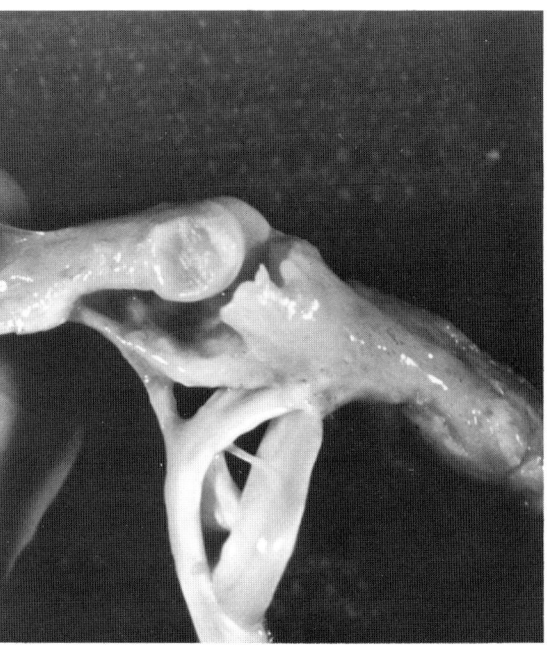

Fig. 1.14 The 'critical corner' attachments of the collateral ligament and volar plate are shown. In addition, the twin tailed proximal attachment of the volar plate and its relationship to the vincular system can be appreciated.

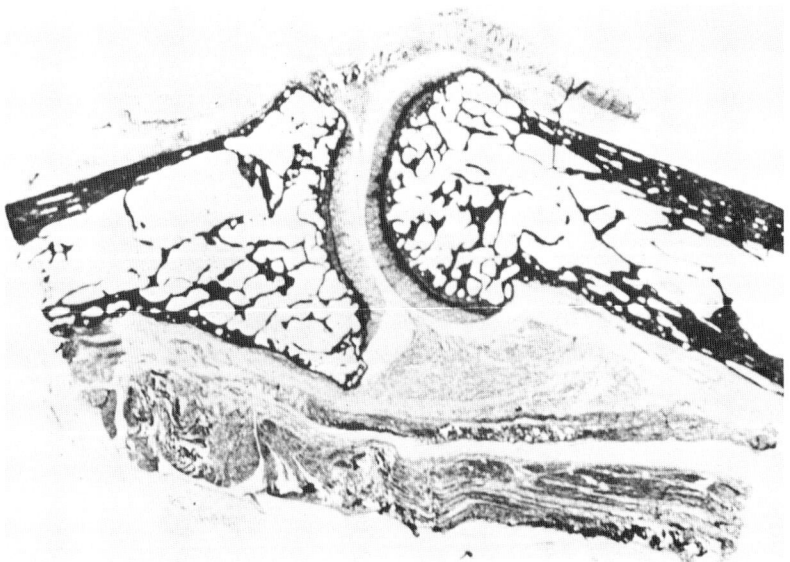

Fig. 1.15 This histological section emphasizes the meniscal recess between the volar plate and volar articular facet of the middle phalanx (MP) at the PIP joint. The structure of the plate and its thin attachment on the volar metaphysis area of the MP is shown (compare with Fig. 1.16). (Reproduced from Eaton, R G Joint injuries of the hand 1971, courtesy Charles C Thomas, Publisher, Springfield, Illinois.)

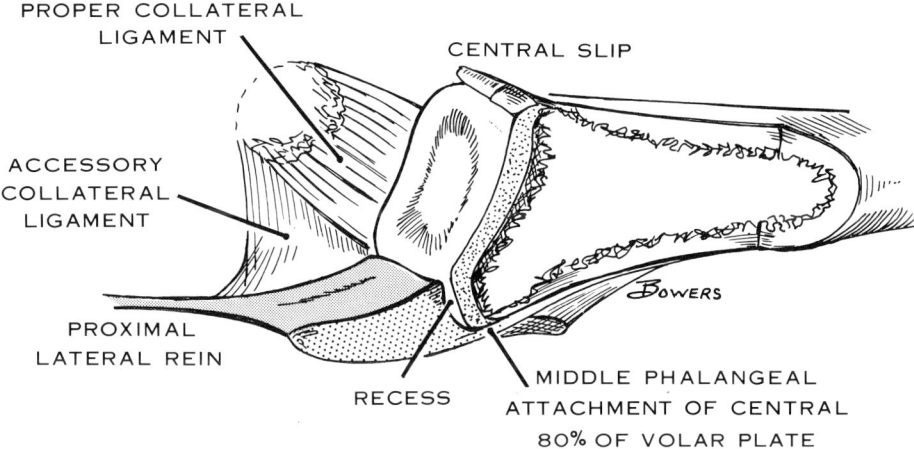

Fig. 1.16 Hemi section of volar plate. In addition to the meniscal recess separating the thick portion of the volar plate (VP) and the volar articular facet, the insertion of the central 80% of the VP on the metaphyses of the middle phalanx is well shown. The 'suspensory' nature of the ACL is depicted (compare with Figs. 1.10 and 1.15).

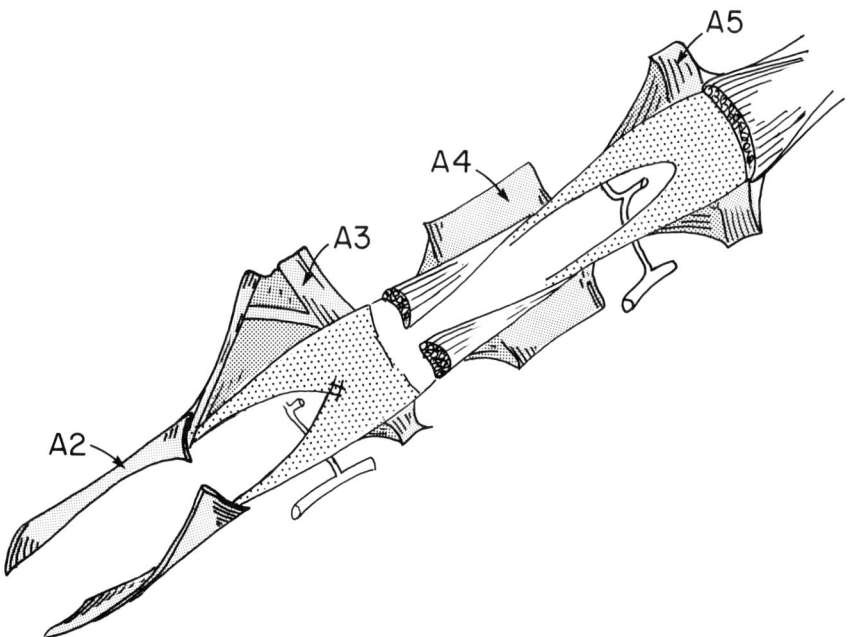

Fig. 1.17 The entire two joint volar plate–flexor sheath relationship is seen face on. (Reproduced with permission of Bowers, 1983.)

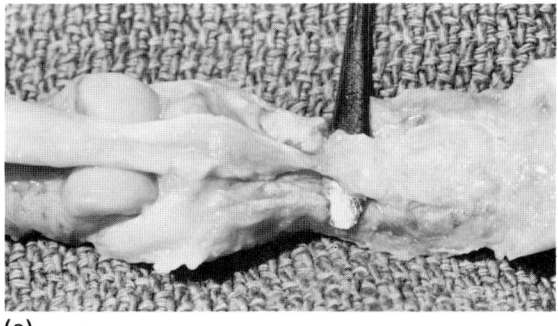

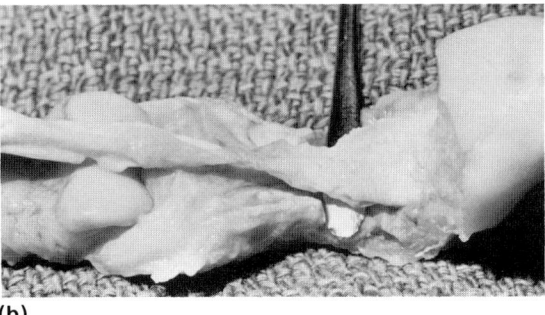

Fig. 1.18 If one dissects the FDS insertion carefully from bone in the floor of the A-4 pulley, it is possible to continue the dissection distally such that the two terminal slips of the FDS seem to flow uninterrupted into the proximal reins of the distal joint volar plate. This provides a specimen such that one can produce distal joint flexion by traction on the FDS—the pull delivered to the DIP by the volar plate. The usefulness of this anatomic potential to convert a middle joint flexor into a terminal joint flexor has not been clinically tested. (**a**) No traction, DIP extended; (**b**) Traction on FDS, terminal joint flexes.

blends completely with the volar plate at the distal joint, fanning over the plate from one of its lateral insertions to the other and extending distally onto its extensive distal phalangeal insertion. The profundus tendon is variable in its division into two slips over the plate.

INNERVATION

Schultz et al (1984) described the capsular innervation of the proximal interphalangeal joint. The joint is innervated by a constant branch that arises from the palmar proximal digital nerve at the level of the middle of the proximal phalanx. This articular branch is accompanied by an arterial articular branch that arises from the digital artery proper at about the same level. The articular nerve adopts a dorso-lateral course, passes superficially to the digital artery, bifurcates near the capsule and enters the PIP joint in a midlateral plane and at the junction of the palmar plate with the capsule. Within the joint capsule, the nerve fibres are initially distributed in bundles located in the lateral and infero-lateral part of the capsule. They then distribute themselves along the lateral capsule across the palmar plate. The nerve fibres are also found in the synovium. No contribution of the innervation of the PIP joint was found to arise from the nerves that provide sensibility to the dorsum of the finger, either as branches of the radial, dorsal cutaneous, or collateral branches of the palmar digital nerve proper. The articular innervation of the PIP joint appears to be congruent with the palmar sensory cutaneous distribution of the finger and has no relationship with the dorsal cutaneous sensory distribution.

SHEATH RELATIONSHIPS

The sheath relationships of the volar capsule may be appreciated by reviewing Figure 1.17. The volar plate structures resemble one another in providing attachment for the A-3 and the A-5 pulleys and in providing a subsheath approach for the vincular feeder vessels. Both volar plates are suspended from the phalangeal condyles by the accessory collateral ligament. The general nature of the 'suspended sheath' concept put forward by Landsmeer (1976) can be appreciated by considering that the third suspended segment is at the metacarpophalangeal joint and A-2 pulley. There is, in fact, a sheath system that resembles a suspension bridge which is held tight to the phalanx only in such areas as the A-2 and the A-4 pulleys. The importance of this concept, of course, transcends the subject of interphalangeal anatomy; however, the present author wishes to point out its interdependent nature with the joint structure.

REFERENCES

Barnett C M, Davies O V, MacConaill M A 1961 Synovial joints, their structure and mechanics. Longmans, London

Bogumil G P 1983 A morphologic study of the relationship of collateral ligaments to growth plates in the digits. Journal of Hand Surgery 8:74–79

Bowers W 1983 Management of small joint injuries in the hand. In: Wilson R L (ed) Orthopedic Clinics of North America. Saunders, Philadelphia, p 793–810

Bowers W, Wolf J W, Nehil J L, Bittinger S 1980 The proximal interphalangeal joint volar plate. I. An anatomical and biomechanical study. Journal of Hand Surgery 5:79–88

Eaton R G 1971 Joint injuries of the hand. Charles C Thomas, Springfield, Illinois, p 15–32

Gigis P I, Kuczynski K 1982 The distal interphalangeal joints of human fingers. Journal of Hand Surgery 7:176–182

Kuczynski K 1968 The proximal interphalangeal joint. Journal of Bone and Joint Surgery 50B:656–663

Kuczynski K 1975 Lesser known aspects of the proximal interphalangeal joints of the human hand. The Hand 7:31–34

Landsmeer J M F 1955 Anatomical and functional investigation on the articulations of the human finger. Acta Anatomica 25 (suppl 24):p 1–69

Landsmeer J M F 1976 Atlas of anatomy of the hand. Churchill Livingstone, Edinburgh p 189–199, p 239–249

Santos L 1968 Rôle du jeu agoniste—antagoniste dans l'analyse vectorielle de l'action musculaire pendant la flexion. Comptes rendus de l'Association des Anatomistes 52:1085–1087

Schultz R J, Krishnamurthy S, Johnston A D 1984 A gross anatomic and histologic study of the innervation of the proximal interphalangeal joint. Journal of Hand Surgery 9A:670–674

Stern P J, Kiefhaber T R, Grood E S 1985 Lateral stability of the proximal interphalangeal joint. (Presented at the American Society of Surgery of the Hand Las Vegas 1985). Journal of Hand Surgery (in press)

J. W. Littler and J. S. Thompson

2

Surgical and functional anatomy

'The book of Nature is written in characters of geometry'

GALILEO

INTRODUCTION

The classical anatomy of the interphalangeal joints has been beautifully presented in the preceding chapter. The purpose of this chapter is to introduce selected anatomy and geometrical concepts of interphalangeal joint function in the normal and disabled digit. The chapter is not meant to be comprehensive, but rather to highlight certain aspects of interphalangeal function that, in the present authors' opinion, deserve emphasis. Disturbed anatomical components that frequently result in interphalangeal dysfunction will also be discussed. These aims will allow a brief discussion of both functional and anatomical features, plus a review of the rationale and philosophy influencing surgical treatment of the interphalangeal joint structures. The functional contingency of the distal joint upon that of the proximal one will also be emphasized.

It is important to consider the proximal interphalangeal joint as a prime anatomical and functional region rather than simply an articulation. The transitional movement of soft tissues, in many instances, may be more important than the static normal osseous or articular anatomy. (See Ch. 3 for expansion of this concept.) Interphalangeal joint movement (so critical to finger function) is exquisitely sensitive to alterations in the elastic and gliding characteristics of the surrounding soft tissue components. Reconstructive surgery (controlled trauma) of the interphalangeal joint structures should be conceived and executed in a manner offering the greatest potential for improvement with the least possible dissection. Intact soft tissue anatomy that must be traversed or displaced during reconstruction, must be guarded by the utmost atraumatic technique in an attempt to prevent any loss of interphalangeal joint excursion. The ideal surgical solution is one that corrects the pathoanatomy with the least disturbance to the normal anatomy. This ideal is not always possible.

FLEXION–EXTENSION ARC

The importance of normal function of the interphalangeal joints, especially the proximal one, cannot be overemphasized. The metacarpo-interphalangeal flexion–extension curve (Fig. 2.1), executing an equiangular spiral, is the basis of adaptability of the human hand (Littler 1973). This universal grasp ability is markedly altered by any limitation of interphalangeal joint movement. Examination of the flexion–extension path reveals that it is divided into two distinct components: (1) the metacarpo-phalangeal (MP)—tip (pulp) placement arc; and (2) final or total encompassment. The placement arc is formed by full metacarpophalangeal extension and flexion (Fig. 2.1). The placement arc is that component of the curve lost with absence of extrinsic extensors and intrinsic MP flexors, i.e. complete radial nerve palsy. Final or total encompassment is that vital component of the curve dependent upon extrinsic

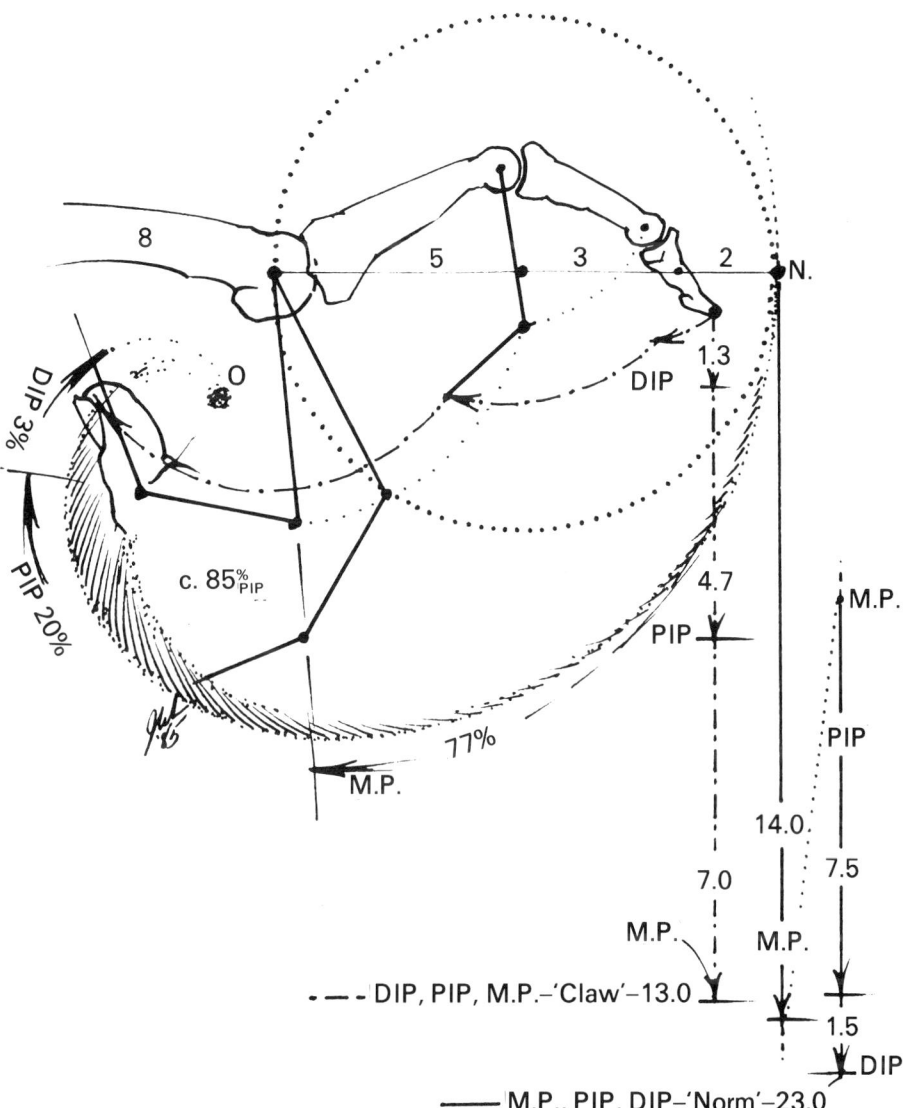

Fig. 2.1 Composite figure illustrating (1) the flexion–extension spiral arc. (2) The skeletal lengths of the phalangeal segments (closely corresponding to the ratio 1/1.618—(the golden mean), approximated by the Fibonacci series.) (3) The axis of PIP rotation as the centre of the digit (dotted circle). (4) Comparative finger tip evolute pathway lengths of the normal (N) and claw hand (———: normal pathway; ·—·—·—: Claw pathway). Total evolute lengths: 23.0—normal, 13.0—claw. Without the stabilizing force of MP flexors (i.e. intrinsic muscle paralysis) the MP joints hyperextend and the IP joints rest in the variable degrees of flexion (loss of intrinsic interphalangeal extension force). Interphalangeal extension is lost and no effective phalangeal grasp (encompassment) is possible. The claw pathway is simply that provided by possible MP flexion–extension. Normal finger extension–flexion allows the greatest area of encompassment with the MP, PIP and DIP joints flexing progressively through an equiangular pathway from full finger length to full closure at the distal palmar crease. (5) Relative areas provided by individual joint flexion are illustrated: MP = 77% flexion by intrinsics or 'intrinsic' flexion; PIP = 20% flexion by extrinsic flexors; or DIP = 3% 'extrinsic' flexion. The 77% of the total encompassment provided by MP flexion is the placement arc. The 23% of total encompassment area provided by IP flexion is the vitally important final encompassment. The PIP joint contributes 85% of the final encompassment. (It is obvious that this most important functional range should not be jeopardized by attempts to restore DIP flexion which represents only 15% of final encompassment. 0 = polar axis of the normal flexion–extension spiral pathway.

16 THE INTERPHALANGEAL JOINTS

interphalangeal flexion (Fig. 2.1). If final extrinsic encompassment is analysed, it is found that the proximal interphalangeal (PIP) joint contributes 85% and the distal interphalangeal (DIP) joint 15% (Fig. 2.1). Therefore, in terms of functional limitations with interphalangeal restriction, the PIP joint is the critical finger joint.

An excellent clinical illustration of this fact is the effect of arthrodesis of the PIP joint on the flexion–extension path. PIP arthrodesis, although a satisfactory solution in some cases where pain relief and stability are desired, is not a functional solution when adaptability is the goal. However, even though the 15% of final encompassment that results from the DIP range of motion remains important, complete loss of the DIP range of motion (such as surgical arthrodesis in proper position) will result in a satisfactory digit, as long as the PIP range of motion is normal. Therefore, a surgeon contemplating a procedure to improve the DIP range of motion must be acutely aware of the possible PIP jeopardy involved. Loss of the PIP range of motion is an unacceptably high price to pay for any significant gain at the DIP level. A prime and tragic clinical example of this (still frequently encountered) is the failed primary flexor tendon repair distal to the flexor digitorum superficialis (FDS) insertion or the failed flexor tendon graft in a digit with an intact FDS and full preoperative PIP range of motion.

STRUCTURAL RELATIONSHIPS

Interaxial finger length (MP joint to centre of finger pulp) approximates a unit of ten in accord with the Fibonacci series of 2, 3, 5*. This sequence of numbers progresses at a ratio of 1:1.618 from each number to the next (each number is the sum of the previous two numbers). Therefore from distal to proximal, each interaxial length is the sum of the previous two bone lengths. Thus, the length of the proximal phalanx approximates the sum of the lengths of the middle and distal phalanges (Figs. 2.1 and 2.2). The PIP joint axis resides exactly at the mathematical centre of the finger

* After the discovery by Leonardo da Pisa (1202 AD) of the numerical series: 0, 1, 1, 2, 3, 5, 8, 13, 21, 34, ... (Fibonacci, son of Bonacci).

(Fig. 2.2) and is the anatomical and functional locus of finger function. PIP joint structure, location, and critical geometric contribution to the equiangular spiral combine to make it the nucleus of finger anatomy and function.

Use of the Fibonacci series allows a simple calculation of normal phalangeal or metacarpal bone length, if the length of any one bone in the series is known. The metacarpal length is the sum of the lengths of the proximal and middle phalanges or 1.618 times the proximal phalangeal length. Clinically, this understanding can be extremely useful in determining the amount of bone lengthening or shortening to achieve proper anatomical relationships, i.e. correction of congenital or traumatic metacarpal or phalangeal shortening. It is

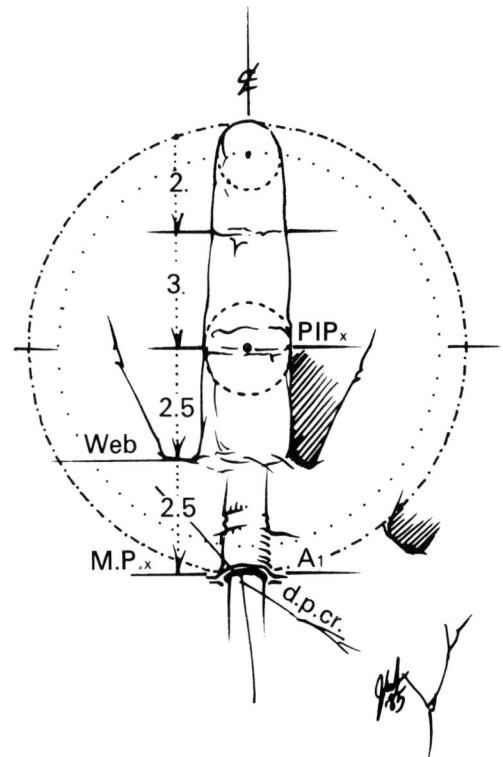

Fig. 2.2 Mathematical relationships of phalanges and web. The distal palmar web is located directly at the midpoint of the proximal phalanx, one quarter of the finger length proximal to the PIP joint. The PIP axis of rotation (PIPx) is the anatomical and functional centre of the finger. The interaxial phalangeal lengths follow the Fibonacci series 2, 3, 5, ... It is interesting that the proximal edge of the A_1 pulley can be located at one-half the total finger length proximal to the PIP joint. This level corresponds with the MP axis of rotation (MPx). d.p.cr.: distal palmar crease.

also of some clinical interest that the level of the finger skin webs lies directly at the midpoint of the proximal phalanges (Fig. 2.2). This small piece of anatomical mathematics may be useful in situations requiring reconstruction and placement of web spaces, i.e. syndactyly or burns.

THE VOLAR PLATE

The volar plate represents an extremely important tethering structure influencing both functional and surgical anatomy of the interphalangeal joints. Although a static structure, it has great influence on the dynamics of interphalangeal balance. The contribution of the volar plate in preventing interphalangeal hyperextension and the maintenance of proper function of the extensor mechanism is not always appreciated.

With its restraining tether into the flexor sheath and periosteum (Littler 1960, Bowers et al 1980), the volar plate provides powerful resistance to the final stress of interphalangeal extension. The extrinsic finger extensors, inserting primarily on the dorsal tubercle of the middle phalanx, exert powerful stress on the volar plate/check ligament system in final extension. If that system becomes incompetent, recurvature of the PIP joint will occur with resultant imbalance of finger dynamics.

In each of the classic finger deformities, i.e. the boutonnière and the swan neck, the volar plates are involved. In the boutonnière deformity, the volar plate of the DIP joint under lateral band extensor stress becomes increasingly insufficient and the terminal phalanx progressively hyperextended. In the swan neck deformity, laxity of the volar plate at the PIP level allows progressive PIP hyperextension followed by compensatory DIP flexion, secondary to dorsally displaced relaxed lateral bands plus increased flexor profundus tendon tension.

The volar plate restraint system functions at both levels (PIP and DIP) and represents a structure of prime importance in finger function and balance. In general, the interphalangeal volar plate tends to be stronger at the PIP level than at the distal joint. Also, in some individuals, there is greater passive hyperextension for the interphalangeal joints and, in these fingers, the volar plate may play an even more important role since less trauma is necessary to produce a functionally disabling abnormality of finger balance. An example of this situation would be a patient with 20° of passive PIP joint hyperextension, who sustained a hyperextension injury of the joint. This patient might be a more likely candidate to develop a locking swan neck deformity than a patient with tighter volar plates at the PIP joint limiting extension only to the neutral position.

Eaton & Malerich (1980) have clearly shown that the volar plate can be a satisfactory structure when advanced for soft tissue biological arthroplasty of the PIP joint in intra-articular fracture/dislocation of the volar base of the middle phalanx.

THE RETROCONDYLAR SPACE

The PIP retrocondylar space represents an anatomical area of extreme importance. It is in this space that the major vincular systems (brevum and longum) to the superficial and deep flexor tendons originate (Bowers et al 1980, Eaton 1971). The neurovascular supply of the tendons passes collaterally beneath the check ligaments of the volar plate and enters the vinculum brevum in the retrocondylar space. Any disruption in this region, causing scarring dorsal to the flexor digitorum superficialis (FDS) tendon in the retrocondylar space, may lead to a severe flexion contracture of the PIP joint (North & Littler 1980). The retrocondylar spaces of both interphalangeal joints are often the site of extension of giant cell tumours of the tendon sheath (xanthomas) originating either from the vinculum, flexor sheath or the intra-articular synovium (Moore et al 1984). This tumour may extend beneath the check ligaments of the volar plate and cause pressure necrosis of the phalanx. Occasionally in these cases, the intra-articular tumour extension from the retrocondylar space will necessitate resection of the joint and arthrodesis.

Any damage to the FDS tendon or its removal in the area of the retrocondylar space will greatly increase the likelihood of an extremely difficult proximal interphalangeal flexion contracture (North & Littler 1980). In primary flexor tendon

18 THE INTERPHALANGEAL JOINTS

surgery, it is prudent to repair the FDS at this level to restore its continuity and not allow a stump of the superficialis to become tethered across the PIP joint. In secondary surgery, however, if a lacerated stump of FDS spans the joint but imposes no extension restraint, it should be left in place. A tendon graft can be performed in the presence of that dorsally lying tendon which now acts as volar plate augmentation. If a tendon graft has been done in the absence of an active FDS, the characteristic position of the finger is slight recurvature at the PIP joint. This can be prevented by simply leaving the stump of the superficialis in place at the PIP joint to act as further resistance to any possible hyperextension deformity at the end of extension (North & Littler 1980). This PIP hyperextension restraint permits the extensor tendons to act more effectively on the terminal phalanx.

OBLIQUE RETINACULAR LIGAMENT

The oblique retinacular ligament (ORL) (Landsmeer 1949) is a variable and underemphasized anatomical structure which, in certain instances, may have a profound influence on the interphalangeal range of motion (Littler 1966). The ORL (Figs 2.3 and 2.4) originates volar to the PIP axis of rotation from the proximal phalanx and flexor sheath and passes dorsally and distally to join the terminal extensor tendon (Shrewsbury & Johnson 1977, Milford 1968). The ORL may act as a dynamic tenodesis assisting in DIP extension as the PIP joint is extended and relaxing with PIP flexion to allow full DIP flexion (Haines 1951, Eyler & Markee 1954, Zancolli 1979). PIP extension, the key to action of the ORL, is initiated by the long extensor acting principally to extend the PIP joint which tenses the ORL, assisting DIP

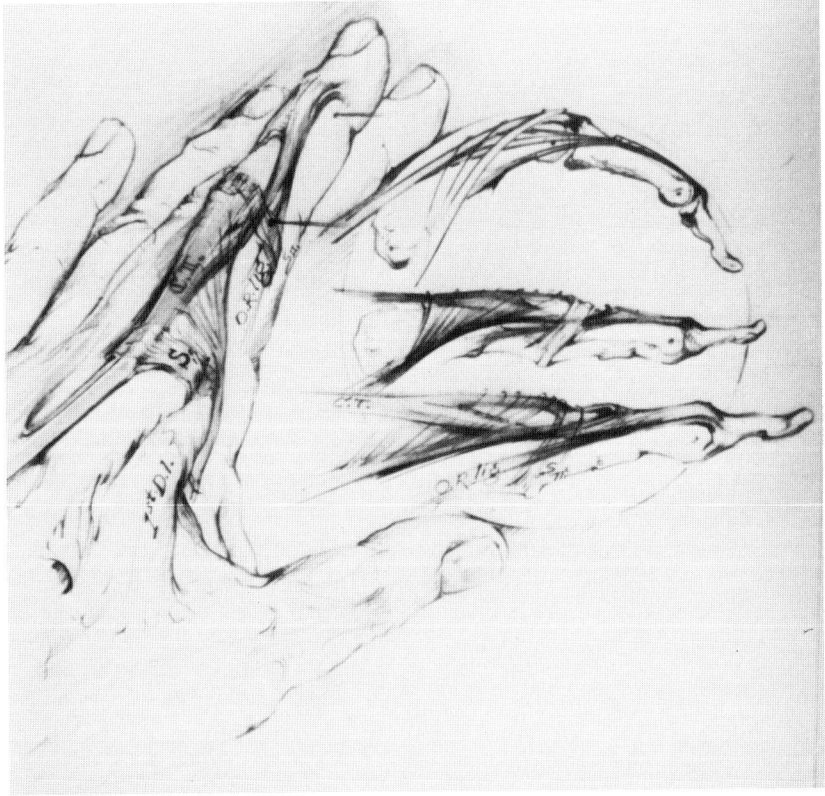

Fig. 2.3 Relationship of the extensor mechanism to the oblique retinacular ligament (O.R. lig.). The oblique retinacular ligament tenses with PIP extension to assist DIP extension and relaxes with PIP flexion to allow complete DIP flexion. C.T. = central extensor tendon; S = sagittal fibres at MP joint. 1st D.I. = first dorsal interosseus; l = lumbrical.

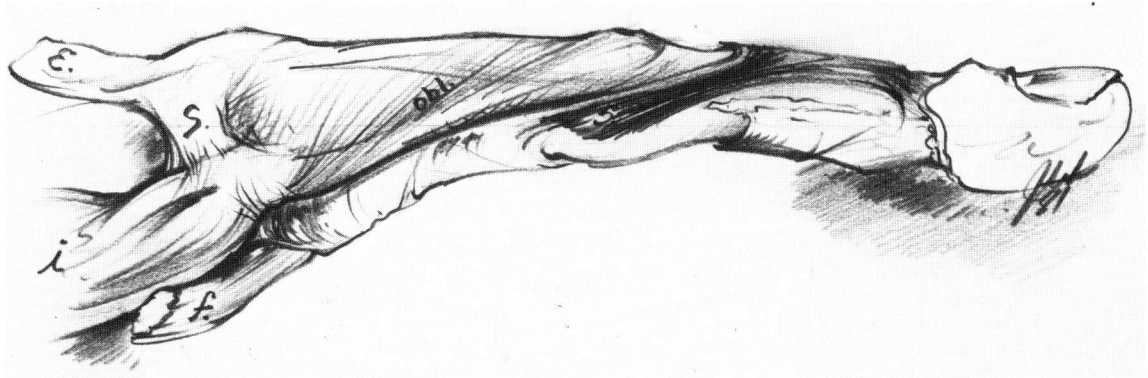

Fig. 2.4 The oblique retinacular ligament (ORL) is labelled no. 5. This figure is redrawn from Walsh (1897) who described the ORL as 'Lateral edge of the tendon of the common extensor; ... is also joined by a process of filaments (5) coming from a bony ridge on the lateral aspect of the shaft of the first phalanx, just below its articulating surface.'

extension which is completed as the lateral bands rise dorsally and finally reach the same tension as the central extensor tendon itself (Fig. 2.3).

Contracture of the ORL can be seen in Dupuytren's contracture, contributing to the boutonnière deformity occasionally seen in severe digital Dupuytren's contracture, especially in the little finger (Littler 1966). The tightness of the ORL can be tested by checking the resistance to passive flexion at the DIP joint in PIP flexion and then PIP extension. A marked increase in resistance to passive DIP flexion with the PIP in the extended position indicates abnormal tightness of the ORL (retinacular plus finger). ORL tightness may occur after trauma and may present as limited DIP flexion. It should be kept in mind when one evaluates a finger for a decreased interphalangeal range of motion.

Understanding the anatomy and dynamics of the ORL has contributed to the successful reconstruction of this anatomical structure for interphalangeal deformities (Thompson et al 1978, Kleinman & Peterson 1984).

This chapter has been a brief exposition of several rather underemphasized concepts and anatomical entities which should be recognized by hand surgeons as important in the understanding of the interphalangeal joints. Successful restoration of a painless stable range of motion in the interphalangeal joints remains one of the most difficult surgical challenges. The difficulties encountered are well known to hand surgeons and, indeed, have contributed to the development of hand surgery as a speciality. The importance of preservation of motion at these critical articulations cannot be overstressed.

REFERENCES

Bowers W H, Wolf J J, Nehil J L, Bittinger S 1980 The proximal interphalangeal joint volar plate. I. An anatomical and biomechanical study. The Journal of Hand Surgery 5: 79–88

Eaton R G 1971 Joint injuries of the hand. Charles C Thomas, Springfield, p 15–32

Eaton R G, Malerich M M 1980 Volar plate arthroplasty of the proximal interphalangeal joint: A review of ten years' experience. The Journal of Hand Surgery 5: 260–268

Eyler D L, Markee J E 1954 The anatomy and function of the intrinsic musculature of the fingers. The Journal of Bone and Joint Surgery 36A: 1–9

Haines R A 1951 The extensor apparatus of the finger. Journal of Anatomy 85: 251–259

Kleinman W B, Peterson D P 1984 Oblique retinacular ligament reconstruction for chronic mallet finger deformity. The Journal of Hand Surgery 9A: 399–404

Landsmeer J M F 1949 The anatomy of the dorsal aponeurosis of the human finger and its functional significance. Anatomical Record 104: 31–44

Littler J W 1960 The physiology and dynamic function of the hand. Surgical Clinics of North America 40: 259–266

Littler J W 1966 Restoration of the oblique retinacular ligament for correcting hyperextension deformity of the proximal interphalangeal joint. GEM L'Expansion Editeur no 1: 39–42

Littler J W 1973 On the adaptability of man's hand (with reference to the equiangular curve). The Hand 5: 187–191

Milford L W Jr 1968 Retaining ligaments of the digits of the hand. Gross and microscopic anatomic study. W B Saunders Co, Philadelphia, p 23

Moore J R, Weiland A J, Curtis R M 1984 Localized nodular tenosynovitis: experience with 115 cases. The Journal of Hand Surgery 9A: 412–417

North E R, Littler J W 1980 Transferring the flexor superficialis tendon: technical considerations in the prevention of proximal interphalangeal joint disability. The Journal of Hand Surgery 5: 498–501

Shrewsbury M M, Johnson R K 1977 A systematic study of the oblique retinacular ligament of the human finger: its structure and function. The Journal of Hand Surgery 2: 194–199

Thompson J S, Littler J W, Upton J 1978 The spiral oblique retinacular ligament (SORL). The Journal of Hand Surgery 3: 482–487

Walsh J F 1897 The anatomy and functions of the muscles of the hand (and extensor tendons of the thumb). Charles H Walsh, Philadelphia

Zancolli E 1979 Structural and dynamic bases of hand surgery. 2nd edn. J B Lippincott, Philadelphia, p 45–51

P. W. Brand, D. E. Thompson and J. E. Micks

3

The biomechanics of the interphalangeal joints

INTRODUCTION

The complexity of the human hand as a mechanical device becomes evident when one realizes the many components that must be described in engineering terms. Some of these components are the phalanges and their internal structures, the tension in the tendon apparatus, the viscoelastic properties of the joint capsules, the tendons and their sheaths, the skin, scar tissue, the sensory and motor nervous system, and many others. Biomedical engineers are wont to gather all the analytical information available, use it to define mathematical models, encode these into a computer, preferably in conjunction with an interactive graphics simulation, vary the parameters in the models, and 'answer' all the questions. It must be remembered that at times assumptions used to produce a mathematical model will oversimplify a complex problem, limiting the model's usefulness in some clinical situations.

This is a challenging analytical problem that is compounded by the complexity of living systems having redundant controls and multivariable interdependence. For example, in the static analysis of the human hand, questions about the proximal interphalangeal (PIP) joint cannot be answered without considering the distal interphalangeal (DIP) joint, the metacarpophalangeal (MP) joint, and in some cases the wrist joint. Each of these joints is, in turn, dependent on the others as well as the non-linear properties of the biological materials that one finds in human hands. In spite of the difficulties of this approach, it is in the language of the mathematician that information can be properly preserved and new knowledge and understandings shared.

Description of the interphalangeal joints

The interphalangeal (IP) joints of the fingers are the terminal links of a kinematic chain of which the MP joint is a key element. It is possible to describe the anatomy of each interphalangeal joint on its own and to summarize its individual movements and limitations. However, the active biomechanical function of the IP joints cannot be described or understood in isolation from the metacarpophalangeal joint. The position of the fingers, the mechanics of application and dissipation of load, and the mechanics of the muscles relating to the IP joints are all directly affected by the MP joint.

The term kinematic chain refers to a sequence of articulating solid members, like the phalanges. A closed chain refers to a sequence whose starting and ending member are the same. Thus, the forefinger and thumb form a closed kinematic chain when they meet at their tips in a pinch, with the bones of the carpals and metacarpals helping to close the chain. The chain is also closed during the grasping of a solid object. A general rule for kinematic chains is that open chains are inherently unstable, and closed chains are marginally stable. Such chains may be analysed either in equilibrium situations, a 'static' analysis, or in non-equilibrium, a 'dynamic' analysis. Because the natural movements of human hands and their digits are so slow, the inertial effects are usually felt to be negligible, allowing one to assume a static analysis.

When contemplating the terms force and torque, one must think of the tension in a tendon as a force. The effect it has on a joint, however, is to produce a moment (torque) that is the product of the force (tension) in the tendon and the moment arm through which it acts. The moment arm is the shortest distance between the tendon and the axis of rotation of the joint. Generally, the moment arms change with the degree of articulation of the joints. The magnitude of the angular change may be expressed in degrees or in radians. This unit of angular change is the circular arc subtended when a disc is rolled on edge for a distance equal to one-half of its diameter (Fig. 3.1). There are approximately 60° in one radian.

AN ANALYSIS OF THE FORCES, MOTIONS, AND TORQUES AT THE IP JOINTS

When analysing the forces in a finger (where a chain of phalangeal segments are joined end to end) a tendon exerts the same force at each of the joints, even though it attaches only to the distal segment (see p. 24: Analysis of flexion–extension moment). This concept applies to a body in which forces are being applied to both the flexor and extensor sides. Ketchum et al (1978) included this concept in discussing the participation of the extrinsic flexor muscles in the forces across the MP joint.

A physical analogue model was constructed to show that a series of joints will react according to the extensor–flexor moment ratios even though there is no tendinous attachment to the intermediate segments. This model was not constructed as a functional replica of the human finger but only to illustrate this concept (Fig. 3.2). Three bone segments were represented, joined by two single axis hinge joints. Each joint was supplied with two pulleys, one twice the diameter of the other. This, in effect creates two moment arms (levers), one twice the size of the other. Two strings were attached only to the most distal segment, one at the top and one at the bottom, and then carried over the distal and proximal pulleys. A weight was then attached to the flexor string. In the model, the flexor weight has an equalizing effect on the flexor force across the two joints. Otherwise, gravity alone imposes a much greater force at the proximal joint. This model provided a direct mechanism for studying the balance of motion and torques of the phalanges.

When applying a force to the extensor using the largest proximal pulley and the smallest distal pulley, the central segment extended to its constraint prior to any movement of the distal segment. If the extensor was placed on the small proximal pulley and the large distal pulley, then the distal segment extended to its constraint before extension of the central segment began. This relates directly to the effects of the extensor on the phalanges whenever the moment arms change relative to one another.

Balancing of moments between the MP and PIP joints

In the intrinsic minus finger, moment ratios favour extension at the MP joint over extension of the IP joints. Therefore, the equilibrium of the three concurrent forces is reached before the IP joints can be fully extended. This claw configuration can be overcome and the moment ratios equalized by including the intrinsics which supplement primarily the flexor moment at the MP joint (Flatt 1961, Landsmeer 1976) (Fig. 3.3). Since in the unloaded hand the interossei do not fire either in extension or flexion, one must attribute their balancing effect in this condition to their viscoelastic force. The lumbricals function primarily to stabilize the MP

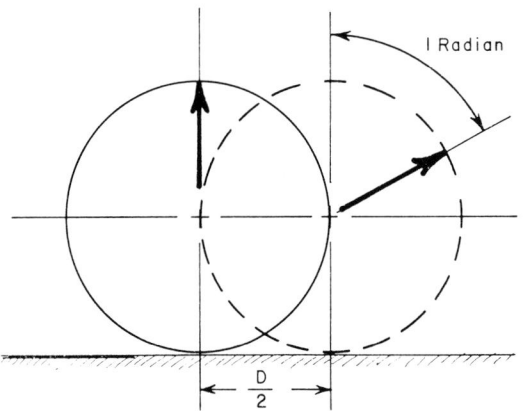

Fig. 3.1 A diagram to illustrate the concept of a radian. A radian is equal to 57.296°.

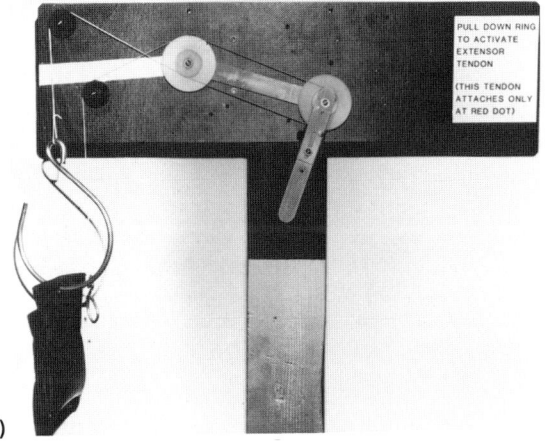

(a)

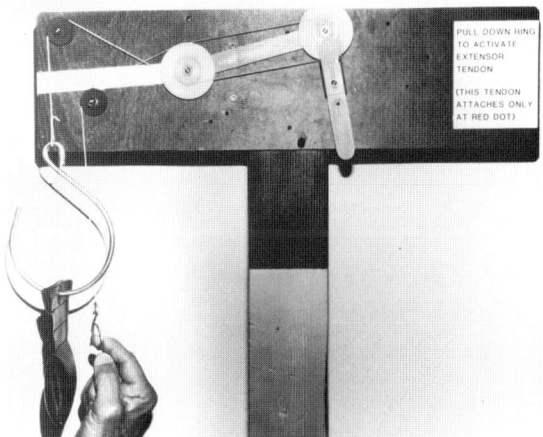

(b)

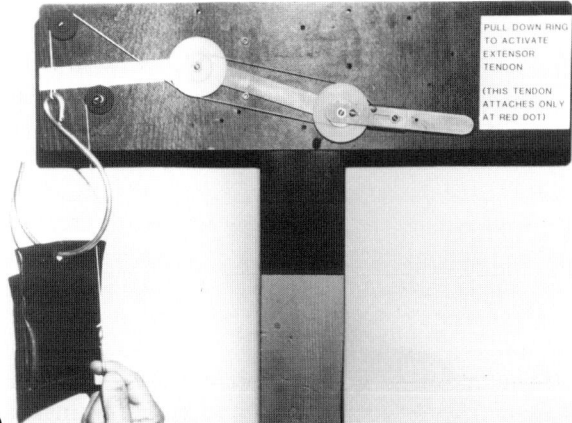

(c)

Fig. 3.2 Model demonstrating that intercalated segments joined by pin axes behave according to the ratio of moments on each side of the joint even though the attachment of the forces is only to the last or distal segment (Micks et al 1978). A load ring was attached to the extensor string so that an extensor force could be applied by the investigator and two strings properly directed. When force was applied to the extensor string with this string on the largest proximal pulley (**a**), that is, the largest lever or moment arm, and on the smallest distal pulley (**b**), that is, the smallest moment arm, the central segment extended to its constraint before extension of the distal segment began even though there was no attachment of the extensor string to the central segment. If the extensor string was placed on the small proximal pulley and the large distal pulley (**c**), then the distal segment extended to its constraint before extension of the central segment began.

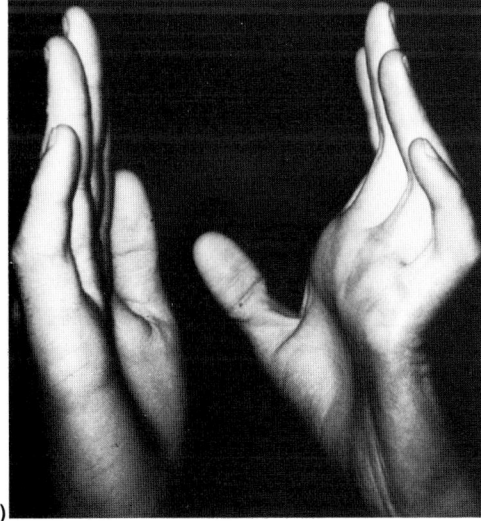

(a)

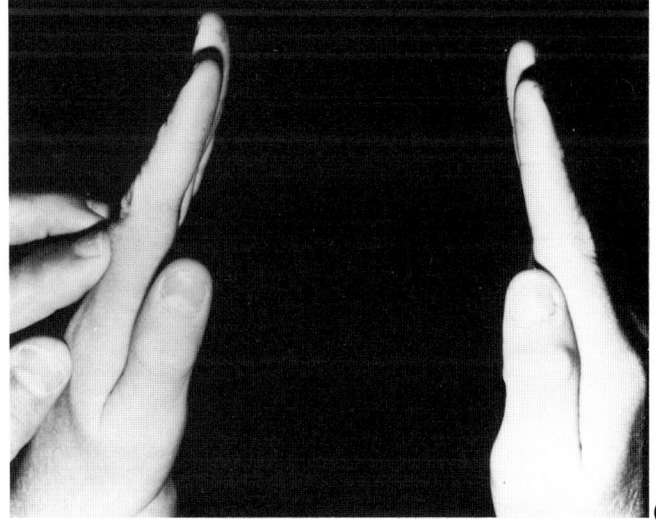

(b)

Fig. 3.3 (**a**) This patient, with an intrinsic minus left hand (visualized from ulnar aspect), is making a full voluntary effort to extend the digits. (**b**) If hyperextension at the MP joint is prevented by a passive flexor force (same hand visualized from radial aspect), then the extrinsic extensors are capable of fully extending the IP joints. The passive flexor force is helping to balance finger extension by substituting for the viscoelastic force of the interossei and the firing force of the lumbricals. (In the normal hand, the intrinsics also assist in extension of the IP joints.)

joint (Eyler & Markee 1954). However, it has been speculated that they are expending most of their energy countering the viscoelastic force of the profundii (Thomas et al 1968). Such speculations may be strictly relevant only in the unloaded hand.

The balancing of motion between the IP joints

The lateral fibres of the extensor assembly that derive from the extrinsic extensor tendon are able to bypass the axis of the PIP joint through their lateral path which crosses very near to the axis. They separate because of the increasing width of the trochleae with their overlying collateral ligaments. These fibres continue on across the DIP on the dorsum of the joint. Although the two joints normally move simultaneously, the actual angular velocities are different. The lateral fibres and the central fibres move in synchrony, however, due to the stiffness of the fibres in the longitudinal direction. Thus, when the muscle moves 1 cm, both the central and lateral fibres move 1 cm. Several factors or theories have been offered to explain this exquisite fibrous mechanism:

1. Littler feels that the communications between the central and lateral extrinsic fibres of the extensor assembly near the PIP joint prevent excessive volar movement of the lateral fibres because this area moves distally as the joint flexes
2. Gaul states that the distal spiral fibres of the extensor assembly are essential in controlling the descent of the lateral portion of the extensor assembly at the PIP joint when the finger flexes
3. The criss-cross pattern of the fibres of the assembly as described by Schultz et al (1981) is a plausible factor providing that one assumes the presence of some sort of bonding at the intersection of the fibres. Without such bonding, the criss-crossing fibres would slide by one another and the descent of the most lateral fibres could not be controlled in acute flexion
4. The cross-sectional configuration of the head of the proximal phalanx clothed by the collateral ligaments demonstrates a 'slope' which the lateral fibres traverse. In extension, these fibres converge as they move dorsally and in flexion they separate as they move volarly (Harris & Rutledge 1972)

(Figs 3.4, 3.5 and 3.6). However, when near full flexion of both IP joints, the lateral fibres will drop excessively volarward if the above described tissue connecting the lateral and central fibres is divided.

The extensor mechanism which acts at the PIP joint is a matrix of elastic and non-elastic fibres which conforms to the head of the proximal phalanx and the collateral ligaments during PIP joint flexion and extension. As this joint extends, this matrix necessarily adapts longitudinally in the relatively thin areas between the central and lateral fibres.

An analysis of flexion–extension moments

As previously noted, a static analysis may be employed since the motions of the fingers are not rapid enough to generate significant inertial loads. There are, however, forces generated during motion due to the viscous effects of distending the muscles, the motion of tendons in their sheaths or across gliding surfaces, friction in the joints, or viscoelastic effects resulting from deforming the soft tissues of the finger. These effects will be discussed in a later section.

The basis of current knowledge of the interphalangeal joints results from the studies of Landsmeer and others as well as from the fresh cadaver studies and analytical work at the National Hansen's Disease Center (NHDC), Louisiana. One of the objectives of the NHDC studies was the definition of 'effective' moment arms for each tendon at each joint throughout its range of motion. Using a special mathematical optimization technique, the parameters of a mathematical joint model are evaluated for each joint. The results for the intact thumb, reported by Ou (1979) and Thompson (1981), show good agreement between the model and the experimental results. These data, combined with the static analyses of pinch and grasp functions, and other tendon orientation models (Chao & An 1978, An et al 1979, Cooney et al 1981) provide a substantial knowledge base for further analysis and modelling.

A simple static analysis of the interphalangeal joints can now be formulated based on our current knowledge. Emphasis will be placed on the assumptions required to make the problem tractable. It

THE BIOMECHANICS OF THE INTERPHALANGEAL JOINTS 25

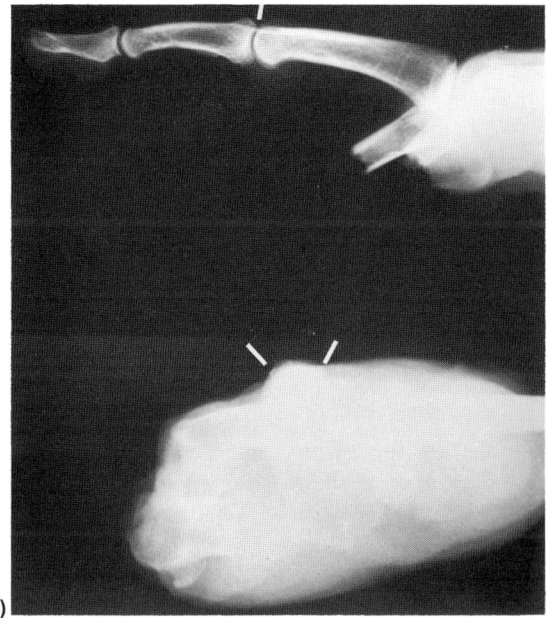

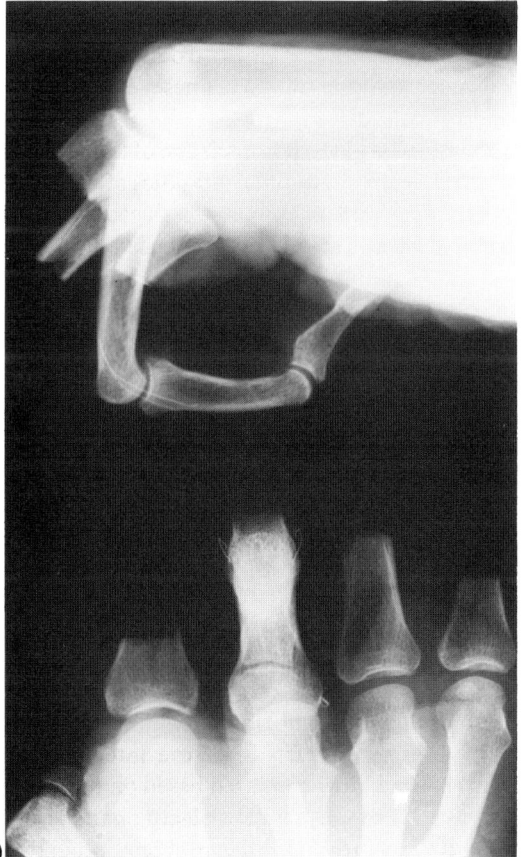

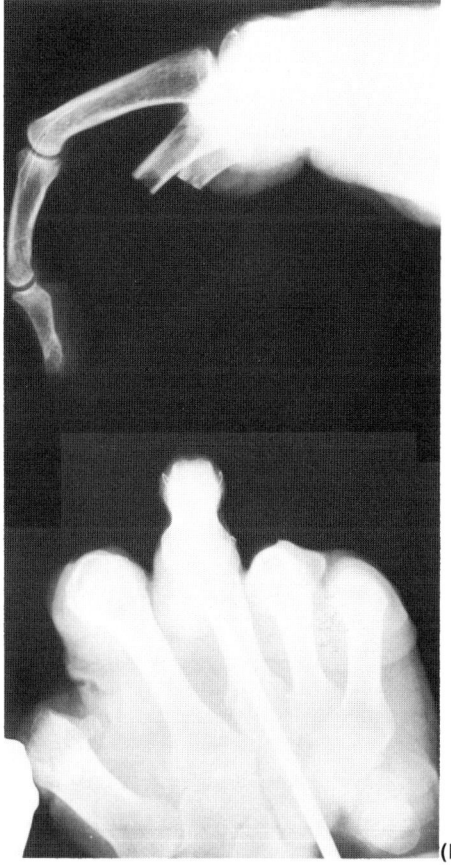

Fig. 3.4 (a) (b) (c) These lateral and axial radiographs are of the long finger of a fresh cadaver. The tendons were loaded so that the finger would simulate three **a**, **b** and **c** video stop frames of a normal living hand. (The white lines localize the wires in the lateral fibres.)

should be noted that the essential analytical work on the IP joints is just beginning. A greater understanding of joint function will come to fruition only when analytical methods are rigorously applied in concert with clinical research.

The objectives of this section are to relate an understanding of:

1. Three-dimensional free-body diagrams applied to the fingers
2. Requirements for definition of kinematic chains
3. The needs for assumptions and the limitations that go along with them
4. The relevance of the results of such analyses to further interpretation

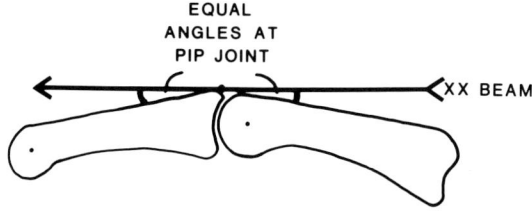

Fig. 3.5 Diagram showing the direction of the beam when taking the axial radiographs.

A free-body analysis is used to study how rigid bodies respond to forces applied to them. The equations used are based on Newton's laws of motion. This field generally includes statics and dynamics. Static systems are those in equilibrium, having no acceleration or deceleration. Many of these systems are analysed using static analysis when the accelerations are small. Dynamic systems are those which have large rates of change in velocity (acceleration) resulting in inertial effects. Dynamic analysis encompasses all of the forces considered in static analysis, but it also includes other terms related to rates of change that cannot be neglected.

When applied to man-made systems, free-body diagrams normally result in a set of equations that yield solutions directly. When applied to living systems, however, there are usually more unknowns than equations, yielding an indeterminate set of equations with many possible solutions, but no unique one. This occurs when modelling the joints of the hand because there are more muscle tendon units than are necessary to provide motion and force control of joints with two or three degrees of freedom. For example, the control of a rod mounted on a spherical joint requires only three cables and motors to affect motion about three orthogonal axes. Many of the joints in the hand have redundant controls of this nature as well as complex structures like the extensor hood mechanism that cannot be directly described with a simple force diagram.

A simplified free-body diagram for the middle finger is shown in Figure 3.7. The forces in the tendons are represented by vectors which themselves vary with the positions of the phalanges. Each phalanx can be analysed independently or in concert with others as indicated in the lower half of the figure. The separate free-body diagrams for the three phalanges include the forces that act on these segments. Note that between any two phalanges, the joint reaction forces and tendon forces are of equal but opposite direction. No attempt has been made to include all possible forces; for example, all the viscoelastic forces have been omitted.

The problem of defining the internal force structures which result from an external load requires the equations to be written in such a way that they depend on the position of the joint. A three-dimensional frame of reference for each skeletal segment in the kinematic chain must be defined, and the positions of each tendon and structural unit involved must be known within that frame of reference. The modelling research at NHDC uses matrix methods and a specialized graphics computer to define the translations and rotations applied to the skeletal segments, so that they may be analysed and visualized. This was developed by Buford (1984) along with methods for analysing tendon transfers. An optimization method is applied to the equations and the moment arm data to compute the physical dimensions in a two point model for each tendon at each joint (Ou 1979, Thompson 1981). This provides an 'effective' description of the line of action of each muscle acting on a joint. An et al (1979) defined a normative model of the hand using biplanar X-rays to define tendon and joint orientations.

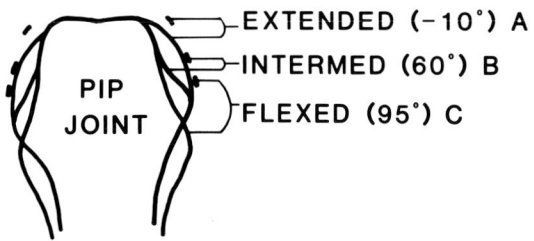

Fig. 3.6 In this drawing, tracings of the axial radiographs for positions A, B and C have been superimposed. The metal sutures in the lateral fibres are observed to separate and move volarly as the finger flexes. The cross-sectional slope of the PIP joint favours this movement. Apparently the separating of the lateral fibres does not offset the volar detour; otherwise flexion of the DIP joint would not be possible.

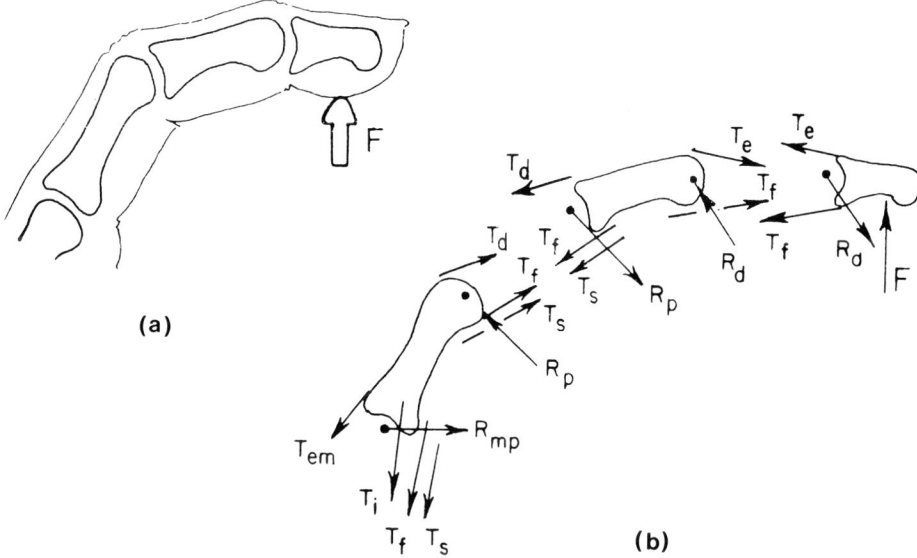

Fig. 3.7 A free-body analysis of a kinematic chain in the human hand. The chain shown depicts the phalanges and includes an abstraction of the types and locations of forces which normally act on them. (**a**) The physical situation; (**b**) free-body diagrams. F, External load; R_d, Joint reaction DIP; R_p, Joint reaction PIP; R_{mp}, Joint reaction MP; T_d, Tension extensor PIP; T_e, Tension extensor DIP; T_{em}, Tension extensor central slip; T_i, Tension wing tendons; T_f, Profundus; T_s, Sublimus.

Typically, once the equations of equilibria are set up, the number of unknowns must be reduced in an attempt to make the system determinate. Often, simple factual relationships or assumptions can serve to reduce the redundancy. Otherwise, mathematical methods involving optimization and search techniques must be employed to arrive at a set of possible solutions. These methods are dependent on the formulation of some criteria to enable the search to converge upon a solution.

Figure 3.8 shows a free-body diagram of the distal phalanx and the forces which act on it. Each of the two tendon forces are shown along with their effective moment arm. An externally applied load is also shown, along with the ever-present joint reaction force. Again, no viscoelastic forces are shown, although in free motion of the finger or as the finger approaches its range of motion limit they become dominant terms.

Thus, the moment balance may be written as:

Summation of torques
$$= -F \times R + Tf \times rf - Te \times re = 0 \qquad (1)$$

An example of a simple estimate of the resultant force in the profundus tendon comes when we assume that the force in the terminal extensor is negligible and that the viscoelastic forces and other constraint forces and moments at the DIP are also zero. Using these simplifying assumptions we can solve for the force in the profundus for a given force at the fingertip. Newton's law for equilibrium states that the net moment at the joint must be zero. Thus, an external force, F, applied at a distance R from the joint axis produces an extension moment which must be exactly countered by a flexion moment produced by the profundus. In the preceding equation, the positive moments are for flexion, and the profundus produces a tension in its tendon of Tf which acts at a moment arm rf. The force Te is the effective force which would act

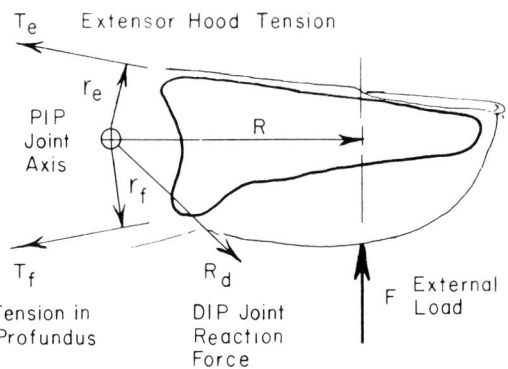

Fig. 3.8 A free-body diagram of the distal phalanx.

at a distance *re* to have an equivalent moment to the sum of all of the extensor hood fibres acting at their respective radii from the joint axis. Also note that by summing moments about the joint axis, the reaction force, *Rd*, does not contribute to the torque equation. This is because it acts through the axis of the joint and has no moment arm relative to it.

Thus, the equation simplifies to the relation:

$$Tf = F \times \frac{R}{rf} \qquad (2)$$

If any three of the above four variables are known, it is possible to use this equation to solve for the fourth. This is of value in functional testing of fingers, where one may estimate moment arms, measure the external force, and use these data to estimate the tension produced in the profundus. Because of the poor accuracy of the estimate of the moment arm for the profundus and the questionable value of maximal voluntary effort of the terminal phalanx against a transducer, this method does not yield accurate or repeatable results. The errors involved in the experimental determination of the distances and forces in this situation are in excess of any errors introduced by neglecting the viscoelastic forces.

Because of the assumptions used, the free-body analysis of even a simple moment balance must therefore be interpreted with caution. The static loading analyses by Chao et al (1976), for example, include both the interphalangeal joints of the forefinger and thumb in tip pinch and grasp. Table 3.1 presents results from a simple pinch and grasp analysis. These results show the trends of increasing joint constraint forces at the more proximal joints produced by a unit force applied to the fingers to simulate pinch or grasp.

The results are valid only for the specific positions studied. The information has more general value in that it provides data about the distribution of forces between the active muscles in pinch and grasp.

OTHER FORCES INTERNAL TO THE MUSCULOSKELETAL SYSTEM

The musculoskeletal system has many other forces which act on it directly. These include forces due principally to the viscoelastic behaviour of the joint structures and the soft tissues surrounding the joint. There are also viscoelastic forces which are internal to the muscles. A block diagram of such forces is given in Figure 3.9. In this figure, it is seen that the muscle has both an elastic and a viscous character. The tendon sheath interacts with its surroundings in a viscoelastic manner as well. The joint capsule provides another source of elastic and frictional losses, and the bone and ligament structures provide non-linear limits to the joint. The compression and distension of the soft tissues surrounding the joint and phalanges during flexion and extension result in additional forces.

Resistance to passive motion of the IP joints

Active motion of joints is provided by muscles. This active motion is alternately augmented (during contraction from the stretched position) and diminished (while a muscle is nearing full contraction) by viscoelastic forces. Passive motion may also be caused by external forces and loads. However, before the joints can actually move in response to any motive force, the restraints of friction and the elastic resistance of passive soft

Table 3.1 Averaged constraint forces of a joint resulting from an applied unit load to simulate pinch or grasp. (Abstracted from Chao et al 1976)

Finger	Hand function	DIP Compression	Subluxation	PIP Compression	Subluxation	MP Compression	Subluxation
Index	Pinch	4.46	−3.30	4.70	−3.70	8.00	−2.70
	Grasp	1.95	−2.40	3.25	−2.88	11.46	−4.29
Long	Pinch	4.00	−1.10	7.03	−1.97	0.0	−0.44
	Grasp	2.94	−1.19	6.59	−2.65	13.84	0.43
Little	Pinch	4.53	−1.80	5.55	−3.31	5.65	−3.58
	Grasp	2.93	−1.55	5.04	−3.29	11.66	−8.59

THE BIOMECHANICS OF THE INTERPHALANGEAL JOINTS   29

on the underlying skeletal structures. Since this is unacceptable in a living hand, one must strive to achieve mechanical evaluations of the intact hand with sufficient precision to allow quantification of progress or regress in treatments to mobilize joints and tendons.

Injured or diseased interphalangeal joints often become stiff. A unique combination of factors are operative in these conditions. These factors are related to:

1. A closely fitting hinge joint
2. Tendons running in a long sheath
3. Flat tendons with a large bone interface
4. Complex sheets of tendon fibres that move on each other
5. Limited room for fluid

In order to evaluate these issues separately as well as when they act in concert, one must have a system for quantifying torque and range of motion simultaneously. The important factors are reviewed in the following sections.

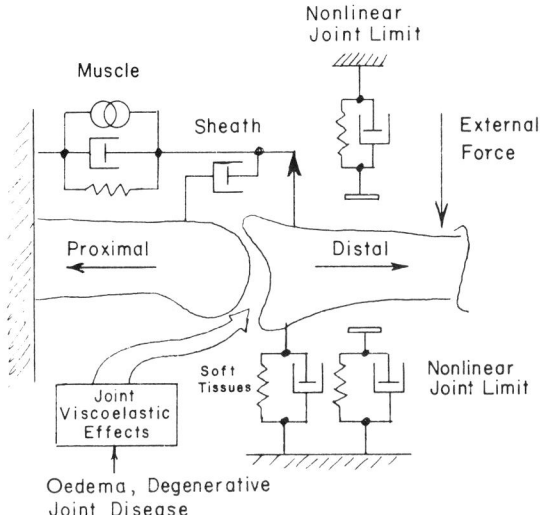

Fig. 3.9 Block diagram of some of the forces and torques acting at a joint. Only the extensor muscle is shown for clarity.

tissues have to be overcome as well as the viscous restraint of fluids that move around in the tissues.

These restraints may be referred to collectively as 'drag'. Our understanding of this subject is poor. There have been very few attempts in the literature of hand surgery to quantify or to attempt an analysis of this subject. The problems of stiffness of joints and the failure of tendons to move constitute perhaps the greatest cause of failure in hand surgery. There has been some attempt to study the nature of scar tissue, and to look at the chemistry of collagen and the patterns of its formation and removal. However, there is no satisfactory way of clinically monitoring the biomechanical effects of stiffness in any actual hand, joint, or muscle tendon unit. Since it is the mechanics of scar and stiffness that is the enemy of motion, this is a subject which must be studied. Most bioengineers shy away from it because there is no way to be precise about measuring the elasticity or viscosity of any tissue or structure without opening up the hand to gain a solid grasp

Closely fitting synovial hinge joints

Normal healthy human cartilagenous joints are lubricated by synovial fluid. They are some of the most efficient and frictionless joints in existence. When engineers first began to study synovial joints with the idea of building total joint replacements, they found it hard to understand how normal human joints could have a coefficient of friction of around 0.02 when the best figure that could be obtained between polished metals, lubricated with standard boundary lubrication, was five times as high, at about 0.1. They finally found that this extraordinary freedom from friction depended upon hydrodynamic lubrication which, while still relatively new in engineering, seems to have been routine for thousands of years in animals.

Hydrodynamic lubrication is a term which indicates a system whereby the relative motion between two curved surfaces may generate a pressure so that they are lifted apart and actually float while moving. This is in contrast to boundary lubrication which occurs when a film of oil is allowed to coat a surface, filling in irregularities and minimizing contact friction.

The essence of boundary lubrication is that

metal surfaces must be engineered to the finest tolerances, allowing space for only a thin film of oil. The joint must fit perfectly to spread the contact stress evenly. In hydrodynamic lubrication, it is essential that the joint surfaces must *not* fit perfectly, because this would deprive the joint of the mechanism to generate the pressure to separate them.

There are two mechanisms by which human joints ride on fluid while moving. Both require that there be room, and that the radius of curvature of the convex surface be smaller than the radius of the opposing concave surface as shown in Figure 3.10.

The first mechanism depends upon the fact that hyaline joint cartilage is a porous material similar to a sponge. It may be thought of as having a compressible texture traversed by fine canaliculi, full of synovial fluid and synovial gel. When the convex head rolls over the concave socket, the relatively small area of cartilage in contact is compressed, and synovial fluid squirts out all over the surface, lifting the surfaces apart. As the head rolls on, a new area is compressed while the previous area expands again and the resulting drop in the pressure within the cartilage matrix draws the fluid that is loose in the cavity back into the cartilage.

The second mechanism depends upon the viscoelastic character of synovial fluid. This fluid has unique properties derived from very strong intermolecular attractions and weak polymeric bonds. This prevents the synovial fluid from spreading out infinitely over a surface, and pulls it together into a globule. It is rather like egg-white that sticks to the egg shell and bounces up and down in a string of semi-fluid that is almost elastic. An automobile wheel that rolls over fluid on a road has a tendency to push the fluid aside, or to roll over it if the wheel is moving fast and the fluid deep. This is termed 'hydroplaning' and results in loss of control because of the dramatic reduction in friction between the wheel and road. The special character of synovial fluid enhances this transition

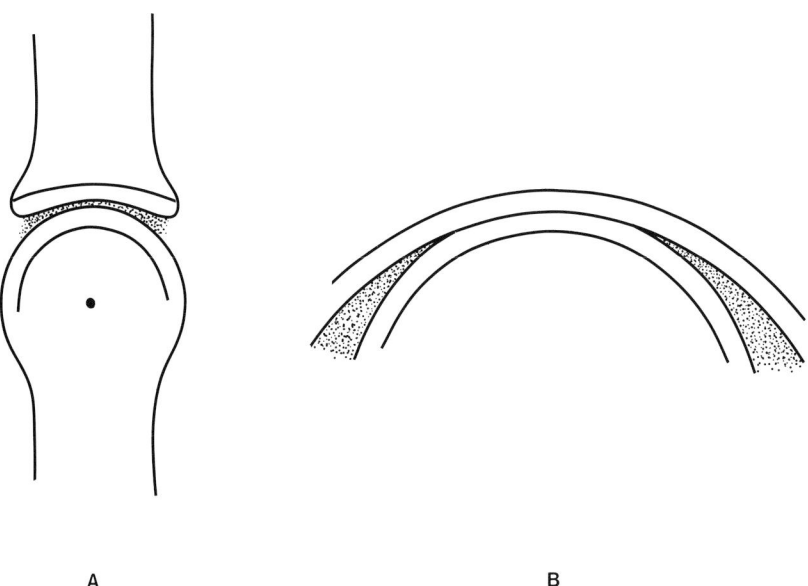

Fig. 3.10 Hydrodynamic lubrication. Note the wedge of fluid on each side of the area of contact of cartilage. The compression of the cartilage under stress causes synovial fluid to be squeezed out of intracartilage canaliculi. (From Brand 1985, by permission.)

and the 'fluid' becomes trapped so that the joint rolls over it, preventing contact between the two cartilage surfaces and thereby reducing the friction even when the motion is slow.

Both of the above mechanisms work most efficiently when the joints are moving fast and freely. They have no effect when the joint is stationary. They also have minimal effect when the joint is in total contact. The IP joints have much smaller clearances than most other joints. The radius in the concave surface is larger than that of the convex, but the contrast is not as great in the IP joints as in others. In the IP joints, the lubrication approaches pure boundary lubrication. This is especially true in the DIP, and less so in the MP joints.

The relative narrowness of the joint space of the cartilage may also predispose the joint to stiffness when other factors, such as old age, result in a thinning of the cartilage. This may also be due to irregularities which occur following injury or in rheumatoid arthritis, or because of the loss of thixotropic qualities in the synovial fluid which occurs in older people.

Thus, there is a trade-off between the mobility and the stability of a joint. The very stable, closely fitting nature of the IP joints may predispose them to more stiffness in states of disease and injury in old age.

Tendons in a sheath

The behaviour of flexor tendons in synovial sheaths is very well known, as are the problems of adhesions between the tendon and sheath in tendon or bone injury. These factors will not be enlarged on here except to comment that the IP joints may, of course, suffer a limitation of motion from tendon adhesions which may be proximally located in the hand or forearm.

There are marked differences between the lubrication of tendons in a sheath and in synovial cartilage joints. In the former there is no hydrodynamic lubrication, because there is no cartilage to hold fluid and squirt it out. Also there is no 'rolling-over' of a convex sphere or cylinder that can trap thixotropic fluid. The 'cylinder' of tendon does not roll; it slides longitudinally. Therefore it can only use boundary lubrication. The resultant friction during fast repetitive motion of tendons in sheaths may result in tenosynovitis, whereas fast repetitive motion in a synovial joint seems not to suffer such problems.

Tendons with a large bone interface

This problem is at the root of much distal stiffness affecting the IP joints. It is important to distinguish between true gliding as occurs in a synovial sheath cavity and apparent gliding between two surfaces which have an interface of paratendinous soft tissue which is attached to both surfaces.

Where tendons run through areolar connective tissue, as in the forearm, and are not subjected to lateral stress (going around a curve) there is usually no tendon sheath. The areolar connective tissue around the moving tendon becomes specialized to allow stretch. The individual fibres of this tissue are attached at one end to the moving tendon, and at the other end to some other tissue, such as fascia or bone. The unique quality of this 'paratenon' is that the fibres are folded, coiled, and loose. They have a mucopolysaccharide ground substance that looks gelatinous. They carry fine blood vessels that are also loosely coiled. Thus the whole tissue moves with the tendon while still being attached and fixed to motionless parietal structures. It is rather like a mesentery (but more dispersed) which sustains and nourishes the bowel without restricting its movement.

When a muscle or tendon is transferred in the forearm or palm, it is possible to lay it in a bed (or to tunnel it through a bed) that is largely composed of compliant fatty or areolar tissue. This bed of tissue soon adapts to become similar to paratenon in its response to stretch, permitting a smooth motion, comparable to gliding.

The tendon sheaths of the dorsal expansion, lying on the dorsal aspects of the phalanges, are not true gliding tendons because they have no synovial cavity or bursa except at critical areas where they cross a joint. In the region between joints, there is a thin layer of areolar tissue between the skin and tendon and between the tendon and bone. This is satisfactory unless the integrity of the layer is disturbed by a burn, an injury, a surgical operation, or even by prolonged immobilization that allows tissue fibres to shorten. This limitation is more severe in the presence of inflammation and inflammatory oedema.

One critical factor that spoils efforts at reconstruction of the dorsal apparatus following boutonnière or swan-neck deformities and that hinders movement after a fracture in this area, is the occurrence of scar tissue that forms across the bone–tendon interface on the dorsal surface of the proximal two phalanges.

If the original paratenon tissue between the flat tendon and flat bone is destroyed or denatured, the only tissue that can replace it is scar tissue. That scar is not specialized in any way, but joins tendon to bone directly by dense collagen fibres.

Collagen fibres become longer in response to tension and then immediately shorten when the tension is removed. The mechano-physiology by which collagen fibres actually increase their resting length in response to the stimulus of repeated stretch over a period of time is not well understood. However, it seems clear that when lengthening occurs it does so by a change along the whole length of each fibre in which the old collagen is absorbed and new collagen is laid down with updated bonding patterns, allowing for greater length. Whatever length is gained, and by whatever chemical change, it is not a totally new structure that can start all over again with a reassessment of biomechanical needs. It is a gradual replacement, molecule by molecule, within the overall fabric that was there before. Therefore the lengthening of any collagen structure cannot be measured by the addition of new units, but only by a proportional lengthening which could be thought of as a percentage change of the length that was there before. Thus if it takes a week of effort to change a 10 mm fibre to become an 11 mm fibre, then the same week of effort will be needed to turn a 1 mm fibre into one that is 1.1 mm in length. When scar forms between the sheet of dorsal expansion and the bone on which it rests, the fibres may be of the order of 0.5 mm or less in length. A 10% lengthening, achieved through great labour, will not be perceived as any improvement at all by the patient or by a therapist, because it will be unmeasurably small. Moreover, the area of attachment of tendon to bone is very large. The possibility of providing effective lengthening of any biological structure must be thought of as proportional to its length divided by its cross-sectional area. There is, perhaps, no area in the body where this ratio is as unfavourable as between the extensor tendon and the bone along the dorsum of a digit.

This subject has been stressed because it is the principal cause of many surgical failures when attempting to free a dorsal expansion. At one time, the standard practice of the author was to pass a blunt dissector between bone and tendon to release the adhesions. This would result in immediate release of the joints and the tendons would again move freely. Unfortunately, during the postoperative period the adhesions reform, perhaps more densely than before. The best that may have been achieved was a new position of a joint that became stiff at a more functional angle. Riordan (1984) now specifically treats most dorsal expansions conservatively, even the boutonnière deformity. The results leave more motion than any radical solution which exposes naked bone to naked tendon.

The problem of dorsal tendon adherence may have been overstated here because until it is taken seriously and measured with precision, advances in treatment will be small. The excursions that must be measured are in the order of 0.2 mm of lengthening. The resulting joint angular variations for this small increase in tendon motion are approximately 4°. Such accuracy is only possible if one exercises great care. A special instrument to measure the torque-angle (T-A) relationship may provide the necessary precision (see below). Unless one utilizes torque-angle measurement, it will not be possible to evaluate the rival claims of interpositional plastics, free grafts, early postoperative movements under local anaesthesia or any other method. It is important to note that any small residue of the original tissue that may remain between bone and tendon offers much more hope of becoming restored to part of its first mobility than any scar tissue that may take its place after surgery. Whenever one is tempted to 'free up' a flat tendon that lies on a flat bone, one maxim to be remembered is: 'Freeing up now, means binding down later'.

Sheets of tendon with relative motion

The following section discusses the function of the differing elements of the dorsal expansion. Agee &

Guidera (1980) refer to this as a 'torque tube' which has numbers of muscles sending fibres into it at various levels. Additionally, it has fibres which diverge distally to attach to bones and proximally to attach to sagittal bands and capsules. Most of the interdigitating and criss-crossing fibres are on their way from some muscle to some insertion. Seen in a preserved specimen they look just like a sheet of tendon. Seen at operation in a normal finger, while the patient is awake and able to move, the whole sheet is seen as a living matrix of fibres that each have some freedom to move on each other. With a fresh cadaver hand one can sit for hours, pulling on different interossei and lumbricals, flexing and extending joints while attempting to recognize simple patterns of interaction out of 1000 moving fibres. Each of these fibres has its own individual, firm relationship to one of a variety of muscles and joints. It also has a more loose, semi-fluid relationship to the fibres adjacent to it in the sheet composing the torque tube. It is often impossible to say what a given fibre in the sheet could accomplish at a given joint without first asking about the effect of the fibres on each side of it, because each fibre has only a limited independent motion. If one fibre has to move 3 mm, then the fibre next to it must move at least 1 mm in the same direction, and the fibre beyond that may remain stationary but must not move backwards.

This fine interplay between adjacent fibres in the torque tube and their mobility on each other may also be lost. Injury, infection, burn or surgery may result in a panus of inflammation that turns a whole area of dorsal expansion into an inelastic, impliable sheet. The sheet may still be mobile as a whole, and may transmit force from a major origin to a major insertion, but the fine interplay of differential fibre movement is lost. The condensations of fibres into thickened bands, such as the lateral band, may not be affected to a great extent because a band is much like a tendon. The fibres that feed into it and away from it, however, may lose some of their independence.

Limited room for fluid

Oedema fluid in any limb is a hinderance to rapid free motion. At the level of the IP joints of the fingers, fluid swelling is especially productive of stiffness. This limitation of range of motion due to fluid is seldom absolute. It is, however, time related. Fluid in the tissues has a shock-absorber quality, and will slowly yield to persistent torque or pressure as the fluid moves about in the tissues. It is important to remember that there is more than one mechanism that results in joint stiffness from oedema.

The first is a reorientation of loose connective tissue fibres in a perpendicular direction that ordinarily are parallel to the line of movement of the tendons and skin. Weeks & Wray (1973) demonstrated this factor in relation to loose skin, showing how skin loses much of its mobility when it rides over fluid. This is not just due to the skin becoming tight as it has to surround a larger volume of hand, it is also due to tissue fibre orientation. In Figure 3.11, a ship at anchor is used as an example to demonstrate that as long as the water is shallow in relation to the length of the anchor chain, the ship may retain a wide range of motion. When the tide rises so that the water is nearly as deep as the chain is long, the ship has very limited mobility because it is tethered to the earth by a now vertical chain. Mobile structures in the hand all owe their range of mobility to the length and elastic range of the individual fibres that make up the connective tissues anchoring them to their surroundings. Most tendons are surrounded by paratendinous tissue traversed by long fine strands of collagen and elastic tissue that are pulled distally and proximally as the tendon moves. If the space around the tendon is blown up with fluid, the fibres are forced into a transverse orientation, and the longitudinal range of motion of the tendon is limited.

A second cause of stiffness, which is especially applicable to the IP joints, is that if skin and fascia are distended with oedema then the finger becomes stiff in the same way that an empty rubber glove finger is stiff when distended with air or water. A similar effect in a finger is due to the fact that the skin and fascia have to stretch further, in bending, than is usual. Figure 3.12 shows how a 5 mm increase in the diameter of a finger results in the need for the skin to stretch longitudinally an additional 7 mm during flexion. Figure 3.12c shows how the joint may finally flex without so much skin lengthening by flexing slowly enough to allow the

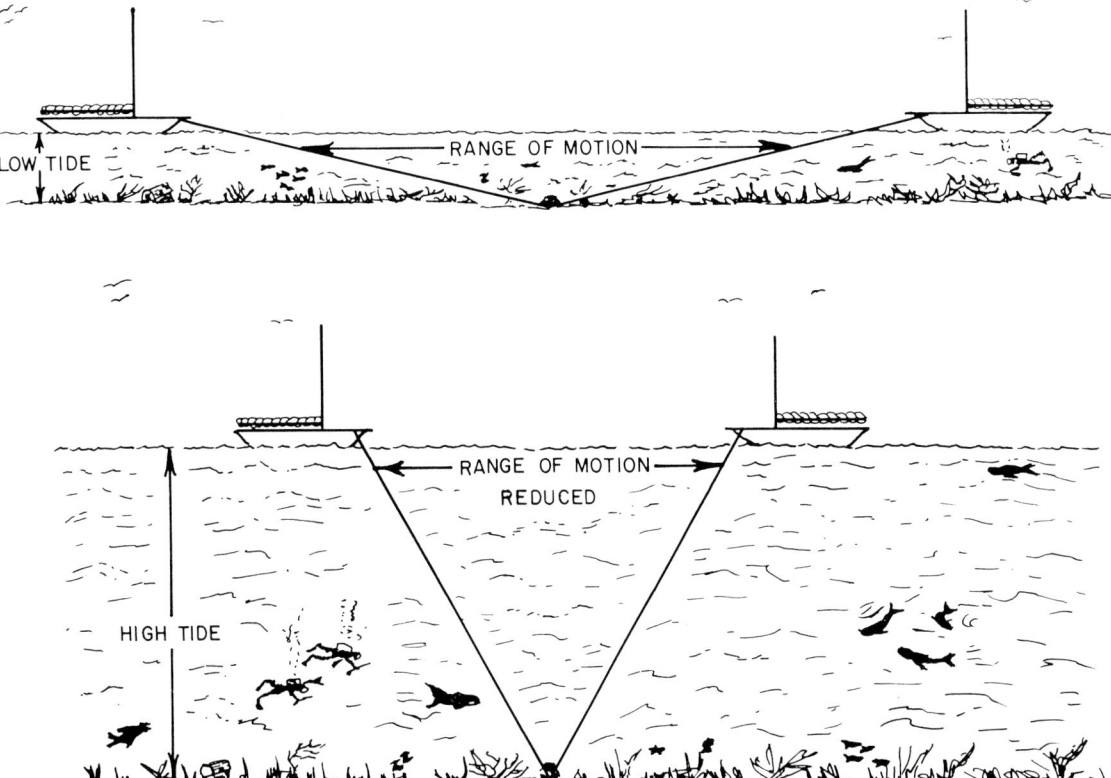

Fig. 3.11 Every sailor knows that a ship at anchor has a wide range of mobility at low tide and much less mobility at high tide. This is because water (oedema) has lifted the boat. The anchor chain (connective tissue fibres) is then orientated vertically, limiting its range horizontally. (From Brand 1985, by permission.)

fluid to disperse to areas where it is under less pressure. This dispersal of fluid may be helped or hindered by gravity as well as by local pressure differentials. A more serious stiffness occurs when the fluid in a finger has a high molecular weight created by the presence of a high protein and cellular oedema. This fluid moves very slow and there is a tendency for it to become organized into a fibrous matrix, forming permanent stiffness.

It is not our intent to discuss this more fully here because knowledge of the whole phenomenon is limited. The chemistry and basic physics of fluid movement in the tissues are not well understood, but the biomechanical implications are still more poorly documented. The present authors urge surgeons and therapists to develop and use various means of numerical evaluation of these physical parameters so that they may be used to develop techniques to manage these crippling causes of stiff hands.

Joint torque-angle measurements

There are several factors which contribute to the relationship between the articulation of a joint and the forces which act on the joint. Some of these include the passive distension of muscles, the viscous effects of tendons sliding within their sheaths, the compression of soft tissues on one aspect of the joint with distension of the tissues on the opposing surface, stretching of the joint capsule, displacement of both fluid and gel components of the interstitium, and finally, at the outer limits of the range of motion are the restraining forces imposed by the collateral ligaments and palmar plates. In the normal joint, there is a balance between these forces which allows the joint to remain supple, while at the same time keeping the joint surfaces in alignment. In degenerative joint diseases, this balance is destroyed. The joints may be restricted in total range of motion,

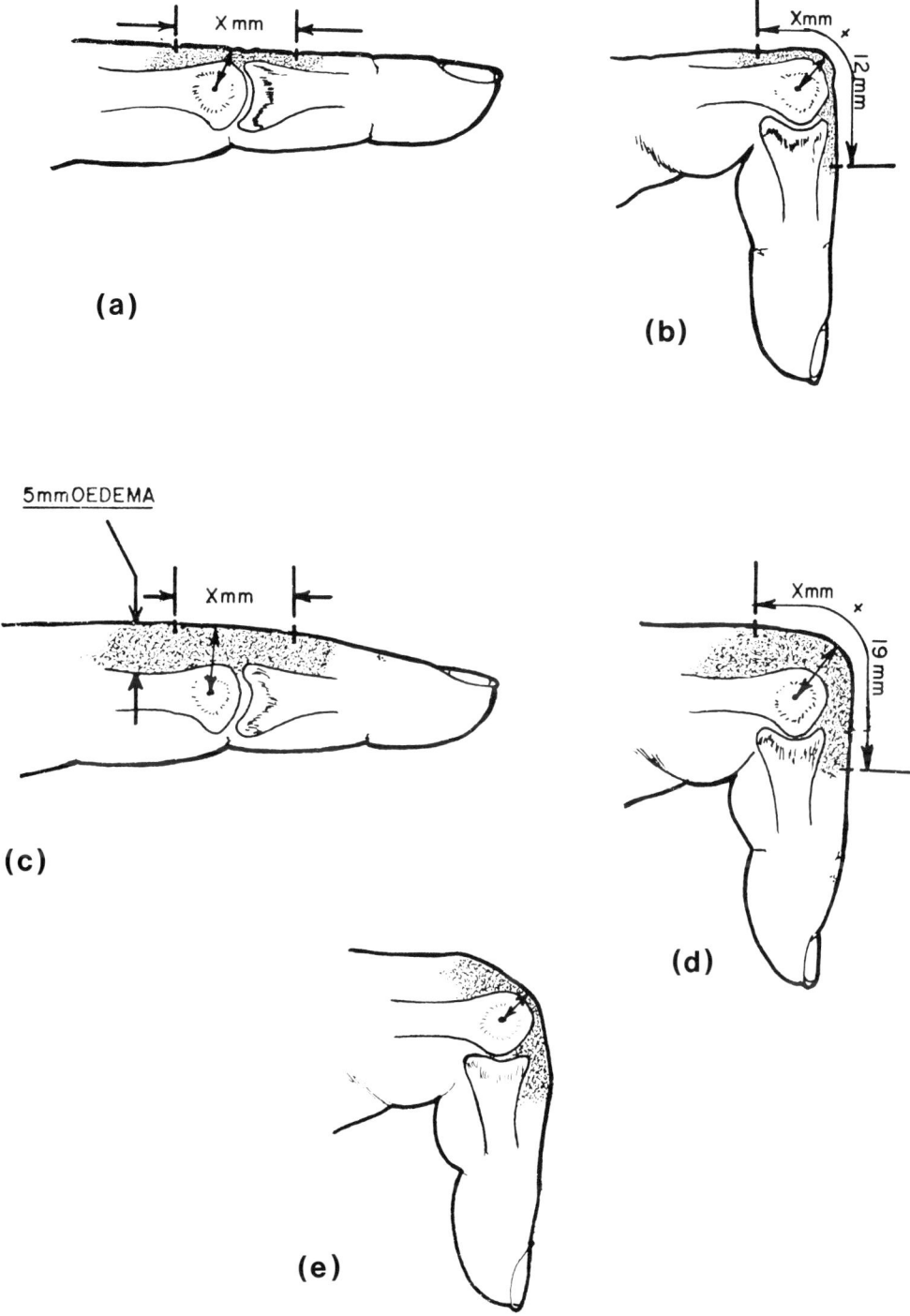

Fig. 3.12 (a) and (b) Dorsal skin requires 12 mm of lengthening for 90° of flexion. (c) and (d) With 5 mm of thickness of oedema, the skin requires 19 mm of lengthening for 90° of flexion. (e) With continuing torque, slowly applied, the oedema fluid moves around, permitting the skin to cross closer to the joint axis and require less stretch. (From Brand 1985, by permission.)

the torque required to move the joint may be modified, and the joint dysfunction may even progress to total lack of motion and misalignment of the digits. If the collateral ligaments are involved in the degenerative process, the joint surfaces may be eroded resulting in subluxation of the joint. In the treatment of such cases, the physician lacks the means to assess the severity of the pathology or the progress of any treatment modalities he uses.

Joint torque-angle measurements are windows into the mechanics of joints. Through careful clinical measurements, one may gain significant insights into the aetiology and treatment of joint disease. Although much needs to be done to improve the measurement and interpretation techniques, the following sections describe simple clinical tests which are of great value. The section on dynamic measurements describes results from state-of-the-art instruments which illuminate the importance of viscous effects in the balance and motion of the hand.

Static measurement of torque-angle relationship

The IP joints of the hand lend themselves to precise measurement of angle changes related to torque. We are increasing the understanding of all the above factors by following clinically a sequence of T-A curves using simple measurements.

The measurement of IP joint angles should be accomplished using standard torque values in routine measurements of joint angle. It is less important that the exact torque be measured than to use exactly the same technique every time a measurement is taken. For speed and simplicity, one should not attempt to measure the lever arm (moment arm) at which force is applied (except sometimes for the first application). By using the same anatomical markers on the first and every subsequent measurement, repeatability is assured. For measurements of torque at the PIP joint, it is recommended that one always apply standardized loads at the joint crease of the DIP joint for moving the joint into extension. The loads should be applied to the dorsum opposite the joint crease for movement into flexion. It is suggested that the force be applied at the centre of the pink nail bed or at the pulp level opposite to that point for the DIP joint.

Although the lever arm is not repeatedly measured, the force or load must be known, and the direction of application of force must be at right angles to the segment of the digit that is to move.

With the wrist and all other joints in a neutral (straight) position, a series of torques are applied to the joint, using the standard lever arm as previously described. Weights or loads (Fig. 3.13) of, perhaps 200, 400, 600, 800 and 1000 g are applied and the joint angle measured at each torque. The resultant data may be plotted to demonstrate the elastic profile of the tissues that resist full joint motion.

Most normal IP joints become straight (0°) half way through the sequence of torques. The curves then become steep or nearly vertical. Normal metacarpophalangeal joints, by contrast, will usually continue to hyperextend under increasing torque and their curves rarely end steeply.

When joints are under treatment for stiffness, the shape of the curve may alter week by week, giving information about the elastic qualities of the restraining tissues as well as documenting the effectiveness of therapy which is increasing the range of motion of the joint.

Evaluation of viscoelastic constraints

Torque-angle curves of IP joints may be made under the following conditions:

1. Wrist in neutral position
   a. MP joints extended to 0°
   b. MP joints 60° flexed
2. As above, but with the wrist 45° extended
3. As above, but with the wrist 65° flexed

The resulting curves should then be compared by superimposing them together (Fig. 3.14). Since the tissues immediately around the IP joints will not have changed, all recorded variations must be due to the increase or decrease in motion or tensions of the long flexors and extensors alone or by the intrinsic muscle and proximal dorsal expansion tightness or laxity.

These studies provide a great deal of information about the causes of limitation of motion, especially after operations such as tendon transfer. It may also point the way to better management of stiff joints.

THE BIOMECHANICS OF THE INTERPHALANGEAL JOINTS 37

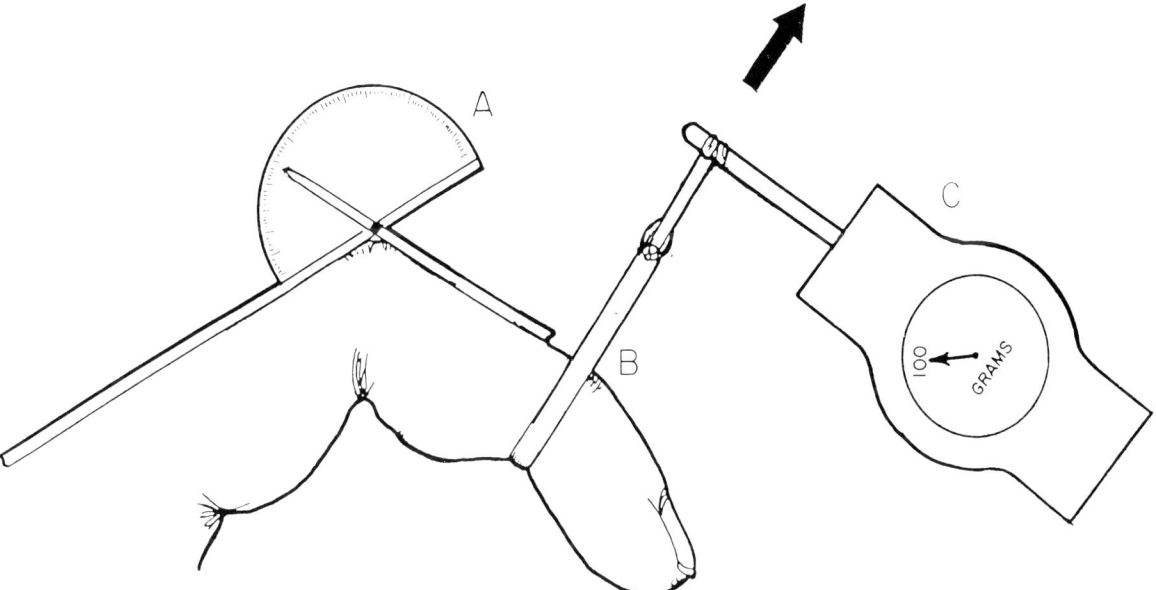

Fig. 3.13 Clinical evaluation of torque-angle of PIP joint, moving into extension. (A) Goniometer on back of finger. Held by therapist's hand, which also stabilizes the proximal segment of finger. (B) Narrow sling or loop of string at the joint crease. This loop must pull at a right angle to middle segment of finger. (C) Calibrated spring gauge to determine the tension applied to the loop.

Evaluation of viscous tissue factors

Torque-angle data may prove to be significant in the mechanical analysis of swollen hands. They are also important in older patients who often have a diurnal variation in the mobility of finger joints. This generally manifests itself in joints that are stiff in the morning but which may gradually increase in range of motion through the activity of exercise throughout the day. This is probably due to the presence of a high molecular weight fluid in and around the joint structures.

A special test procedure is proposed that utilizes a constant torque of perhaps 600 g applied at the level of the crease, and measurement of the angle of the joint every 15 seconds. The resulting time response of the joint to a constant torque provides a measure of the mobility of the fluids within the finger. Normal fingers adapt quickly to the applied load, with very little secondary creep. Oedematous tissues will typically respond much more slowly, especially if the tissues are filled with high molecular weight infiltrates. One may use this technique to follow the course of treatment of a hand for oedema, performing such a test before and after elevation or exercise of the hand.

Dynamic measurement of torque-angle relationships

The joint torque goniometer is a device built specifically to assist in the management of joint diseases. The mathematical modelling is an attempt to understand the experimental results obtained with the device. At the present time, this device is experimental. It does, however, provide insights into the viscous as well as the elastic character of joints.

The device. The joint torque goniometer is shown in Figure 3.15. It is of lightweight construction, and uses strain gauges on its active-arm to monitor the torque applied to a digit. The unit has a miniature potentiometer in the central housing which is used to measure the joint angle. The unit is clamped to the proximal and distal phalanges of the joint to be evaluated and the unit is manually rotated back and forth over the desired range of motion and with the desired torque. The output from the transducers is fed to a two-channel strip chart recorder.

Mathematical model of the joint. The mathematical model used in this pilot study is based on experimental observations and has several parameters that are relevant to joint biomechanics. A

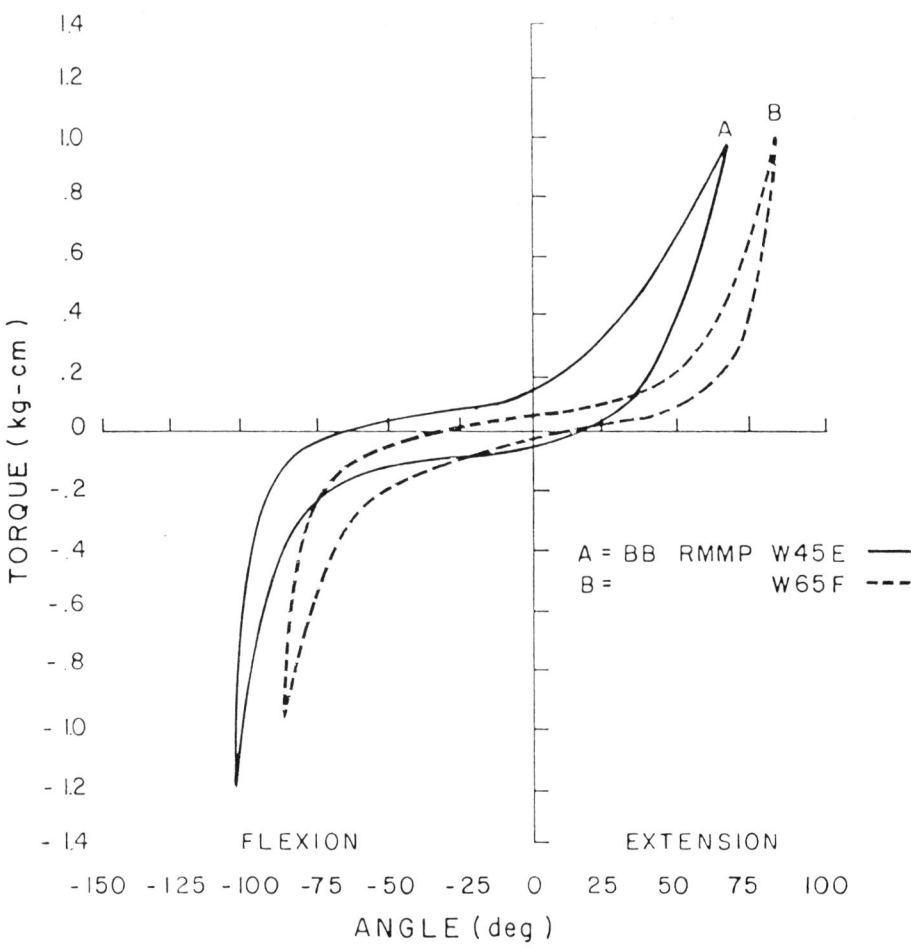

Fig. 3.14 Static torque-angle curves for an MP joint with the wrist in 45° of extension (A) and then repeated for a wrist position of 65° of flexion (B). Note the more gradual change in the torque as the extension limit is reached compared with the more rapid increase in the magnitude of the torque as the flexion limit is approached.

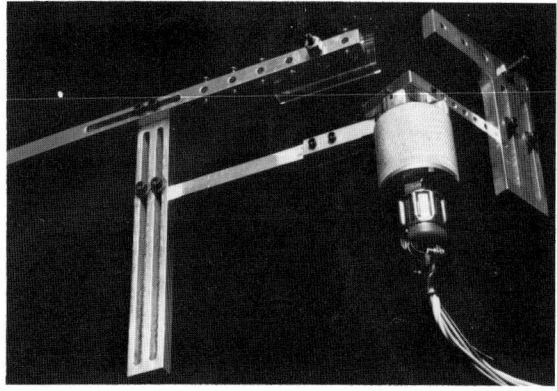

Fig. 3.15 Photograph of a prototype joint torque goniometer for dynamic measurements of the viscoelastic behaviour of joints. The device monitors both torque and angle for the joint simultaneously. The cable leads to a recording instrument.

typical experimental readout from the two-channel recorder is shown in Figures 3.16. The resulting flexion and extension angles and associated torque values may be found from these tracings. A plot of the torque versus joint angle is shown in Figure 3.17 for two different rates of joint angular velocity. These different rates of joint motion were achieved manually and produce different hysteresis curves. Hysteresis is a term used to describe the magnitude of the difference between the angular changes obtained as one increases the load and those produced during decreasing loads. It is usually sensitive to the rate of application of the loading and is attributable to viscous effects. The first feature to be noted from the torque-angle relation-

THE BIOMECHANICS OF THE INTERPHALANGEAL JOINTS   39

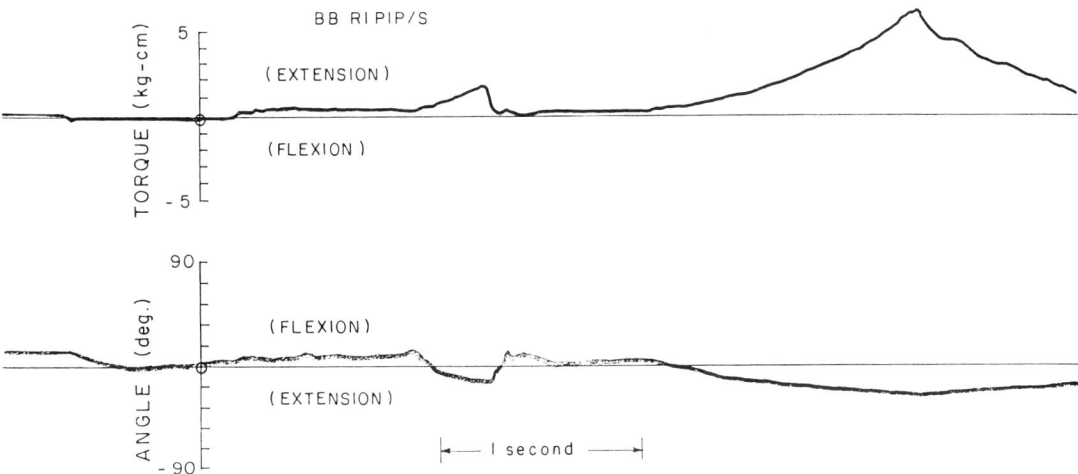

Fig. 3.16 A strip chart recording of the output of the joint torque instrument. The upper trace is the torque and the lower is the angle. The direction of paper travel was from left to right.

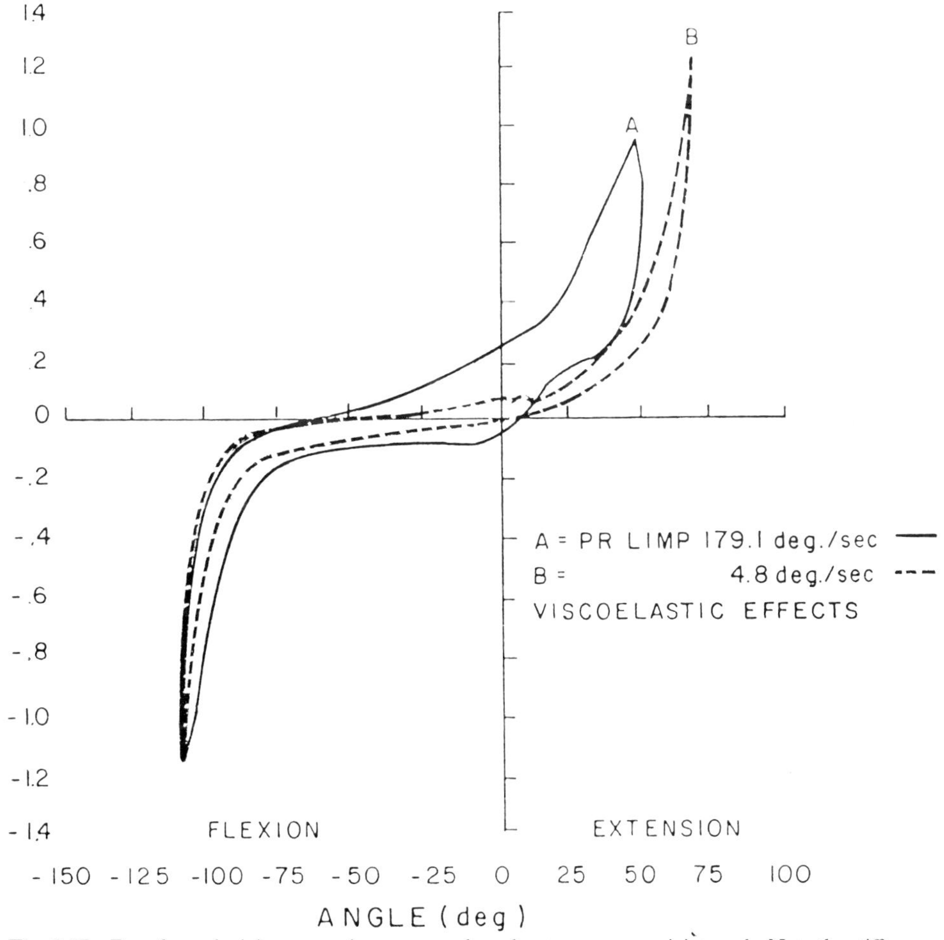

Fig. 3.17 Data from the joint torque instrument plotted as torque versus joint angle. Note the stiffness of the flexion limit and the greater range of joint extension for the same torque when it is applied slowly (– – –) rather than fast (——). This hysteresis is due to the viscous nature of joint motion.

ship shown in figure 3.17**b** is the smooth, low-torque motion described by the mid-range of both curves. In this range of the motion, there are few elastic structures that are under stress and thus few forces acting on the joint. The soft tissues are not stressed, the muscles are in their mid-range resulting in a low torque requirement to elicit joint motion over most of its range of motion.

A second important feature is the sharp increase in the torque required to move the joint at the ends of its range of motion. At these limits, many structures contribute to the increase in joint torque. As described previously, these include stretching muscles, joint capsules, paratenon and compression and elongation of soft tissue as well as tendon drag. The representation of these factors must be included if the behaviour of the joint is to be simulated with any realism.

The third significant feature is the hysteresis associated with the motion (Fig. 3.17**a**). It is noteworthy that the larger hysteresis is directly related to the velocity of the joint. In general, there are three factors contributing to this phenomenon. These include the following:

1. Drag of the joint surfaces on each other. In the normal joint, the smooth, sliding action of the articulation is lubricated by the synovial fluid and results in very low friction. In a diseased joint, this action diminishes and is lost, with subsequent wearing away of the articular cartilage and, finally, bone-to-bone rubbing friction.
2. Viscous drag due to the distension of muscles and the motion of tendons in their sheaths. The distension or elongation of muscles forces a redistribution of the fluids within the muscle. The motion of these fluids results in viscous drag within the muscle tissues.
3. Distortion of the soft tissues. As the joint flexes and extends, the soft tissues must change volume and readjust their fluid distribution. The motion of the interstitial fluids between the various compartments within the finger results in viscous torques applied to the joint.

The importance of the joint T-A curves depicted in this section lies in the wealth of useful information they contain:

1. The steepness of the slope of the curves near the ends of the range of motion infers whether the restriction to motion is an elastic structure, such as skin or muscle tissue, or a more rigid structure such as scar tissue or the normal joint constraints.
2. The area within the hysteresis loop indicates the magnitude of the work required to return the joint to its original position
3. The effects of the angulation of more proximal joints infer where the source of joint motion restriction is located
4. The angular change between two standard torque limits is the range of motion of the joint. These and many other factors may be read from torque-angle curves

It is common for many surgeons and therapists to track the range of motion of joints pre- and postoperatively, Figure 3.18 shows the variability that humans may interject into these measurements. This is largely due to the fact that even trained evaluators each use different levels of torque while making their measurements of range of motion. The simple measurement techniques described earlier can be used to avoid such gross errors. While the dynamic measurement technique may be far more useful and faster, it is still a research tool. The static torque angle measurements are possible for anybody who has a calibrated spring and a goniometer.

FLEXION OF THE IP JOINTS

Each joint can be considered to have an axis about which it rotates. In some joints, this is very nearly a fixed line in space, while in others it may be multiple axes that rotate and migrate as the joint moves. Fortunately, the IP joints are simple hinge joints with a single fixed axis of rotation. First, let us consider the balance of the moment arms and the muscle forces that act around the axis of each joint and then consider the vector analysis by which one can resolve all of the forces at each joint at certain functional joint positions. The balance of forces can best be understood by examining each of the muscles and their action at the joints for which they provide motive power.

The flexor digitorum profundus (FDP) is the only flexor of the DIP joint of each finger, and it is

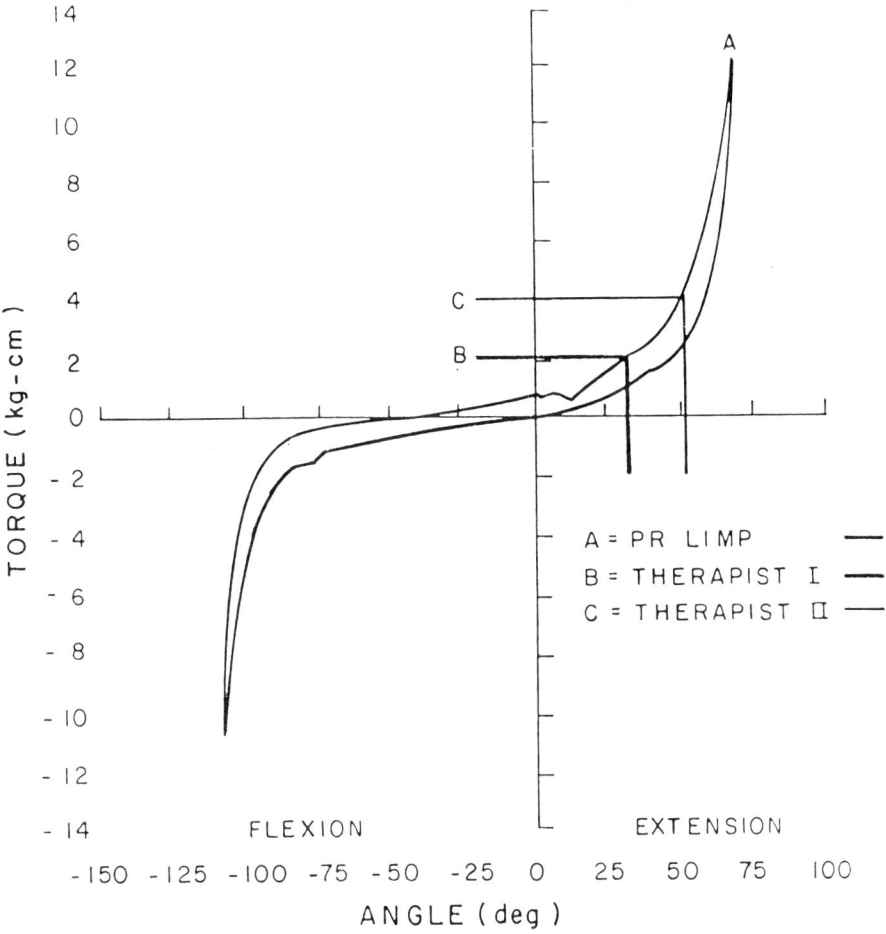

Fig. 3.18 A typical normal torque-angle curve recorded by an electronic device. Two therapists evaluated the angle of the extension limit noted as B, C. Without some reference torque measurement, the results cannot be repeated or used to quantify progress or regress of treatment.

one of the two flexors of the PIP joint. Since the tip of the finger is the point of application of a high proportion of the skilled activities of the hand, it seems strange that the only flexor of the DIP joint is the flexor profundus which has the least degree of independence between fingers. The thumb and index fingers can each move their deep flexors independently, but the middle, ring and little fingers have very limited independent motion.

A pianist or typist is constantly having to flex and extend alternating fingers at high speed and independently move every digit. How is this done? The answer is that the commonality between profundus segments is not in the nerve supply or in the muscle fibres but in the connective tissue and tendon structures. Careful dissection at the muscle belly area of the FDP demonstrates that almost all fibres are dedicated to one tendon or another. The innervation is distinct enough and sufficiently rich to give good independent control for the fingers. By careful observation of the hands of pianists, harpists, typists and flautists, it can be observed that the greatest range of independent movement needed between fingers that strike a key and those lifted away is within 4 cm at the finger tip level. The joints that are used for most of this individualized motion are the MP joints. For a digit 10.0 cm long to flex 4.0 cm at its tip requires an angular motion of 20° at the MP joint. This is about one-third of a radian and would require about 3 mm of movement of the flexor profundus tendon in an average finger. This is well within the free independent range of excursion within the various segments of the profundus (Table 3.2).

The finger whose independent profundus stretch is put to the highest test is the little finger of the left hand of a violinist who has to flex and abduct the MP joint while the PIP joint is extended and the DIP flexed on the G string at the time when the other fingers are in a contrasting flexion at the PIP joints (Bendz 1985) (Fig. 3.19). This requires nearly 1 cm of differential FDP excursion. Even this is small when compared with the 6 or 7 cm of total profundus excursion which is used in common wrist motion and coordinated finger flexions. However, when real strength is required in flexion of the terminal joint of a finger as when pinching pulp-to-pulp against the thumb, only the index finger can use its maximum force when the other fingers are extended. Even in the strong 3-jawed-chuck pinch of thumb against index and middle fingers, the pinch is strengthened when the two other fingers are flexed into a fist. The wrist is also usually stabilized at or near its neutral position to avoid using up finger excursion at this most proximal joint.

The flexion strength of the DIP joints

In an average adult middle finger, when an opposing force is applied at the distal pulp at right

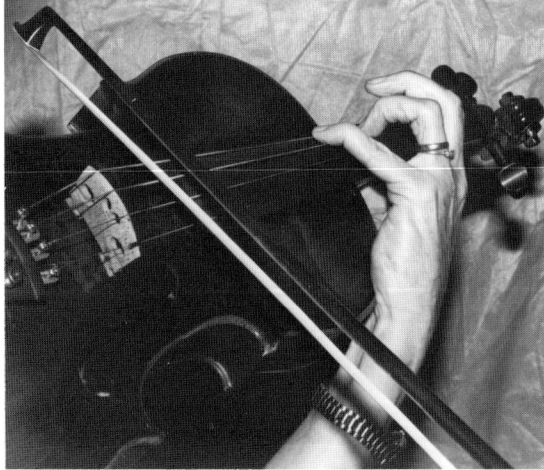

Fig. 3.19 The female violinist's little finger is stretched forward and the flexed fingertip is pressed on the G string with the PIP joint maximally extended. (Based upon Bendz 1985.)

Table 3.2 Moment arms, ranges of motion, and required excursions of profundus tendons. These figures are approximate and rounded off to give numbers that are easy to remember

Joint	Moment arm (cm)	Range of motion (degrees)	Required excursion (cm)
Wrist	1.25	120	2.50
MP	1.00	90	1.50
PIP	0.75	100	1.25
DIP	0.50	60	0.50
Total required excursion			5.75

angles to the finger length, it is 2.0 cm from the axis of the DIP joint. Since the profundus tendon has a moment arm of approximately 0.5 cm at this joint, the muscle must contract with a tension that is four times the opposing force for equilibrium (refer to Equation 2, p. 28). In measurements utilizing fresh frozen cadaver hands, the profundus to the middle finger has a cross-sectional area of 3.4% (Brand et al 1981) of the cross-sectional area of all muscle fibres below the elbow. Thus its 'tension fraction' is 3.4%. To relate the physiological cross-section to the maximal force potential of a muscle, Steindler (1950, 1955) showed the proportionality constant to be 3.6 kg/cm^2. If a person of moderate strength had 200 cm^2 of total cross-sectional area of all muscles below the elbow, his middle finger profundus tendon would have 6.8 cm^2 of cross-sectional area (200×0.034) and might exert 24.5 units of tension (3.6×6.8). It could flex against a load of approximately 6 kg (24.5/4) at right angles to his pulp near the end of his finger. This is approximately 2 cm from the axis of the DIP joint (Brand 1985). The variations of the tension fractions in other fingers would be in the ratio of 2.7 index, 3.4 middle, 3.0 ring, and 2.8 little, which are the relative cross-sectional areas of their profundus muscles.

Note

The index finger is stronger than the little finger mainly because of the contrasting contributions of the two tendons of the flexor digitorum superficialis (FDS). The profundus muscles to the four fingers have tensions that are not very different from each other. The FDS, however, has a very wide variation on the order of 0.9 (little finger) to 3.4% (middle finger) tension fraction (Brand et al 1981).

The flexion strength of the PIP joints

The flexion capability of the PIP joint is based on the FDP and the flexor digitorum superficialis (FDS) together. In the extended position, both tendons hug the skeletal plane. The profundus, being superficial, has a slightly larger moment arm. The two slips of flexor superficialis flatten and diverge to their insertions. As the PIP joint flexes, the profundus bowstrings, but this motion is restrained by the flexor tendon sheath. The two slips of the superficialis also bowstring and rise up off the bone on each side of the profundus. Long (Long 1960, Landsmeer & Long 1965) in his electromyographic studies of hand motion showed that when the hand opens and closes without resistance, the profundus is the only active flexor of the IP joints. The superficialis plays no active part in this motion. However, as soon as resistance is encountered or when finger independence is important, the superficialis carries its part of the load.

Considering the resistance to a given external force at the end of the finger, the moment at the PIP joint is much greater than that at the DIP, since the moment arm is approximately 5 cm. Since the moment arm of the profundus is about 0.75 cm at the PIP joint, the mechanical advantage of the external force is 6.67 (5.0/0.75). The profundus can maintain the equilibrium of the distal joint with a tension of only four times the external force. It unavoidably provides the same tension at both the DIP and PIP joints. Therefore, an additional 2.67 units of tension is required to provide enough moment for PIP equilibrium. This can only be provided by the superficialis.

Thus the ratios of profundus/superficialis tension at the PIP joint in response to a distal load on the finger is determined entirely by the ratios of the lengths of digital segments and of the moment arms of the tendons at the two joints. In the case of the middle finger, which has a strong superficialis, the two muscles have approximately the same cross-sectional area. The superficialis can exert a larger proportion of the total tension if needed.

This would occur if the load was applied to the middle of the terminal segment. The load, at a moment arm of 1 cm would have twice the moment arm of the profundus at the DIP joint. Such a load would be 4.0 cm from the PIP joint and would require a higher tension from superficialis than from profundus.

In the index and ring fingers the profundus muscles are almost as strong as the profundus muscle in the middle finger. The superficialis muscles are weaker than the profundus by the ratio of 2:3. Thus, when a hand carries a heavy load across the ends of the fingers, it is most efficiently placed when it crosses near the end of the ring and index fingers, but a bit further back on the middle finger. This, in fact, is how it would naturally lie when the fingers are nearly extended, and all the muscles would be fully utilized. The little finger has a much weaker superficialis muscle with a tension fraction of 0.9% and is more inclined to have an extended PIP joint and to flex its DIP joint at maximum effort. This may be observed in a violinist's left hand during high notes on the G string (see Fig. 3.19). The question arises: Is the superficialis weakness in part responsible for the observed greater tendency for DIP flexion contractures in the little finger when compared to the other fingers?

EXTENSION OF THE IP JOINTS

Extension moments of DIP joints

It is relatively easy to determine the moment arm of the extensor tendon at the axis of the DIP joint. There is really only one tendon and it is flat. We have derived a graph of the moment arm by measuring angle change coordinated with the moment (excursion) of the tendon as it crosses the joint. When the flexor tendon moment arm is 0.5 cm, the moment arm of the extensor is about 0.3 cm. Since the joint is rarely hyperextended, the moment arm may also be measured or derived from skeletal measurements in true lateral X-rays and scans because the tendon remains adjacent to the skeletal profile throughout joint motion (Fig. 3.20).

However, when one attempts to determine the details of muscle control of the tendon, all

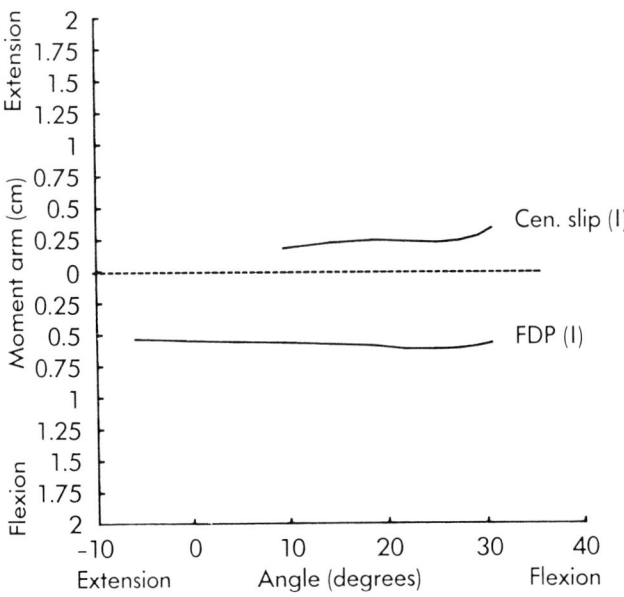

Fig. 3.20 Moment arms for flexion and extension of the FDP and of the central slip (Cen. slip) at the DI joint of the index finger with proximal and metacarpophalangeal joints in extension. The central slip excursion measured by movement of a wire rather than of the tendon itself. (From Brand 1985, by permission.)

simplicity disappears. The ability of the extensor digitorum to exert extensor moment at either the PIP joint or the DIP joint depends upon many factors that are quite independent of the muscle itself. A major factor in this vital question is the posture of the MP joint. In fact, the MP joint is the key to the functioning of all the elements of the extensor expansion. It is quite impossible to give a rational account of the biomechanics of the IP joints without extensive reference to the MP joint.

Biomechanical factors concerning the MP joint

How extension of the MP joint is accomplished

Extension of the MP joint, as with any joint, requires an extensor moment (force times the moment arm). Forces may be exerted by firing the muscles or by a physical property of the muscle known as viscoelasticity. Electrophysiological studies have shown that in unloaded (unresisted) extension of the finger there is motor stimulation of the extrinsic extensor and the lumbrical. In unloaded flexion, there is motor stimulation of the profundus and to some degree the extrinsic extensor. In this phase of motion, the extrinsic extensor appears to be acting as a regulator. The interossei are silent in both flexion and extension when there is no resistance on the finger.

With this information, one can appreciate the importance of the viscoelastic forces in balanced motions of the normal finger. The complexity of firing forces during power grip and precision handling are not known with any precision. They are not discussed here. The viscoelastic response of a piece of tissue following deformation is a slow return to its original shape. Its properties are therefore termed time-dependent. If the flexor tendons are severed, the stored elastic energy and tonus in the extensor muscle results in spontaneous extension of the finger. A gap remains between the ends of the severed flexor tendons even after the finger has been passively returned to its previous position, implying that a viscoelastic force existed in the flexors before they were cut.

The only connections of the extensor tendon to the proximal phalanx which might be effective in MP joint extension are the laminae. However, these structures do not appear to be in a position to do this until extension of the finger is nearly complete. Experiments were performed on fresh cadaver specimens to study the effect the laminae might have in this function. From the fully flexed position of the intrinsic minus finger, increasing weight was applied to the extensor tendon against a constant load on the profundus tendon. Hyperextension of the MP joint was maximum before extension of the PIP joint even began. As more weight was added to the extensor tendon, the PIP joint began to extend. However, extension of this joint ceased before the limit of its full passive extension was reached. At this point, the laminae were divided. There was no drop or loss in hyperextension of the MP joint but there was additional extension of the PIP joint. A ball-bearing pulley was positioned over the dorsal aspect of the joint to prevent spanning or bow-stringing of the extensor tendon across the hyperextended MP joint. The fact that, on release of the laminae, the additional proximal movement of the extensor tendon resulted in further extension of the PIP joint but not of the MP joint, demonstrates that any underlying connection between the extensor tendon and the proximal phalanx could not have been tight. Thus the extension of the MP joint has to be due entirely to the torque produced by the tension of the tendon at the moment arm at the MP joint axis. Neither the laminae nor any hypothetical direct insertion at the proximal phalanx need to be invoked.

Structures limiting hyperextension of the MP joint

The finger behaves according to the flexor–extensor moment ratios within stops or constraints. Constraints may also be classified as forces. For the MP joint, it is theorized that voluntary extension of this joint ceases when there is an equilibrium between three concurrent forces (Micks et al 1978). These three forces are:

1. The restriction imposed by the laminae which extend from the volar plate to the extrinsic extensor tendon and act as fixed-length cords
2. The force of the extrinsic extensor tendon proximal to the laminae
3. The force of the extrinsic extensor tendon distal to the laminae produced by the viscoelastic force of the extrinsic flexors

This equilibrium and restriction of further hyperextension at the MP joint occurs before the mechanical limits imposed by the volar skin, fascia and capsule of this joint (Littler 1967). This is shown pictorially in Fig. 3.21.

Biomechanical factors concerning the IP joints

Significance of the changing moment arms with flexion and extension of the PIP joint

The A3 annular band moves with the volar plate, allowing the flexor tendons to span across the PIP joint as this joint flexes (Fig. 3.22). This spanning progressively lengthens the flexor moment arm during this motion (Spoor & Landsmeer 1976). The change in the flexor moment arm was observed by Idler & Strickland (1984). It seems reasonable that when extending the PIP joint from the flexed position there must be a corresponding increase in the extensor moment arm of the extensor assembly, otherwise extension of this joint could not occur. Landsmeer (1949) theorized that there might be significantly more loading or tension of the central fibres of the extensor assembly as the finger approaches full flexion.

In 1970, Sarrafian et al reported the results of measuring forces by implanting small strain gauges in various components of the extensor assembly of the finger. They found that there is a gradual increase in the relative tension of the middle fibres beyond 60° of flexion. At 90° of flexion of the PIP joint, they reported a total relaxation of the lateral fibres. In 1981, Micks & Reswick reported experiments on fresh cadaver fingers which supported

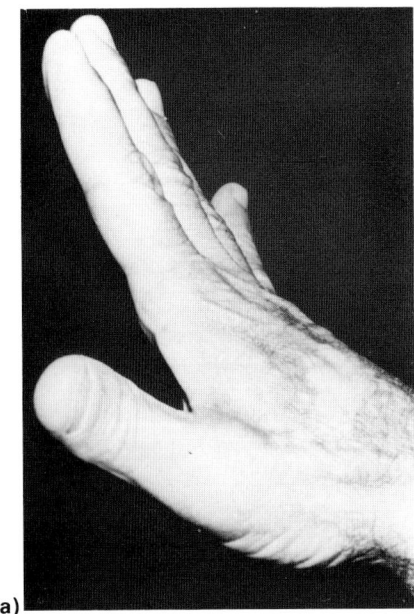 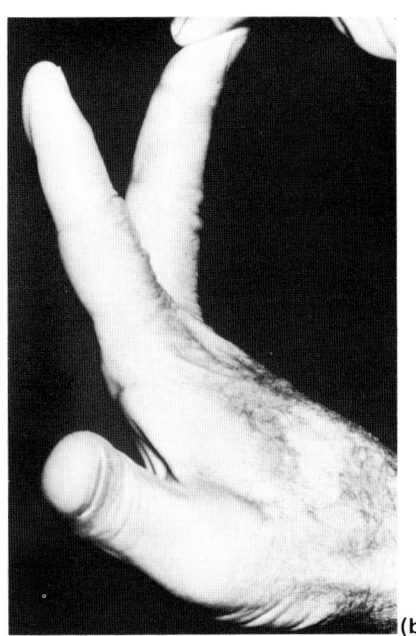

Fig. 3.21 (a) (b) This subject is making a maximum voluntary finger extension effort. Note the additional amount of MP joint hyperextension when the finger is forced to its passive limit.

this differential loading of the lateral and central fibres at the PIP joint as the finger moves. As the load or tension changes from the lateral to the central fibres in the flexing finger, the extensor moment arm increases. These changes are subtle and are constantly adjusting to the demands of the flexor forces (Fig. 3.23). In these experiments, opening and closing of the living hand was stimulated by applying appropriate loads to the cadaver fingers. However, as DIP joint flexion continues to a maximum, the relative loading of the lateral fibres increases.

There are several biomechanical features that operate simultaneously at the PIP joint in order to allow the PIP and DIP joints to move harmoniously together. One is the relationship between two tendons that join proximally to a single tendon and a single muscle, but that cross a joint distally at different moment arms. Fig. 3.24 depicts such a system.

There are two pulley wheels of different radii but fixed to a common axle (axis). When the two ropes (tendons) are independent of each other, the one on the larger wheel will move further, for a given angular motion of the double wheel, whether the movement is distal or proximal. However, if the two ropes (tendons) are joined proximally, they can be at equal tension only in one position of the wheel (or joint) (Fig. 3.24**a**).

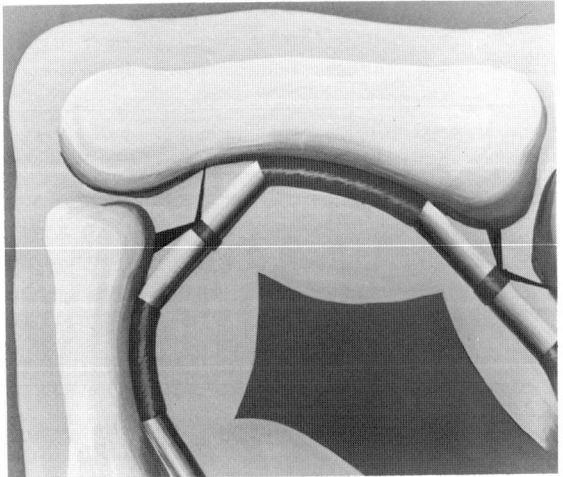

Fig. 3.22 Volar movement of the A3 band with flexion of the PIP joint is demonstrated in this illustration. The volar plate swings away from the axis of flexion–extension as the distance between the attachments of the volar capsule foreshortens. (Illustration from Micks J E & Hager D L 'The A3 pulley: fact or fiction?' presented at the March 1983 meeting of the American Society for Surgery of the Hand in Anaheim, California.)

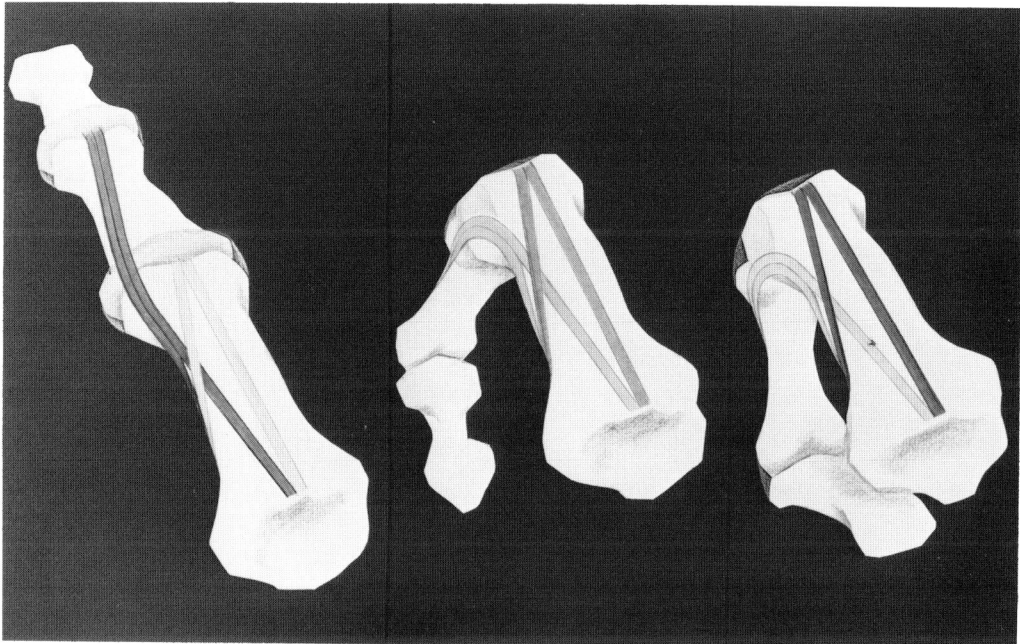

Fig. 3.23 The change in the shading or 'boldness' of the lateral and central fibres indicates the relative load (black indicates maximum load). Note how the maximum load is on the central fibres when the finger is flexed and on the lateral fibres when the finger is extended.

If the common rope is pulled proximally, the rope on the larger wheel becomes slack and only the rope on the smaller wheel will be effective (Fig. 3.24**b**). If the wheel (joint) is turned distally in a manner similar to PIP flexion, it is the rope on the smaller wheel (lateral band) that becomes slack, and only the larger wheel transmits the tension of the common rope (Fig. 3.24**c**).

Applying this principle to the extrinsic extensor tendon, it may be noted that the resting position of the PIP joint is probably between 30–45° of flexion. At this position both the central slip that has the larger moment arm and the lateral band, with the smaller moment arm, could be at equal tension (Fig. 3.24**d** and **e**).

Now, when the extrinsic extensor common tendon is pulled proximally, the central slip, with the large moment arm, would become slack, while the lateral band, with its small moment arm, would extend the PIP joint with its small moment arm. This does not happen because the lateral band is not tethered and can move past the PIP joint and use up its excursion on the DIP joint, allowing the central slip (which crosses only one joint) to share control of the PIP joint. As an example, if the moment arms of the central slip and lateral band are 5 mm and 2 mm at the PIP joint, and if the common extensor tendon caused a 30° (about half a radian) PIP angulation, then the central slip would move 2.5 mm while the lateral band would need to move only 1 mm. However, since both slips are joined proximally, the lateral band may move the same distance as the central band by moving 1.5 mm past the PIP joint, and thus will have 1.5 mm available for the DIP joint. Since the DIP joint in this example would have a moment arm of 3 mm, the DIP joint would also extend half a radian, or approximately 30°.

Thus both PIP and DIP would extend 30° under the influence of one tendon split into central and lateral bands, but crossing the PIP joint at different moment arms.

This is a simplified explanation. There are complexities which make it almost impossible to be precise (see Fig. 3.24**e**). The first complexity is that the lateral band has a variable moment arm. The second complexity is that the distal half of the lateral band has a second group of muscles (the

48 THE INTERPHALANGEAL JOINTS

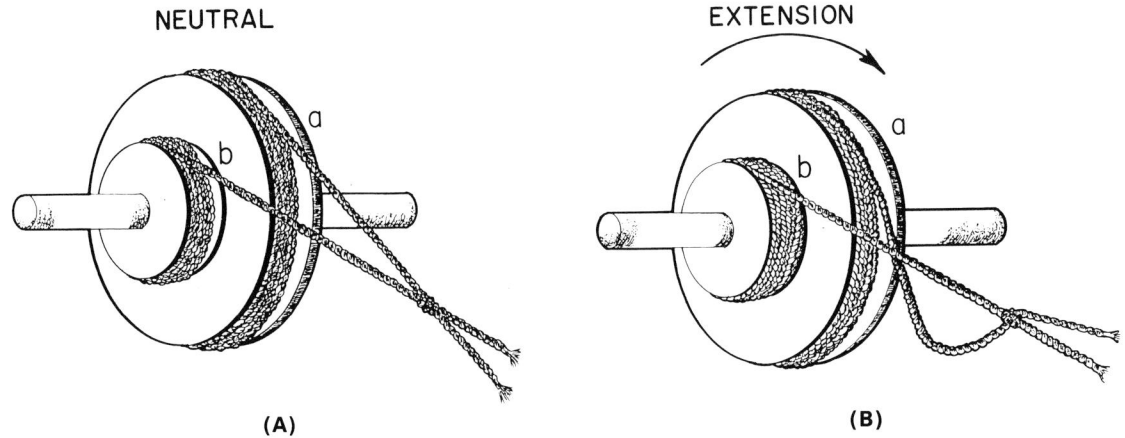

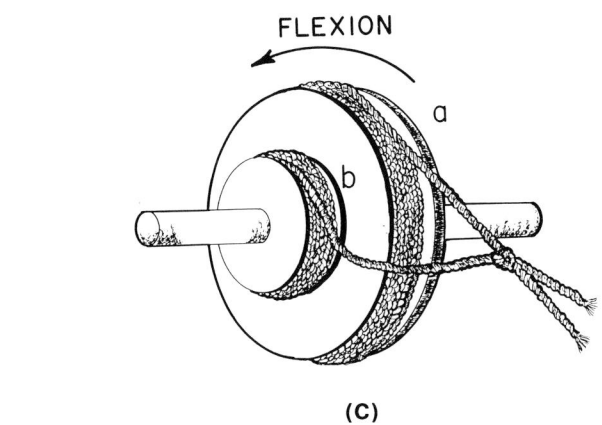

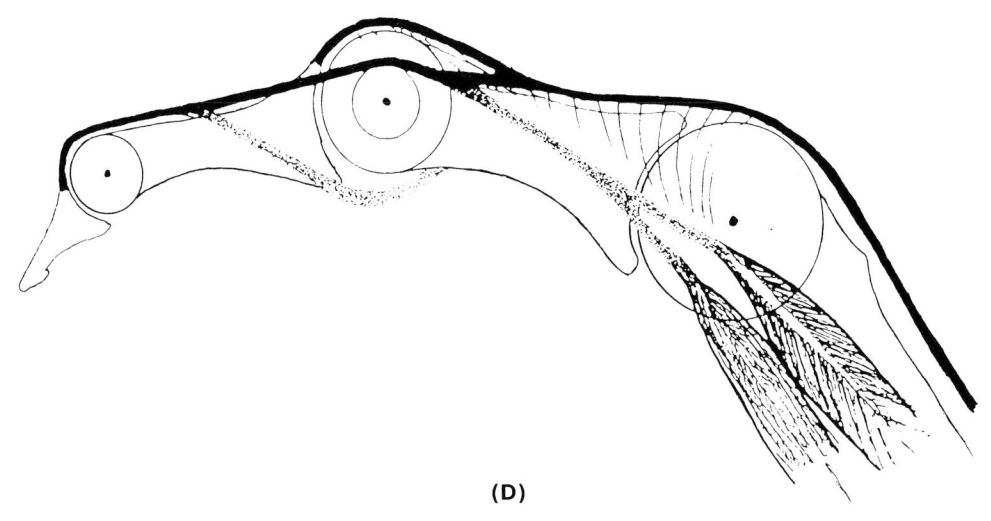

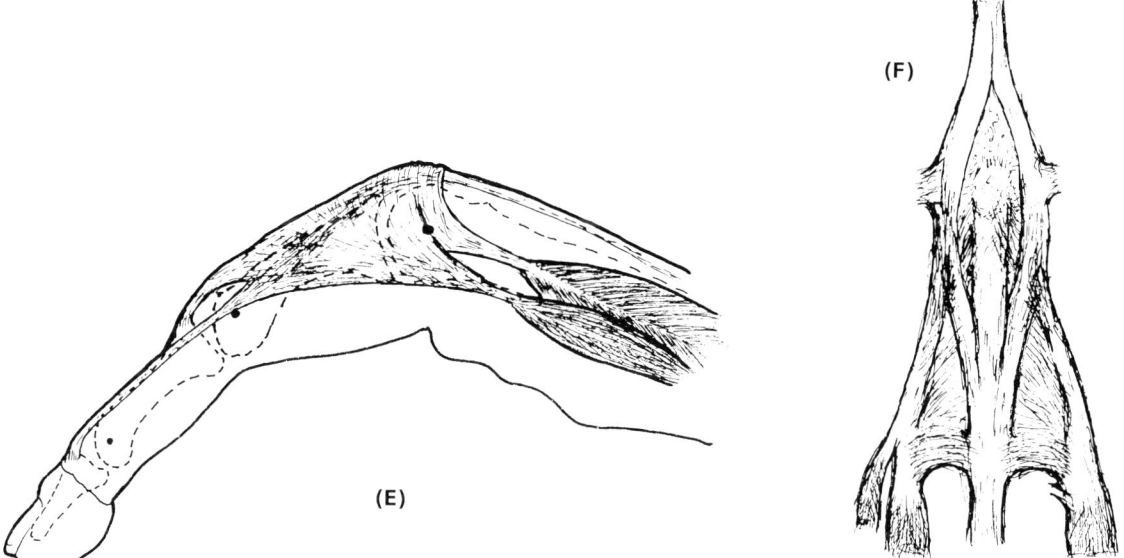

Fig. 3.24 The extensor digitorum (ED) at the interphalangeal joint (Micks & Reswick 1981). Because the ED tendon is single at the MP joint, and splits into central slip and lateral bands before the PIP joint, both parts of the tendon must move through equal excursions or one will become slack and the other alone will work. (**A**) The rope on the big wheel (a) is like the central slip of ED tendon. The rope on the small wheel (b) is like the lateral band, having a smaller moment arm on the same axis. (**B**) Pulling the common tendon extends the PIP joint, but the central band (moving more for the same angular change) would become slack. The lateral band would extend the joint. (**C**) Turning the wheels distally (flexing the joint) pulls tendons distally and the lateral band would become slack. (**D**) and (**E**) But in a real finger the lateral band is free to move past the PIP joint, and use its distal movement to equalize the excursion of the two sides. This allows both central and lateral slips to remain in tension, providing both joints move. (**D**) is a fully diagrammatic lateral view of the dorsal expansion to emphasize double insertion of extensor tendons. (**E**) is a semi-diagrammatic lateral view and (**F**) is a spread-out dorsal view of the dorsal expansion. Thus the ratio of moment arms of the central slip and lateral band at the PIP joint determines how much excursion of the lateral band is made available to the DIP joint. If the lateral band were nearly at the same level as the central slip, the extensor tendon would have minimal effect at the DIP joint. If the lateral band were very near the axis of the PIP joint, the DIP joint would move more than the PIP joint, because the moment arm of DIP joint is smaller than the PIP joint and therefore moves through a greater angle for the same excursion. In fact the ratio of moment arms at the PIP joint varies with the position of the joint.

intrinsics) feeding into it. The distal lateral band may therefore transmit the motor power of the extrinsic or the intrinsic muscles, or both. The third complexity is that the whole dorsal expansion complex (torque tube) is composed of obliquely orientated fibres: it gains length when the tube is narrow and shortens when it is wide, like a fabric woven on the bias. There is a change of diameter of the torque tube while the finger flexes and extends, and this changes the effective length of the segments. The fourth complexity is that the whole moving system of tendons is linked by retinacular ligaments that serve to ensure that the PIP and DIP joints move together. Even when the lateral band is cut at the PIP joint and unable to transmit any muscle tension to the DIP joint, the retinacular ligaments will utilize active extension of the PIP joint to provide a 'tenodesis'-type of extension to the DIP joint. The fifth complexity is the individuality of every finger and of every hand. The two sides of a single finger may differ quite markedly in that the lateral band may have a larger moment for PIP extension on one side of a finger as compared with the other.

Firm figures for the effective moment arms of all the elements of muscles that affect the IP joints are not currently available. The measurement of the action of a given muscle at a given joint in a fresh cadaver hand requires that all other joints be held immobile. This results in restriction of the mobility of the whole complex that crosses both joints. Thus our series of graphs of tendon excursion and of 'effective' moment arms for tendon elements crossing one joint are made while

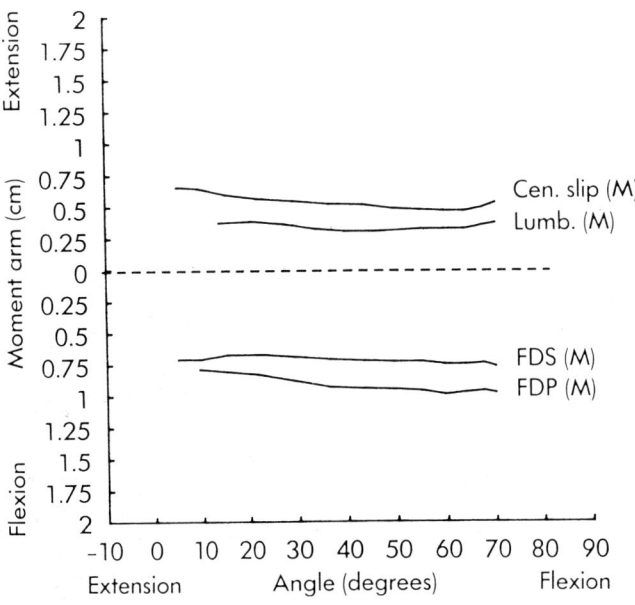

Fig. 3.25 Moment arms for flexion and extension at the proximal IP joint of the middle finger with the MP joint in extension. Note: the excursion of the ED central slip was measured by the excursion of a fine wire running along the tendon, in order to avoid the restraints caused by lateral attachments of the real tendon which vary according to the position of other joints. (From Brand 1985, by permission.)

the other joint is fixed at various positions (Figs. 3.25 and 3.20). This does not match the motions of the human body, however. An electronic system for monitoring two joints simultaneously in the same finger while monitoring tendon motion has not been successfully devised. Our figures should be taken with reservations. Cooney et al (1981) have also tried to measure moment arms of all muscles at all joints and are reticent at citing numbers for these elements at the IP joints.

Structures preventing hyperextension at the IP joints

In addition to balanced moment ratios, the prevention of the zig-zag collapse of the proximal, middle, and distal phalanges requires physical limits, or constraints. The volar portion of the capsule of the IP joints prevents excessive extension. Absence of this predisposes the joint to collapse and assume the well-known swan-neck deformity. This portion of the capsule includes the check ligaments which are an integral part of the dorsal aspect of the flexor tendon sheath, the volar plate, and the volar portion of the collateral ligaments (Bowers et al 1980).

The oblique retinacular ligaments have their origins from the distal portion of the proximal phalanx and from the flexor sheath, and then course distally, volar to the axis of the PIP joint, to converge gradually on the lateral fibres of the extensor assembly. The oblique retinacular ligaments limit flexion of the DIP joint as the PIP joint extends. The normal unloaded finger motion does not seem to be affected by these structures (Harris & Rutledge 1972, Spoor & Landsmeer 1976, Shrewsbury & Johnson 1980).

Passive block to hyperextension of the PIP joint

The torque-angle curves of normal hands show that the PIP and DIP joints have a rather abrupt end to their range of motion. This is in contrast to the MP joints where hyperextension may occur to a considerable extent, and in which a slow loading into hyperextension over a period of minutes will often result in progressive further increase, albeit with some discomfort.

Thus, in the MP joint passive hyperextension may often reach 20 or 30° more than active extension, while PIP and DIP passive extension rarely exceeds active extension by as much as 5°. The limiting factor in PIP extension seems to be due to a firmer attachment of the palmar plate and/or the different orientation of the collateral ligaments.

Bowers et al (1980) demonstrated the significance of these factors by some experiments in which large numbers of digits were loaded into extension at the PIP joints, using forces applied through an Instron testing machine. The forces were applied at the DIP joint level to produce an extension moment to the PIP joint and were increased to the point of rupture in some of the experiments. Using standard torques that were short of that needed for rupture, they showed that for levels of torque that resulted in no hyperextension in the intact fingers, 5° of hyperextension occurred after sectioning of either the accessory collateral ligament alone, or incision of the central 80% of the distal attachment of the volar plate. When, in addition to dividing the central 80% of distal attachment, the major lateral distal attachments of the volar plate were additionally incised, 25–35° of additional extension were noted with the same static loading. This is summarized in Table 3.3.

When the PIP joint was loaded into extension to the point of failure, using a rapid application of load that might be expected in a sports injury, it was the distal attachment of the volar plate which ruptured, sometimes with a flake of bone from the palmar rim of the distal bone of the joint. The force needed for rupture varied from an average of nearly 40 kg for the index finger to 22.5 kg for the little finger.

These studies suggest that the major static resistance to hyperextension is offered by the confluent distal lateral insertion of the volar plate–collateral ligament complex, where it cups the lateral flared margin of the phalangeal condyle. It was noted that instability sufficient to allow dorsal dislocation of the joint did not occur unless there was interruption of the proper collateral ligament as well as the accessory collateral ligament complex in a direction towards its proximal phalangeal origin.

The list of functional contributions exhibited by the palmar plate to the action of the joints includes the following:

1. The palmar plate serves as a mechanism to maintain the moment arms of the flexor tendons of the extended finger preventing them from moving into the intra-articular space during flexion or extension
2. The palmar plate serves as an anchor for the accessory collateral ligaments
3. By acting as a sliding cover for the joint space, the palmar plate reduces the relative motion of these tissues and reduces friction during joint movement
4. The palmar plate serves as an anchor for the flexor tendon pulleys (C1 and A3)

Clinical observations related to hyperextension

Only a minority of adult Caucasians are able to hyperextend their interphalangeal joints. However, among natives of Southeast Asia high mobility of the fingers is common, and is indeed highly regarded as a sign of beauty. The classical dancers of India, and even more so of Thailand, feature an extraordinary ability to place the palms of the hands flatly together while the fingers bend backwards in a curve which involves hyperextension of all joints, so that the terminal phalanges are at 90° to the plane of the palm; (this is called the position of the 'open lotus flower').

Table 3.3 Additional extension resulting from sequential dissection of the joint structures under static loading. (Adapted from Bowers et al 1980)

Structure severed	Additional extension (degrees)
Accessory collateral ligament	5
Central 80% of distal attachment of volar plate	5
Proximal attachment of palmar plate	10
Major lateral distal palmar plate attachments	25–35

This extreme mobility of the finger joints must in part be an inherited feature, common to certain races, but it is also enhanced by a very common habit of 'cracking' the knuckles and deliberate frequent exercises in which each hand exerts mutual hyperextension on the other. It is also enhanced by the habit of washing each hand on its own, without contact with the other.

Hypermobile hands must be treated carefully in muscle balance operations. It is very easy to turn an 'intrinsic minus' into an 'intrinsic plus'. Once the PIP joints are hyperextended, a new feature comes into the muscle balance picture. The lateral bands may rise up dorsally on each side of the central slip, and form ridges across the PIP joint. These tendinous ridges are bowstringing and have a greater moment arm than the central slip, and are thus able to hold the PIP joint in hyperextension even while the profundus is beginning to contract. Since the extensor tendon at the PIP joint is consolidated into a single flat tendon that is inserted on the proximal part of the phalanx, there can be no bow-stringing there. Thus, when the extensors and flexors are contracted simultaneously the profundus maintains its dominance over the extensor at the DIP joint, but loses it at the PIP joint. The result is the ugly swan-neck deformity. This 'trick movement' is not often seen in India and Thailand because, although it is easy to do, it is perceived as ugly. In the USA it is often cultivated by hand surgeons who happen to have hypermobile joints and who like to demonstrate a swan-neck deformity to their students.

Swan-neck deformity

The real pathological swan-neck deformity is common in rheumatoid arthritis where it may follow a loosening of ligaments and joint capsules (Fig. 3.26). Biomechanically it may be a sequel to a primary imbalance at the MP joint, such as the loss of extensor moment arm following slippage of the extensor tendon off the apex of the MP knuckle, or from any blockage to MP extension. This results in the concentration of the effective torque of the extensor tendon to the IP joints. As the patient frequently struggles to extend his MP joints he inevitably constantly produces an extensor moment at the IP joints. This gradually produces a

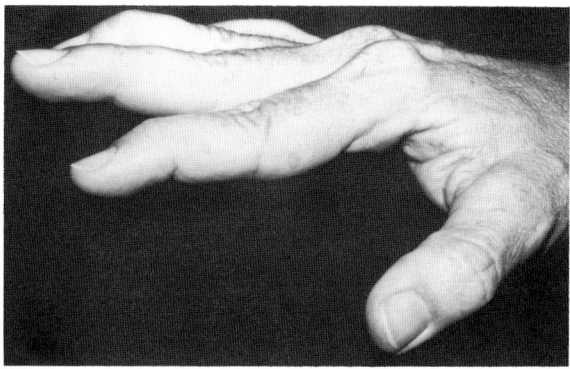

Fig. 3.26 The swan-neck deformity, showing hyperextension of PIP joint with flexion of DIP joint.

stretching of PIP ligaments and palmar plate even in people who have not previously been able to hyperextend their PIP joint.

Another mechanism that may result in PIP hyperextension is due to the loss of the flexor superficialis from its normal position (after a tendon transfer) especially if the superficialis has been transferred to become an extensor of the PIP joint in the same finger, as in the Stiles-Bunnell operation for intrinsic palsy.

Whatever the cause, the result of the imbalance of the PIP joint is hyperextension and consequent increase in the moment arm of the extensor. The patient initiates attempts at finger flexion by contracting the profundus. This results in DIP flexion while the PIP is still hyperextended. Yet another mechanism that results in the same swan-neck deformity is a chronic or constant pull on the lateral band from the intrinsic muscles, such as occurs following ischaemic contracture. This keeps the MP joint flexed and the PIP extended. It should also keep the DIP extended, and does so if the hand is not used much. However, since the attempt to flex the fingers now has more extensor resistance at the PIP than at the DIP joint, a tendency to flex the DIP joint develops which also stretches the retinacular ligament to permit DIP flexion with PIP hyperextension. A later result is a stretching of the extensor expansion over the distal segment leading to the chronic habitual intrinsic plus position, leading ultimately to a fixed swan-neck deformity.

A similar passive stretch of the retinacular ligaments and of the distal dorsal expansion occurs gradually following arthrodesis of the PIP joint, particularly if it is fused in extension. It is difficult to obtain a good PIP arthrodesis without some local adherence between the cut bone and the extensor tendons that run past it. Thus after arthrodesis the profundus flexes freely, but the extensor at the DIP joint is held back. The retinacular ligament is also fixed proximally by the fact that the PIP no longer flexes, so it has to be stretched to allow DIP flexion. Once stretched these dorsal structures are no longer able to restore the extended position to the DIP joint. The result is rigid stiffness of the DIP joint near extension immediately after surgery, followed by a progressive flexion deformity of the DIP joint over a long period of time, finally becoming an ugly right-angled flexion. This occurs faster in the insensitive hand, where the stretching of the dorsal structures is not accompanied by discomfort.

Boutonnière deformity

The biomechanics of this deformity may be inferred from the consideration of all the factors that have already been adduced for the normal finger. The deformity and disability arise from rupture or other failure of the tendon complex over the dorsum of the PIP joint. This may begin by a rupture of the central slip of the extensor tendon due to sudden forced flexion or it may follow an ulcer or infection over the dorsum of the joint, or from attenuation of the dorsal hood, as part of rheumatoid disease.

Whatever the primary cause, the result is a failure of continuity in both the longitudinal and the lateral plane of the tendon fibres over the PIP joint. The name boutonnière is from the French word for button-hole which refers to the way the skeletal joint seems to poke through the hole in the tendon sheath, with the tendon retreating proximally and also falling away laterally.

Once the middle band is ruptured or attenuated, it is free to retract, leaving the lateral bands to carry the full force of the extrinsic extensor tendon. The lateral bands are normally close to the axis of the PIP joint and have a very small moment arm. The defect over the joint allows the lateral bands to fall further palmarwards, sometimes becoming actual flexors of the PIP joint. Thus, the PIP joint is left entirely without extensor tendon, and the effort to extend the PIP joint results only in higher tension on the lateral bands which now hyperextend the DIP joint. At first the DIP joint may not actually hyperextend, owing to the block to hyperextension from the palmar plate and the accessory collateral ligament. However, over a period of time the palmar plate and the ligaments become lengthened and the finger develops the characteristic posture of PIP flexion with DIP hyperextension. Any attempt to extend the PIP joint passively only further hyperextends the DIP joint.

Over a further period of time all tissues of the finger accommodate to the posture. For example the retinacular ligaments become shortened and further resist correction of the deformity. It is not the purpose of this chapter to discuss surgical correction, but it may be noted that it must be done early, so as to avoid the postural adaptation of other structures.

SUMMARY

This chapter has attempted to establish the fundamental issues relative to the biomechanics of the human hand. The theoretical and experimental topics covered should raise as many questions as they answer. This should stimulate the practising clinician to attempt to answer some of these questions through observation of patients or the researcher to attempt to answer other questions via further refinement of the information and measurement techniques presented here. In this way, new insights may be shared by all and the practice of medicine elevated.

REFERENCES

Agee J M, Guidera M 1980 The functional significance of the juncturae tendinae in dynamic stabilization of the metacarpophalangeal joints of the fingers. American Society for Surgery of the Hand, Atlanta, Georgia

An K N, Chao E Y, Cooney W P III, Linscheid R L 1979 Normative model of human hand for biomechanical analysis. Biomechanics 12: 775–788

Bendz P 1985 The functional significance of the oblique retinacular ligament of Landsmeer. A review and new proposals. The Journal of Hand Surgery 10B: 25–29

Bowers W, Wolf J, Nehil J, Bittinger S 1980 The proximal interphalangeal joint volar plate. I. An anatomical and biomechanical study. Journal of Hand Surgery 5: 79–88

Brand P W, Beach R B, Thompson D E 1981 Relative tension and potential excursion of muscles in the forearm and hand. The Journal of Hand Surgery 6: 209–219

Brand P W 1985 Clinical Mechanics of the Hand. C. V. Mosby, St. Louis

Buford W L Jr 1984 Interactive three-dimensional computer graphics simulation of the kinematics of the human thumb. PhD Dissertation, Department of Engineering Science, Louisiana State University, Baton Rouge, Louisiana

Chao E Y, An K N 1978 Determination of internal forces in the human hand. Journal of the Engineering Mechanics Division February: 255–272

Chao E Y, Opgrande J D, Axmear F E 1976 Three-dimensional force analysis of finger joints in selected isometric hand functions. Journal of Biomechanics 9: 387–396

Cooney W P, Lucca M J, Chao R L, Linscheid L 1981 The kinesiology of the thumb trapeziometacarpal joint. Journal of Bone and Joint Surgery 63A: 1371–1381

Eyler D L, Markee J E 1954 The anatomy and function of the intrinsic musculature of the fingers. Journal of Bone and Joint Surgery 36A: 1–9

Flatt A F 1961 Kinesiology of the hand. Instructional course lectures, American Academy of Orthopedic Surgeons, 18: 266–281

Harris C, Rutledge G 1972 The functional anatomy of the extensor mechanism of the finger. Journal of Bone and Joint Surgery 54A: 713–726

Idler R S, Strickland J W 1984 Proceedings of the American Society for Surgery of the Hand. Journal of Hand Surgery July: 595

Ketchum L D, Thompson D, Pocock G, Wallingford D 1978 A clinical study of forces generated by the intrinsic muscles of the index finger and the extrinsic flexor and extensor muscles of the hand. Journal of Hand Surgery 3: 571–578

Landsmeer J M F 1949 The anatomy of the dorsal aponeurosis of the human finger and functional significance. Anatomical Record 104: 31–43

Landsmeer J M F 1976 Atlas of anatomy of the hand. Functional considerations. Churchill Livingstone, Edinburgh, p 326–427

Landsmeer J M F, Long C 1965 The mechanism of finger control, based on electromyograms and location analysis. Acta Anatomica 60: 330–347

Littler J W 1967 The finger extensor mechanism. Surgical Clinics of North America 47: 415–432

Long C 1960 An electromyographic study of the extrinsic-intrinsic kinesiology of the hand: preliminary report. Archives of Physical Medicine and Rehabilitation 41: 175–181

Micks J E, Hager D L 1983 The A3 pulley: fact or fiction? Presented at the 1983 Meeting of the American Society for Surgery of the Hand, Anaheim, California

Micks J, Reswick J 1981 Confirmation of differential loading of lateral and central fibers of the extensor tendon. Journal of Hand Surgery 6: 462–467

Micks J, Reswick J, Hager D 1978 The mechanism of the intrinsic minus finger: A biomechanical study. Journal of Hand Surgery 3: 333–341

Ou C A 1979 The biomechanics of the carpometacarpal joint of the thumb. PhD Dissertation, Department of Mechanical Engineering, Louisiana State University, Baton Rouge, Louisiana

Riordan D 1984 Personal correspondence

Sarrafian S K, Kazarian L E, Topouzian L K, Sarrafian V K, Siegelman A 1970 Strain variation in the components of the extensor apparatus of the finger during flexion and extension: a biomechanical study. Journal of Bone and Joint Surgery 52A: 980–990

Schultz R J, Furlong J II, Storace A 1981 Detailed anatomy of the extensor mechanism at the proximal aspect of the finger. Journal of Hand Surgery 6: 493–498

Shrewsbury M, Johnson R 1980 Ligaments of the distal interphalangeal joint and the mallet position. Journal of Hand Surgery 5: 214–216

Spoor C, Landsmeer J M F 1976 Analysis of the zigzag movement of the human finger under influence of the extensor digitorum tendon and the deep flexor tendon. Journal of Biomechanics 9: 561–566

Steindler A 1950 Postgraduate lectures in orthopedics: diagnosis, and indications. Charles C Thomas, Springfield, Ill

Steindler A 1955 Kinesiology of the human body. Charles C Thomas, Springfield, Ill. p 47

Thompson D E 1981 Biomechanics of the hand. Perspectives in Computing, no. 3. 3: 12–19

Thomas D H, Long C, Landsmeer J M F 1968 Biomechanical considerations of lumbricalis behaviour in the human finger. Journal of Biomechanics 1: 107–115

Weeks P M, Wray R C 1973 Management of acute hand injuries: a biological approach, C V Mosby, St Louis

SECTION 2

Repair and Reconstruction of Injury

4

Injuries and complications of injuries to the capsular structure of the interphalangeal joints

INTRODUCTION

'The skeleton deprived of its ligament dislocates, its form and the power of its muscles negated' (Eaton 1971). The stabilizing function of the interphalangeal ligament structure is herein implied by noting the consequences of its disruption: deformity and loss of power. Interphalangeal ligaments do not provide power or motion. They provide the stable link that allows efficient transmission of muscular force across the joints. This, in turn, permits the digital skeleton to assume varying positions of function.

Capsular structure is differentiated into collateral ligaments and volar capsular ligament (volar plate) with the result that motion in a given plane is either highly, partially, or minimally restricted. Stabilizing demand on the lateral ligaments is continuous throughout the entire range. These ligaments are assisted in their function by muscle tone which compresses the tight-fitting bicondylar joint. The volar capsular ligament becomes tight as the joint nears full extension. It is assisted in its function by the static sheath and retinacular system as well as by tension within the flexors. The ligaments are kept at their optimal length and flexibility by normal joint motion.

Injury and its consequent healing response greatly interfere with this sophisticated restrictive–permissive function (see Fig. 4.1). Depending on the specifics of the structure injured, the type of injury, and the healing event, motion may be allowed in previously restricted planes (instability) or limited in previously unrestricted planes (contracture). Asymmetry of capsular tension as a result of inadequate healing or too much scar may cause uneven joint surface tracking and uneven joint compressive forces. This will eventually result in a loss of full power, a chronically swollen and painful joint, and arthrosis. In this sense, joint laxity, contracture, deformity, arthrosis, pain and loss of strength, job, hobby or happiness may all be complications of digital ligament injury.

Treatment, whether it be 'watchful neglect', immobilization, mobilization, or surgery, is invariably an additional insult to tissue with its own particular consequences. These may include infection, broken pins or wires, injury to uninjured structures, dystrophic pain syndromes, stiffness of adjacent joints, or diagnostic inadequacies leading to the wrong treatment entirely. Thus, the treatment 'insult' must be added to that of the injury itself in order to gain a true overview of a capsular ligament disruption.

In this chapter, injuries to the capsular mechanism alone are discussed. The discussion will stop short of intra-articular fractures or fracture/dislocations unless the fracture is a direct result of tension on the capsule—the so-called 'chip' or avulsion fracture resulting when a ligament–bone interface fails. Thus ligament sprains, attenuation, disruptions and all varieties of dislocations are included along with capsular contracture and capsular instability.

Figure 4.1 depicts the natural history of interphalangeal capsular injury. There is little specific information on this chart. Its value is as a skeleton for the chapter. Table 4.1 lists the capsular elements and their function. In addition, impairment by contracture or instability is listed. This chart may

INJURIES TO THE CAPSULAR STRUCTURE 57

be used in reverse. If the consequences are recognized, structures to be considered for treatment may be found.

EVALUATION AND DECISION MAKING

The age and handedness of the patient are to be considered. At times, the patient's occupation or hobbies can assist in decision making. The mechanism of injury is obtained by specifically directed questioning. The patient's observation of deformity at the time of injury is a critical decision factor. The location of swelling, bruising or skin disruption is an important clue. It is important to X-ray *only* the injured parts. This focuses your attention so that small details are less likely to be overlooked. Roentgenograms should be taken in two planes at 90° to one another with obliques added as necessary. When, because of pain or contracture, the joint cannot be fully extended, the anteroposterior assessment often must by your mental integration of two anteroposterior films, one perpendicular to the phalanx on either side of the joint in question. The neurovascular status is evaluated and recorded. The digital joint structure is then palpated to localize tenderness which is graded and recorded. At this point, if pain appears to be interfering with the evaluation, a metacarpal block is performed and the patient is asked to perform the 'active range of motion (active stability) test' in comparison with an uninjured digit. If the joint deforms or displaces, the injury is classified as a grade III ligament injury which implies more than one major retaining ligament is disrupted (see Table 4.2).

The position at which displacement occurs

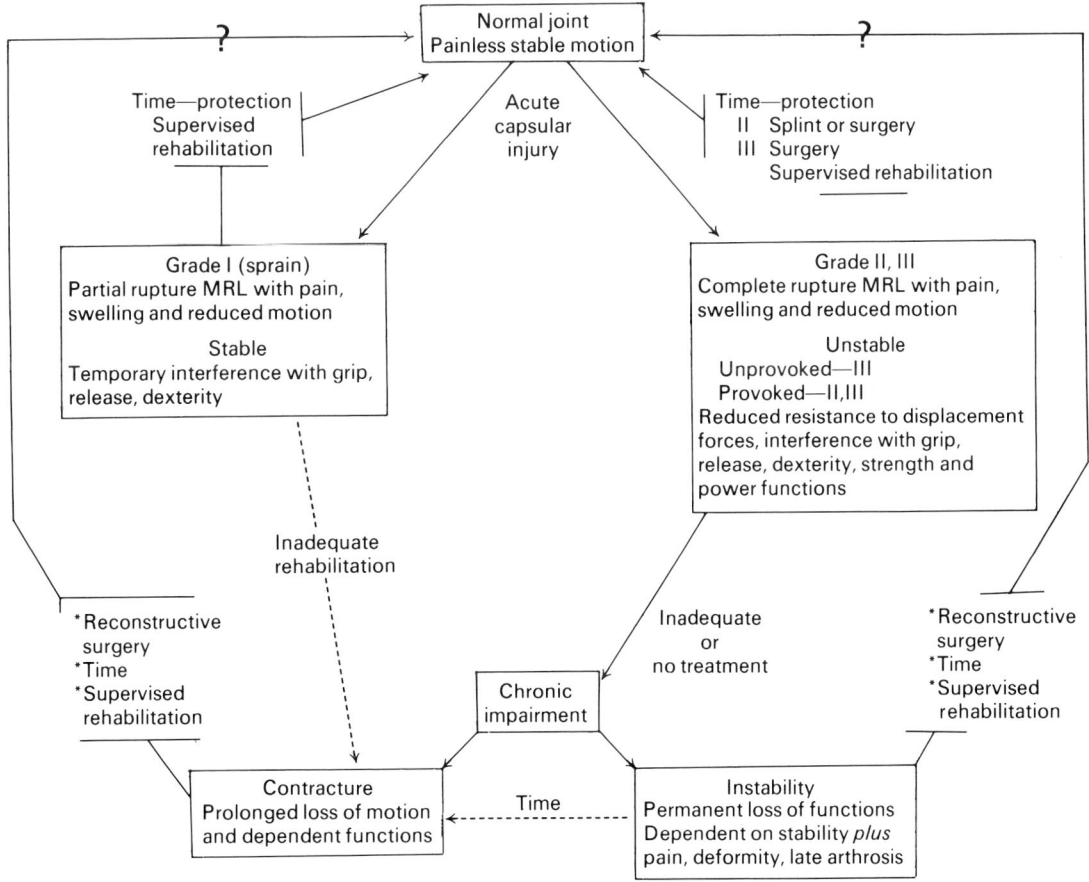

Fig. 4.1 This flow chart represents the various paths a ligament injury may follow. One can appreciate the penalty of inattentive care. MRL—major retaining ligament.

Table 4.1 Capsular ligament function and the consequences of instability or contracture

	Structure	Function	Impairment Chronic contracture	Chronic instability
Proximal interphalangeal joint (PIP)	Radial (ulnar) collateral ligament	Resists lateral displacement in pinch and grip functions Provides stable linkage for force transmission across joint	Extension contracture (Loss of flexion)	Lateral instability in pinch, grip Asymmetric joint tracking
	Volar plate	Static resistance to hyperextension Increases moment arm of flexors Stabilizes joint to lateral stress in full extension	Flexion contracture (Limited extension)	Hyperextension habitus of joint (swan neck) Locking in hyperextension Recurrent dorsal dislocation Extension contracture
	Accessory collateral ligament	Works with volar plate to stabilize joint to lateral stress in full extension	Flexion contracture (Limited extension)	?
	Oblique retinacular ligament of Landsmeer	(see below)	Flexion contracture (Limited extension)	?
Distal interphalangeal joint (DIP)	Oblique retinacular ligament of Landsmeer	Extends DIP joint by static link as PIP joint extends	Extension contracture (Loss of flexion)	?
	Radial (ulnar) collateral ligament	Resists lateral displacement in pinch and grip functions Provides stable linkage for force transmission across joint	Extension contracture	Lateral instability in pinch, grip Asymmetric tracking (deformity)
	Volar plate	Static resistance to hyperextension Increases moment arm of flexors Stabilizes joint to lateral stress in full extension	Flexion contracture	*Rare* hyperextension or dorsal subluxation (strong protection is offered by flexor digitorum profundus)
Both proximal and distal interphalangeal joints	Dorsal capsule	Blends intimately with central slip (PIP joint) and extensor digitorum communis (DIP joint)	Extension contracture	Usually associated with tendon rupture at PIP joint (swan neck) and DIP joint (mallet finger)

suggests the site and degree of disruption. If no displacement or deformity occurs, the joint has 'active stability'. A stress test to determine 'passive stability' is then performed. The joint is stressed laterally in full extension and in 90° of flexion. Instability in 90° of flexion means complete lateral ligament disruption (at least a grade II lesion). If the joint is unstable in full extension as well, the collateral ligament plus a part of the volar plate is disrupted demonstrating a grade III lesion; an X-ray of the stress test may be helpful. If greater than 20° of lateral tilt is present, Stern et al (1985) believe that this comprises a complete and *perhaps* *displaced* collateral ligament rupture. If the joint subluxes or dislocates at *any* position, a grade III lesion is present. The *volar plate* is tested by passive extension. If the joint hyperextends more than an adjacent digit, then there is a grade II volar plate lesion. If the joint subluxes or dislocates, a grade III lesion is present meaning that there is also some collateral ligament injury. If the joint displaces or deforms in a plane other than lateral or dorsal, two major retaining ligaments are disrupted—a grade III lesion. By this combination of methodical testing, a capsular ligament injury can be graded. Accurate selection of the treatment is then possible.

Management principles and decision making

In theory, the rationale for management of small joint injuries is not complicated. In practice, however, inattention to detail, short cuts, treatment modifications and judgement error will combine all too easily to produce unsatisfactory results. Certain *management principles* will help to put the injury in its proper perspective and, if observed, promote valid decisions.

The first of these principles is to recognize the whole injury. The dynamics of injury, inflammation and repair of these small structures are predictable and may be influenced only if recognized for what they are—a non-specific response to injury. The decision to add the insult of treatment to the insult of injury must be approached with this in mind. Collagen and bone formation, maturation and modelling must be considered and utilized.

The second principle is to select objectives consciously. Consider the essential elements of treatment of the injured part itself. Then, modify these, if you must, by considering the particular patient in question. If you begin by 'treating the patient as a whole', you will find yourself immediately compromised on many essential points. The overall objective is a pain free, stable, movable joint as soon as possible. In some situations, these objectives must be placed in order of priority. Several joints function admirably if only stable (thumb metacarpophalangeal joint, carpometacarpal joints of index to ring fingers, distal interphalangeal joints and index proximal interphalangeal joints) whereas others require motion—even at some expense to stability (proximal interphalangeal joints middle to little fingers, metacarpophalangeal joints of middle to little fingers).

The third principle is to inform the patient. As in all physician-managed injuries, an explanation, in advance, of the recovery process is in order. Persistent joint swelling and slow recovery of the extremes of motion are predictable consequences of this injury. It is well to suggest a period of 4–6 months as a reasonable time which must elapse before the patient or physician judge an end result—even when all goes well. If the patient's understanding can be obtained, you will have a cooperative partner in the treatment plan.

ACUTE CAPSULAR INJURY (Table 4.2)

Classification

Capsular injuries are here classified according to degree of injury. The present author considers the major retaining ligaments to be the collateral

Table 4.2 Classification of capsular ligament injury[a]

Grade I: *Partial* disruption of major retaining ligament (MRL) (joint stable to active or passive stress)
   A Collateral ligament
   B Volar plate

Grade II: *Complete* disruption of *single* MRL (joint functionally stable—may be passively stressed beyond usual limits but not to point of subluxation or dislocation)
   A Collateral ligament
   B Volar plate

Grade III: *Complete* disruption of MRL plus one or more adjacent MRL (when seen, the joint is displaced and reducible or irreducible *or* if not displaced, active movement or passive stress easily may do so)
   A Collateral ligament plus volar plate and/or dorsal capsule
      1. Displaced/displaceable—joint can be reduced
      2. Displaced/displaceable—joint cannot be reduced
      3. Ligament displaced—ligament cannot be reduced
   B Volar plate plus one or both collateral ligaments
      1. Displaced/displaceable—joint can be reduced
      2. Displaced/displaceable—joint cannot be reduced
   C Dorsal capsule/central slip plus one or both collateral ligaments
      1. Displaced/displaceable—joint can be reduced
      2. Displaced—joint cannot be reduced

---

[a] This new classification of joint capsule injury attempts to relate the degree of injury to stability and to include all types of injury in the same scheme. Thus, a *sprain* of the collateral ligament (I-A) is in the same classification as a Stener's lesion (III-A, 3) or a 'complex dorsal dislocation' (III-B, 2) or 'complex volar dislocation' (III-C, 2). The word 'complex' has been studiously avoided as inaccurate and confusing.

ligaments and the volar plate. A grade I injury is a partial disruption (0–90%) of the major retaining ligament, but one in which the retaining function of the ligament is intact and the joint is stable to active and passive stress tests. A grade II injury is one in which the major retaining ligament is completely disrupted as a relatively isolated injury—the adjacent quadrant ligaments are intact (for instance, complete volar plate disruption with both collateral ligaments functioning and intact). The joint passes the test of active stability but the passive stress test demonstrates laxity in excess of that allowed by the contralateral or comparison major retaining ligament. The joint cannot be subluxed or dislocated with active or passive stress. A grade III injury represents disruption of two or more adjacent major retaining ligaments. Evaluation may demonstrate failure of both the active range of motion (active stability) and passive stress tests. The joint may be obviously subluxed or dislocated or it may easily assume these positions on active or passive testing. This simple categorization overlaps somewhat but may be uniformly applied to all capsular injuries—dorsal, lateral and volar, reducible or not, stable or not.

Stern et al (1985) have provided valuable insight into the pattern of collateral ligament (CL) rupture and the forces which produce these injuries (see Ch. 1). They have shown experimentally that when the normal collateral system is stressed to rupture at the zero position of flexion, 72% had rupture of both the CL and volar plate (VP) systems (grade III-type A). The majority of this group (73%) had proximal rupture of the CL and distal rupture of the VP. Only 9% of the entire series had an isolated complete CL rupture (grade II-type A) and 17% had isolated incomplete rupture of the CL (grade I-type A). When these ruptures were correlated to radiographic stress tests, 100% of specimens with a stress test of greater than 20° could be shown to have completely ruptured proper collateral ligaments (PCL). Angulation beyond 20° carried an increased chance that the PCL was displaced and would not return to its anatomical position with force dissipation. Angulation under 20° still had a 47% chance that the PCL was *completely* disrupted, but the likelihood was high that the PCL would be found in its anatomic position. Based on these data, they surmised that *early surgery* may have been *beneficial* in the 76% of specimens with greater than 20° angulation and *probably not beneficial* in the 24% with angulation less than 20°.

These data are invaluable in our thinking about pathoanatomy as it relates to surgical indication. To retain perspective, it must be recalled that these are experimental data and all specimens were stressed to a predetermined failure point in a single position of flexion (0°).

Management: collateral ligament injury (capsular injury classification grade I-, II-, III-type A)

Grade I-type A

These injuries are usually termed 'sprains' and represent incomplete tears of the ligament (0–90%). The joint is stable to the active and passive stability tests. The goal of treatment is a quick return to function. This is accomplished by splinting the joint for comfort while the acute injury response subsides. This usually requires 5–7 d in a position of 30–40° of flexion. In the *distal* interphalangeal joint, protected motion is difficult. Therefore, immobilization should continue for 2–3 weeks. Limited motion is inevitable but not disabling. In the proximal interphalangeal joint, however, limited motion *is* disabling and, after a 5–7 d period of rest by splinting, this reduced motion places the joint at risk for re-injury. Re-injury may convert a grade I to a higher grade lesion which might go undetected. At the very least, re-injury adds significantly to the total insult and will prolong recovery. Protected motion is thus necessary and may be easily done using the adjacent digit as a 'buddy'. Three to four weeks of protected motion are usually sufficient for full recovery.

Grade II-type A

The completely ruptured ligament cannot resist passive stress but the joint may be stable to stresses of active motion. Some advise that these injuries be treated as sprains with early protected motion— the rationale being that the joint, if stable to active motion, may be spared stiffness (Carroll 1973). Others advise up to 3 or 4 weeks of immobilization, seeking stability (Curtis 1966, Eaton 1971, Eaton & Dray 1982) and some advise surgical repair (Redler & Williams 1967, Rodriguez 1973, Ali 1984). The present author proposes that once ligament disruption has been demonstrated, the healing process should be allowed to begin with the injured structures firmly in contact, unaffected by stresses which might interfere with the ultimate function of stability. The joint must then be mobilized early enough to avoid prolonged or permanent loss of motion.

Stability is paramount in the distal interphalangeal joint and the index and middle finger proximal interphalangeal joints. Mobility is paramount in the middle, ring and little finger proximal interphalangeal joints. The present author would therefore immobilize the distal interphalangeal joints for 3 weeks at 10° flexion on the index side progressing to 30° in the little finger. He would also immobilize a radial collateral ligament disruption in the index and middle finger and an ulnar collateral ligament disruption in the little finger proximal interphalangeal joint for 3 weeks at 30–40° of flexion. Ulnar collateral ligament injuries in the index, middle, ring and radial collateral ligament injuries in the ring and little fingers he would begin to move after 2 weeks of immobilization. This would be accomplished in the following way: a removable splint is used at night (30–40° of flexion) and 'buddy' splinting is used full time for 1 additional month. Contact sports are avoided for 1 week after full-time immobilization is discontinued but may be pursued thereafter with the digit protected by buddy taping. If this plan is used, stability is assured. There is usually no persisting contracture, although it may be an additional 6 weeks or more before the last few degrees of terminal motion are achieved.

Grade III-type A

In this group, it can be demonstrated that, in addition to the collateral ligament, either the volar plate or dorsal capsule and extensor mechanism, or both, are disrupted. The joint, when seen, is laterally or rotationally angulated, deforms in this manner when active motion is attempted or is easily displaced to this position when passively tested. The contralateral ligament, if uninjured, acts as a rotational axis and resists complete lateral dislocation. If this ligament is also disrupted, the end point of deformity is complete lateral dislocation. If the joint cannot be reduced perfectly (III-A, 2), or the joint deforms with active motion, surgical repair is indicated. The collateral ligament may be trapped in an everted position by periarticular soft tissue (III-A, 3). This is similar to the classic 'Stener's lesion' described at the thumb metacarpophalangeal joint (Stener 1962, Stern 1981). In this case, surgery is imperative (Fig. 4.2). *If* the joint can be reduced *and* can be placed through a full range active motion without deformity *and* the joint is congruous on a post-reduction X-ray, closed management by immobilization is possible. The position is 30–40° of flexion at the proximal interphalangeal joint and 5–30° in the distal interphalangeal joint, depending on the digit (see above). The joint is immobilized for 3 weeks as in grade II injuries.

Based on personal experience, a review of the pathomechanics (see Ch. 1) and the data of Stern et al (1985), the present author favours early operation of the grade III lesion. A more rapid recovery (pain relief and stability) can be achieved through a consistent approach of early surgical intervention (Redler & Williams 1967, Ali 1984). Whether operated on or not, the post-immobilization plan in these injuries is slightly different due to the potentially greater risk of instability. Buddy taping may be applicable when the joint in the adjacent normal finger lies at nearly the same level. If not, the joint may undergo undesirable rotational stresses when forced to track in tandem with its neighbour. An alternative technique is to use 'controlled active motion', a slower but more protective method: after complete immobilization, the digit is splinted at 30–40° in a removable splint. Hourly 3–5 min sessions of active motion are begun and last for 1 week. These progress to active/assistive motion in the fourth postinjury week. At 5 weeks, buddy taping for sport and work exposure is permitted. At 6 weeks, full-time buddy taping is permitted. No dynamic splinting for limited motion is allowed until stability is assured at 6–8 weeks. Films of the joint should be taken during immobilization and after mobilization is begun. If redisplacement is noted, surgery is required without delay.

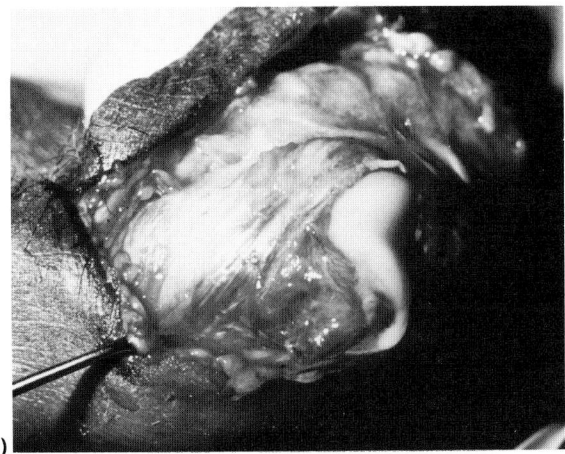

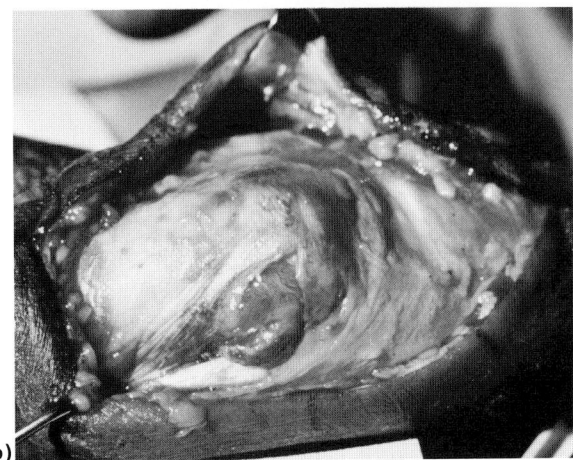

Fig. 4.2 The operative pictures of a III-A, 3 lesion, the so-called Stener's lesion of the joint collateral ligament of the proximal interphalangeal joint. The injured structures are volar plate and collateral ligament which make it a grade III injury. The extent of displacement is seen in (**a**). The middle phalanx is deviated laterally and is not well seen. The main instability following the reduction is lateral, therefore, it is a grade III-A. The joint could be perfectly reduced but it deformed with active motion. The collateral ligament was found everted (**b**) and trapped behind the displaced lateral band which had been split off from the central tendon; thus, the final classification, III-A, 3. This injury pattern is similar to that seen in Figure 4.9, III-C, 1 or 2.

The surgical technique

It should be noted that surgery has two goals—one is to discover and remove obstacles to reduction, the other is to provide for re-establishment of normal stability. Surgery does not accelerate wound healing, it, in fact, adds to the total insult. Surgical trauma should be minimized by a careful plan and utilization of meticulous technique.

Repairs of injuries within the substance of the collateral ligament should be limited to reapproximation of the fragments using as small and as few sutures as possible. When an avulsion fracture exists, the ligament can be restored perfectly with a careful pullout suture technique. The principle is to restore articular congruity with approximation of injured structures using as little foreign material as possible to maintain joint position until immobilization techniques are in place. Occasionally, a transarticular pin must be used to this end. It should be small, placed perfectly the first time, and not expected to be the sole technique of immobilization. The post-surgical joint should be immobilized and subsequently mobilized exactly as the non-surgically treated grade III injury (see above).

Management: volar plate injuries (capsular injury classification grade I-, II-, III-type B)

Volar plate injuries rarely require surgical management in the acute situation. This, in fact, accounts for the relative paucity of information regarding the pathoanatomical nature of these lesions. Exceptions are the open dorsal dislocation (McCue et al 1975, Zook et al 1979), the irreducible dorsal dislocation and the grade III injuries with associated lateral ligament instability.

Acute volar capsular injuries are a spectrum which may end in dorsal dislocation (Eaton 1971, Bowers et al 1980, Bowers 1981). Consider the application of a 'pure' hyperextension stress. As stress increases, tension develops within the volar plate and the accessory collateral ligament. The resultant injury pattern depends much on the rapidity with which the stress is applied. If applied slowly, the proximal attachments or 'swallow's tails' attenuate and ultimately fail. The joint may sublux dorsally, even dislocate, pulling the intact volar plate, flexor sheath and accessory collateral ligament complex over the condyles like a shroud. This slow application of tension is a clinical rarity. Experimentally, it has been shown, and clinically, it has been observed (Bowers et al 1980), that the usual force is rapidly applied. In this case, the ligament fails distally, occasionally avulsing a piece of the volar metaphysis but, just as often, the meniscoid portion will be ruptured without a bony fragment. The critical corner attachments of the volar plate remain intact. Pathoanatomically, this grade I-B volar capsular injury is painful but not destabilizing (Fig. 4.3). If stress continues, the distal lateral attachments of the volar plate fail and the tear extends proximally between the accessory collateral and proper collateral ligament (Fig. 4.4). The middle phalanx may then swing dorsally, hinging on the proper collateral ligament origins and developing stress in its lower fibres (grade II-B). The joint may completely dislocate dorsally without disruption of the proper collateral ligament if the force remains 'pure' hyperextension (Eaton 1971).

Dorsal dislocation is an exception to the grading system. Technically, it is a grade III-B volar plate injury because of the dislocation but, in practicality, it is a grade II-B because the adjacent lateral major retaining ligaments are intact and, once the reduction is accomplished, the joint is stable laterally. In the usual dislocation, the volar plate remains beneath the condyles, stabilized here by its sheath attachments and the accessory collateral ligaments. Reduction is easily obtained by longitudinal traction and a push volarly on the base of the middle phalanx. It is then treated as a grade II injury. If the joint deforms laterally as well as

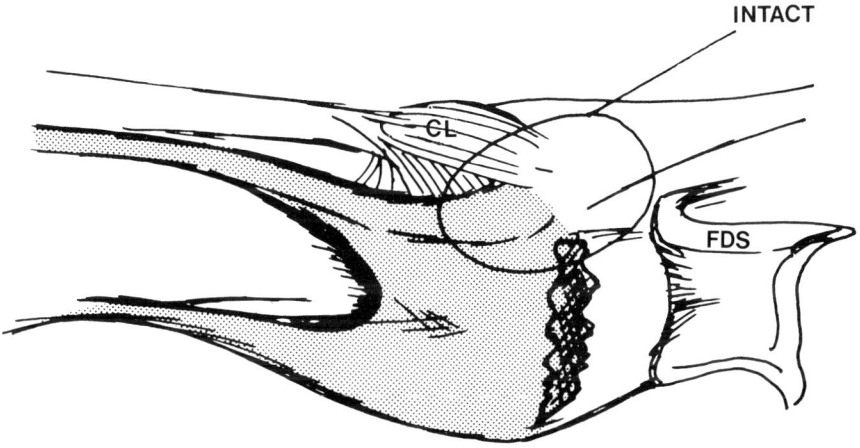

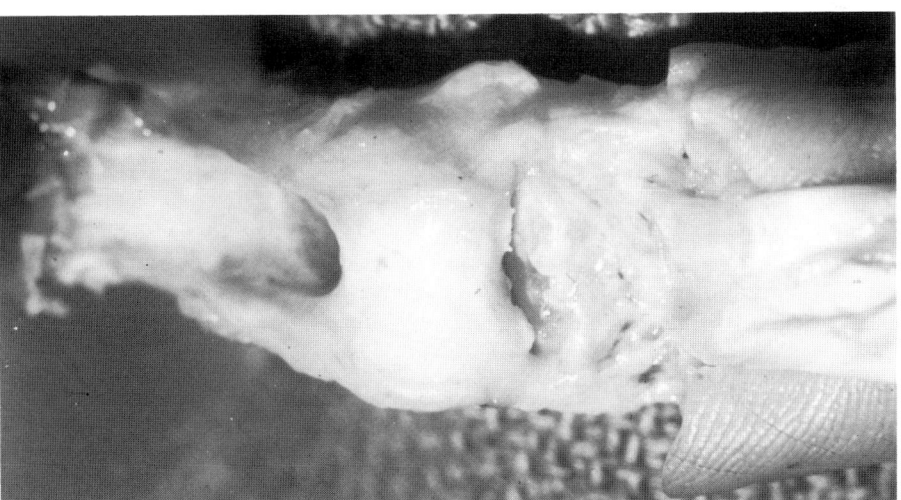

Fig. 4.3 The volar plate is disrupted in its central 80% but the lateral attachments at the critical corner are intact and the joint is not unstable even though painful. It is classified I-B. CL—collateral ligament; FDS—flexor digitorum superficialis.

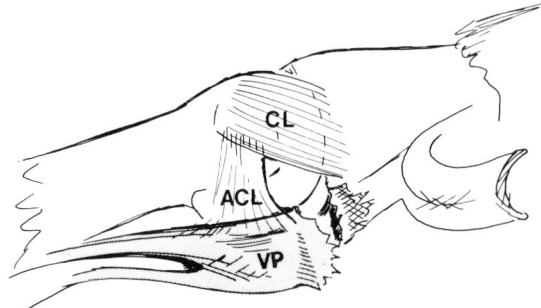

Fig. 4.4 The volar plate is disrupted across the entirety of its insertion on the middle phalanx. The tear has continued proximally separating the accessory collateral ligament from the proper collateral ligament. The joint is, therefore, unstable volarly but stable laterally. Therefore, its classification is II-B. CL—collateral ligament; ACL—accessory collateral ligament; VP—volar plate.

dorsally on the active range of motion or passive stress test or, if after reduction of a dorsal dislocation, the joint is unstable to lateral stress testing, then the lesion is a grade III-B injury and one can infer that torsional as well as hyperextension stress has occurred. The acute injury should be treated as a grade III-A collateral ligament injury expecting the flexion contracture to persist for a longer period. Post-traumatic calcification may occur in one or both of the proximal limbs of the volar plate (Fig. 4.5). This can be associated with a resistant flexion contracture. If the scar process involves Landsmeer's ligament, limited flexion of the distal interphalangeal joint may occur, producing a post-traumatic 'pseudo-boutonnière' lesion (McCue 1975, Lee 1982).

If one encounters an acute dorsal dislocation that is irreducible (III-B, 2), get the camera out for this lesion is rare and worth documenting and reporting. It is possible for the head of the proximal phalanx to 'buttonhole' through the *distal* volar plate disruption and lock itself between the flexors in anatomical dissections. This should, however, be reducible by closed techniques. If not, then operative exploration will allow reduction and visualization of the pathology. If, after reduction, the joint is stable laterally, the injury is still a grade II-B from a treatment standpoint and should be so treated. If one encounters a true dorsal dislocation with the volar plate ruptured proximally and entrapped between the middle and proximal phalanx blocking reduction of the joint—this is a true irreducible dorsal dislocation (III-B, 2) and must be an extreme clinical rarity (Green & Posner 1985). This situation is almost impossible to imagine without an accompanying collateral ligament disruption which, if present, probably preceded the volar plate injury in pathoanatomic sequence and exceeds it in treatment importance. The injury should be treated operatively as a grade III-A collateral ligament injury (see above) after reduction.

Typically, the patient arrives with a history of a rapidly applied force stressing the finger in hyperextension. A true lateral X-ray may be negative, show a small fleck of bone volarly at the proximal interphalangeal joint, or show a dislocation, with or without a fleck of bone (Fig. 4.6). It is essential to recognize that either of the first two may represent the same degree of injury as the dislocation. If maximum tenderness is volarly, specifically at the joint level, we may presume a volar plate injury and determine volar stability by stressing the joint. The patient is asked to perform the active range of motion test after a digital block is applied. It is important also to stress the joint manually, as few completely ruptured volar capsules will allow joint subluxation on voluntary motion. It is equally necessary to discover whether the patient with a 'chip' fracture or negative X-ray is stable laterally and volarly. These grade I volar plate injuries are commonly overtreated. Both the patient with a 'chip' fracture and the patient with a negative X-ray may, however, demonstrate complete loss of volar stability with hyperextension stress. Here, the presence of a 'chip' fracture is of prognostic significance. Proper extension block splinting will oppose the avulsed fragment to its bed, allowing uneventful healing.

The injury that may go unrecognized is the grade II volar plate injury with no visible fracture on X-ray. The diagnosis is usually 'sprain' and perhaps no splint is applied—a serious error. This patient requires dorsal block splinting, for the injury is through a relatively avascular fibrocartilage (Fig. 4.7) and healing without splinting is unlikely (Bowers 1981). This injury is much like the central slip rupture dorsal to the same joint. Eventually, the condyles will buttonhole through

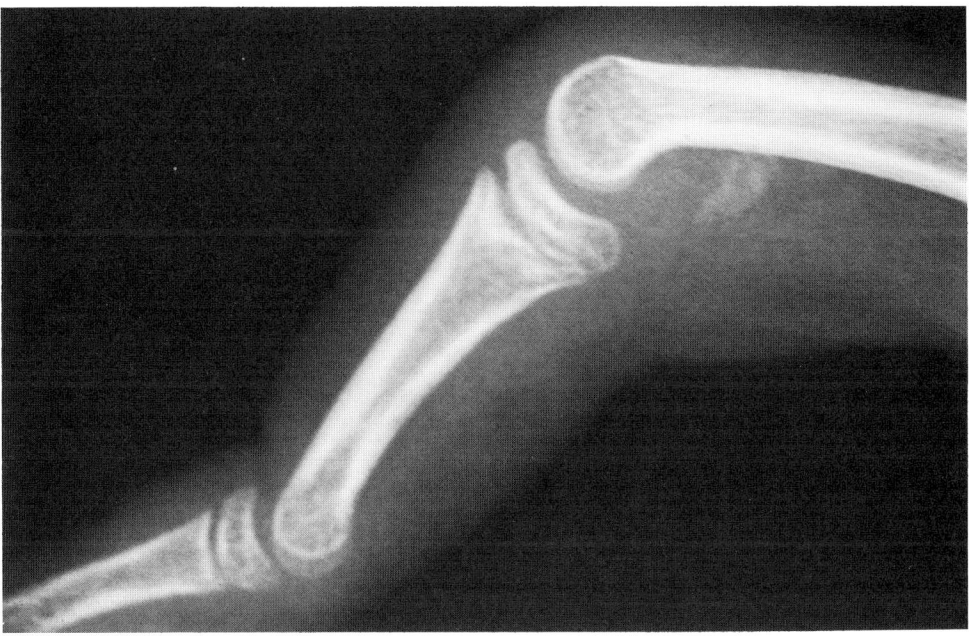

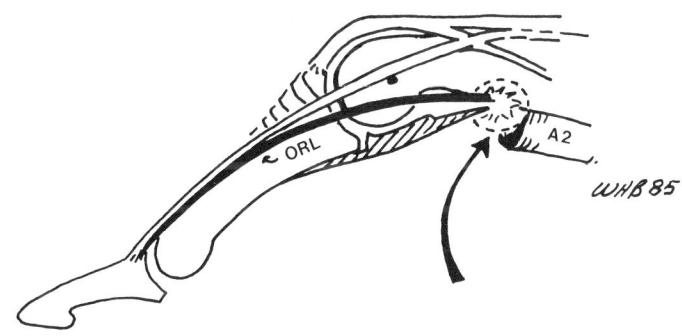

Fig. 4.5 The X-ray shows the calcification in the proximal reins of the volar plate following a hyperextension injury. As shown in the diagram, this injury focus may result in a flexion contracture with some tightness at the distal interphalangeal joint secondary to oblique retinacular ligament involvement in the proximal scar. The terminology is, therefore, 'pseudo-boutonnière'.

the volar capsule and the patient will develop chronic hyperextended deformity—a 'reverse boutonnière' at the proximal interphalangeal joint (Fig. 4.8). At this point, the digit may resemble a chronic mallet finger and a wrong diagnosis may occur (Bowers 1978). This patient must be correctly identified as early treatment is essential in order to avoid problems later. Dorsal block splinting for 3 weeks and buddy taping for an additional 6 weeks is sufficient. Expect a mild flexion contracture to resolve within 2–3 months. Do not use dynamic splinting to treat this contracture until after this time as attenuation of the scar may occur and may result in recurrence of hyperextension.

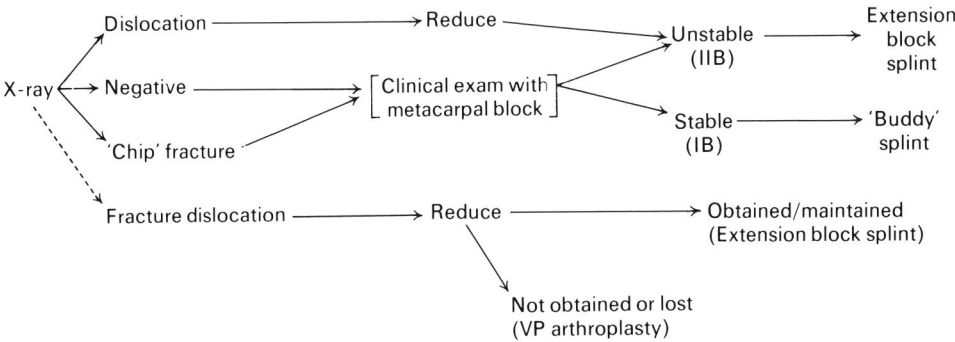

Fig. 4.6 This algorithm of volar capsular injury will help to avoid inaccurate diagnosis and over- or undertreatment.

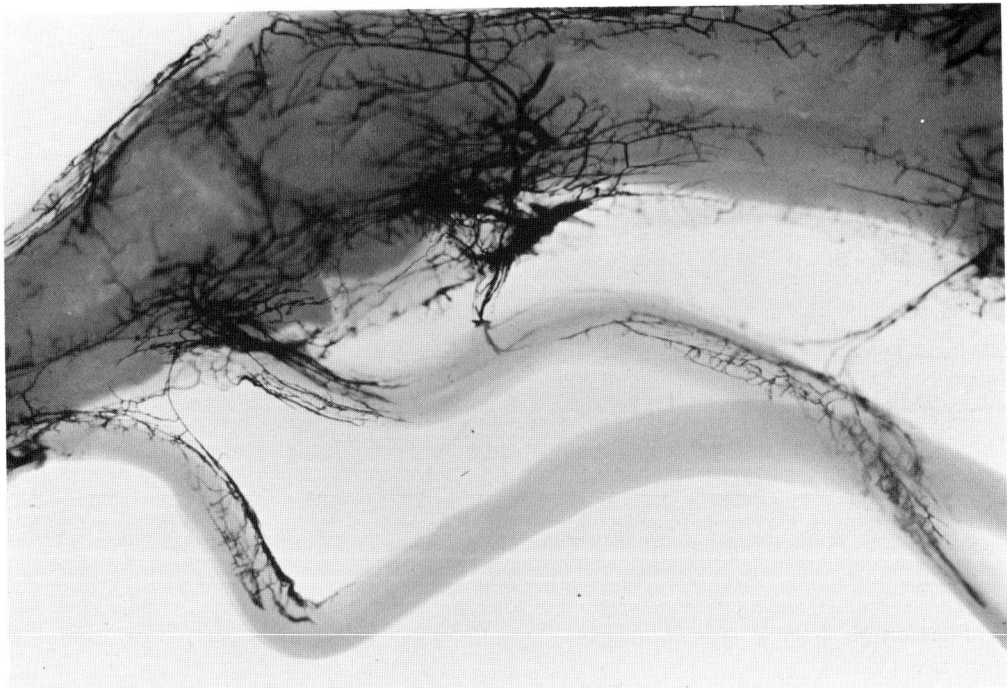

Fig. 4.7 This macrosection of the injected flexor system shows the relative lack of vascularity at the volar plate bone junction while tremendous vascularity is noted in the retrocondylar area and at the flexor digitorum superficialis insertion into bone. This may help to explain the poor healing of a distal volar plate disruption without a fracture avulsion (see Fig. 4.8) and the scarring and tendency to flexion contracture of the volar plate disruption when it occurs proximally (see Fig. 4.5).

Management: volar dislocations (capsular injury classification grade III type-C)

These are rare injuries. The pathology usually, but not always, includes injury to the central slip and one or both collateral ligaments (Meyer 1958, Johnson & Greene 1966, Littler & Eaton 1967, Murakami 1974, Kilgore et al 1976, Spinner & Choi 1970, Thompson & Eaton 1977, Posner & Wilenski 1978, Peimer et al 1984). At a position of

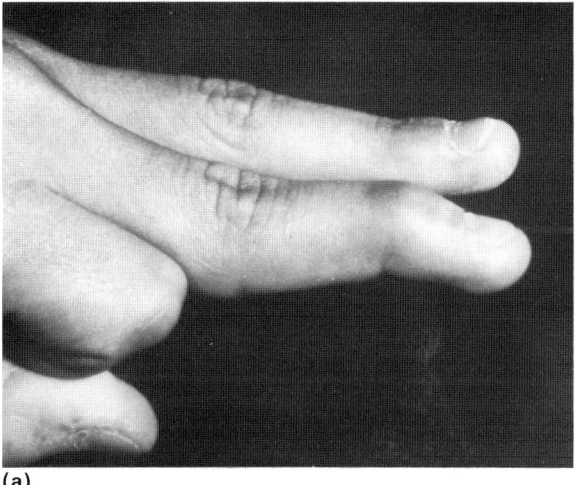

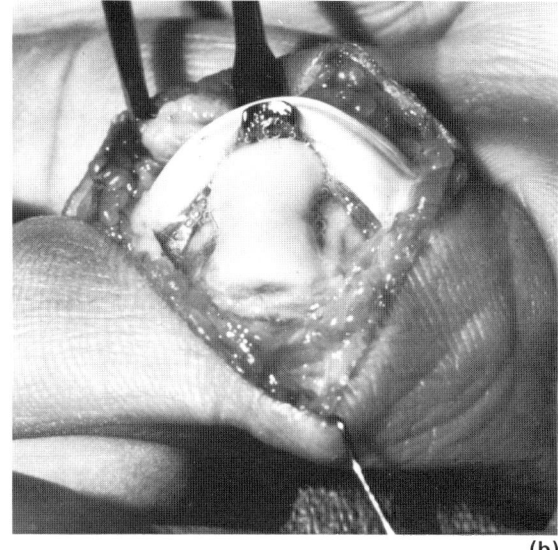

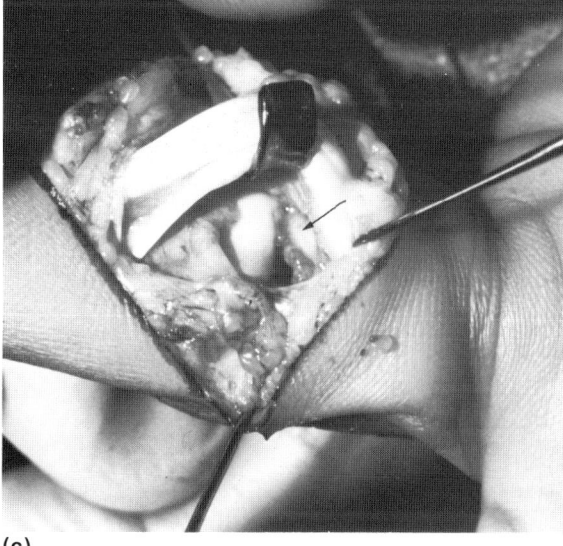

Fig. 4.8 This series shows the (**a**) clinical swan-neck appearance resulting from hyperextension locking or buttonholing of the proximal phalangeal condyles through a tear in the volar plate. (**b**) shows the condyles buttonholed through this tear with the middle phalanx locked in hyperextension. This gives some credence to the designation as a volar boutonnière lesion. (**c**) shows the joint reduced and the ineffective granulations occurring at the distal margin of the volar plate (see arrow).

50–70° of flexion, the lateral band is below the joint axis of motion (Garroway et al 1984). If a torsion force is applied at this position, injury to the collateral ligament and extensor mechanism may occur. The condyles may be caught between the central slip and lateral band and reduction may be difficult or impossible (III-C, 2) (Fig. 4.9). If seen early, closed reduction is attempted and, if successful, is followed by a test of active extension. If there is a lag of more than 30°, then mobilization of the proximal interphalangeal joint in extension for 6 weeks is recommended. Some surgeons suggest immediate repair of the central slip, followed by immobilization. Mobilization may be difficult but results may be very good. If active extension is not tested and a central slip injury exists, the joint may be improperly splinted in flexion and a boutonnière deformity will result. If the injury is seen later, surgical reduction and repair is recommended, but recovery of full motion is the exception rather than the rule. The rehabilitation programme will tax the surgeon and therapist as the combination of repaired dorsal and lateral capsular structure is difficult to manage. Following the requisite immobilization after surgery, active flexion supplemented by careful joint

68 THE INTERPHALANGEAL JOINTS

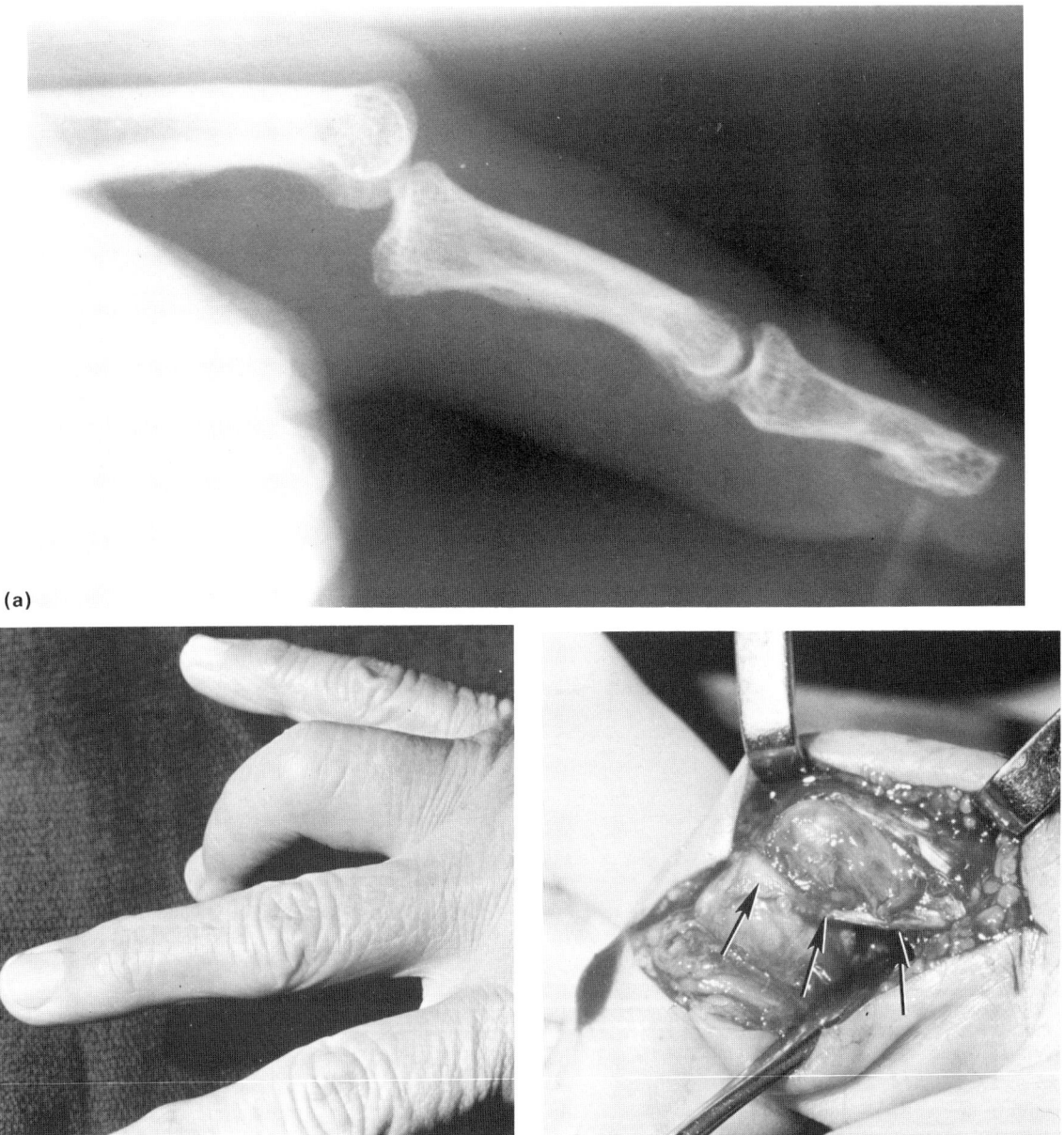

Fig. 4.9 The X-ray (**a**), clinical appearance (**b**) and operative pathology (**c**) of an irreducible volar dislocation. Note the lateral band (arrows) has been split off from the central slip and is interposed between the proximal phalangeal condyles and the displaced middle phalanx, impeding reduction. Note similarity of this to the lesion shown in Figure 4.2, **a**, **b**.

mobilization and interval static splinting is used. Buddy taping may be helpful. If 45° of flexion can be quickly obtained, then dynamic splinting is permissible as joint reaction forces are not excessive in the 45–90° range.

CAPSULAR CONTRACTURE

Loss of motion in this joint severely restricts function. Conversely, if flexion and extension can be maintained in the proximal interphalangeal joint when there is damage in the other small joints of the same finger, satisfactory hand function can be preserved (Green & Rowland 1975). Primary causative factors in postinjury contracture are lack of motion and oedema. The collagen rearrangement that goes with injury will 'cast in stone' the small joint left too long alone in its splint, whatever the position. Neighbouring uninjured joints may also be caught in this well intentioned web. The management of contracture thus begins with the day of injury.

Primary treatment must assure stability and joint congruity in order for the initial immobilization to begin. The injured joints must be elevated, gently compressed, and pain must be eliminated while allowing free movement of all uninjured joints. As soon as the treatment plan will allow motion, it is begun. Rarely is motion withheld for longer than 3 weeks. Often, if stability is present in active range of motion, the joint may be mobilized in a protected way after 7–10 d. Even with this idealized management concept, it may be 3 or 4 months before a full range of motion is obtained especially after grade II or grade III injuries. In this circumstance, it is conceptually better to refer to the joint as having 'limited motion' rather than 'contracture' as the motion will gradually return given time and attention. One should avoid any use of dynamic splinting until full stability is assured (6–8 weeks). During this time, one must encourage active motion, protecting the joint in re-injury exposure periods and using static splints at night to rest the joint in the direction of the most limited range (extension splints for limited extension, flexion splints for limited flexion).

Once stability is insured, the use of serial casting is preferred (see Ch. 15), alternating with periods of active and active/assistive motion. The joints are rested at night in splints designed to maintain the gain achieved. If the joint is not painful or inflamed, the technique of 'joint mobilization' (see Ch. 15) is highly effective. Dynamic splinting is widely used and can be helpful in a *stable* stiff joint if closely supervised by a therapist knowledgeable in this technique. The patient must understand its use and goals. An unattended dynamic splint in a complacent patient can produce pressure sores and undesirable joint compressive forces. Splints particularly dangerous in this regard are the three-point pressure aluminium splints that are tightened by a turn screw and the so-called 'knuckle bender' splints. Contractures that do not respond to this non-operative programme are usually old (more than 6 months) or have undiagnosed elements of articular surface incongruity or capsular instability. The latter two are best managed by joint reconstruction and/or replacement (see Ch. 10). When a stable non-operative programme and the obligatory wait for the joint to return to a stable metabolic state have elapsed, operative release can be considered. One must remember that all successful operative techniques call for the recreation of some element of capsular instability which again requires careful postoperative supervision.

EXTENSION CONTRACTURE

In addition to the joint capsule itself, the surgeon must consider other factors which may participate in limited flexion. These are:

1. Scarred dorsal skin
2. Contracted or adherent extensor tendon or intrinsic tendons
3. Retinacular ligaments adherent to capsular ligaments
4. Bone block or exostosis.

Contracted collateral ligaments, adherent volar plate or scarred volar pouch are the most frequent capsular problems.

Technique

Local anaesthesia with sedation is preferred, so that the patient can actively demonstrate to the surgeon, himself, and the hand therapist, the release of the contracture. If the procedure is performed under other types of anaesthesia, some type of flexor check must be carried out before closure. This can be accomplished by incision and direct traction on the flexor tendon or by hyperextending the wrist and metacarpophalangeal joints. Both should demonstrate flexion of the interphalangeal joints to at least 90°. The preferred incision is a dorsal curved incision (Fig. 4.10). The

70 THE INTERPHALANGEAL JOINTS

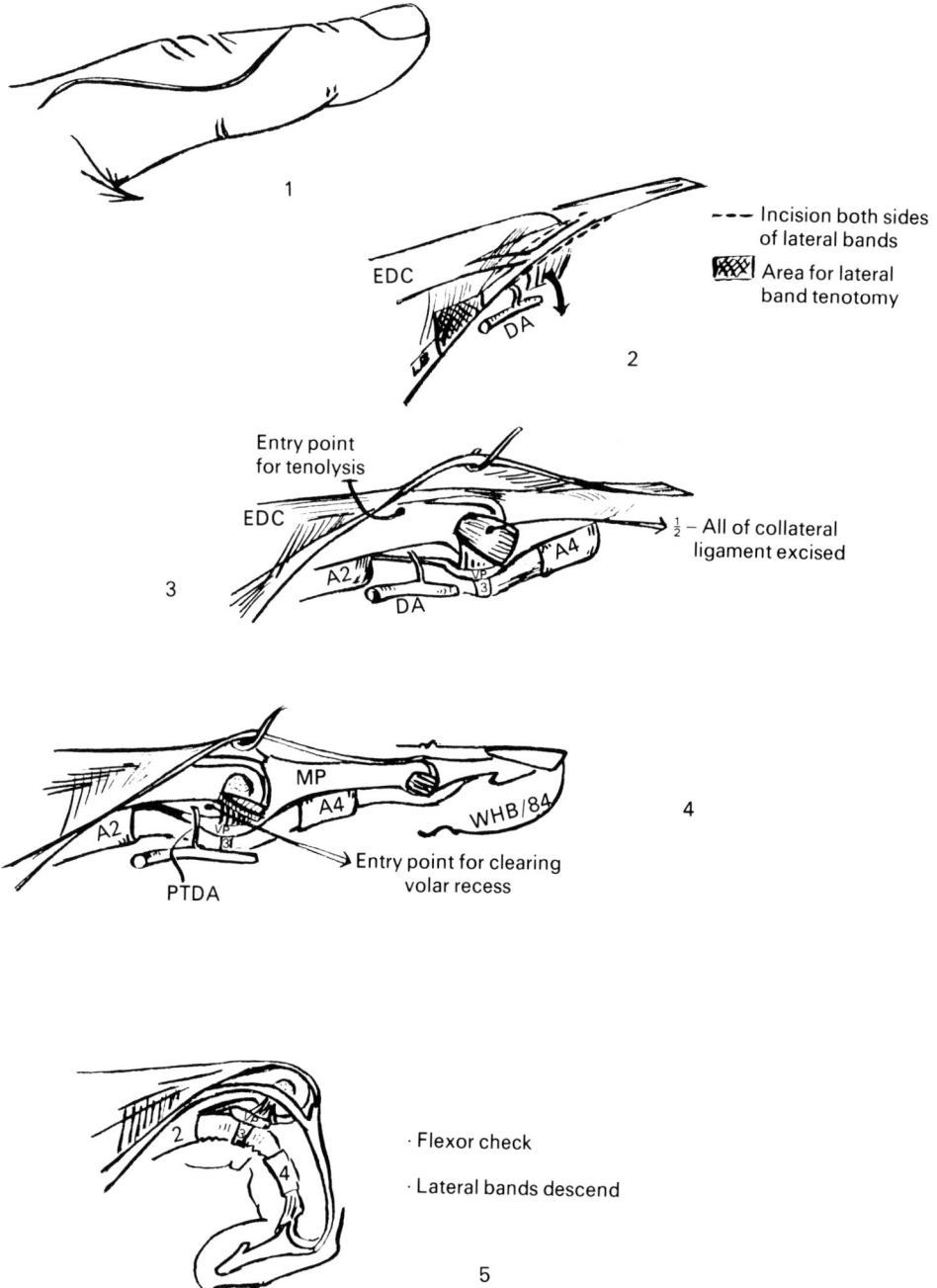

Fig. 4.10 This figure depicts the various steps in the surgical release of an extension contracture. The two major points of emphasis are mobilization or, in some circumstances, release of the lateral bands and excision and/or release of the dorsal portion of the collateral ligaments on either side. It is also important to clear the volar recess (see text).

extensor mechanism is exposed and the volar margins of the lateral bands are identified. A probe identifies their connection to the vertical fibres of the transverse retinacular ligament. This margin is incised and the lateral band is lifted dorsally. The dorsal capsular recess is entered, exposing the articular cartilage, central slip insertion and dorsal margin of the collateral ligaments. An elevator is used to explore and release further the lateral bands and extensor mechanism. The collateral ligaments are isolated and at least the dorsal half of each is resected. A small blade is then passed between the lateral face of the condyle and the collateral ligament to ensure free motion of the remaining collateral ligament and accessory collateral ligament. It is desirable to incise some of the remaining proximal attachment of the collateral ligament. The procedure may end at this point if full motion is obtained.

If the lateral bands do not move volarly past the joint axis of motion at 50° of flexion, an incision is made between the lateral band and the central slip allowing this motion to occur. Lateral bands moving free but tight may be lengthened or tenotomized proximal to the extensor digitorum communis contribution to these bands (Curtis 1954, 1966, Harris & Riordan 1954). If the joint does not move freely into flexion, total excision of the collateral ligament should be carried out (Eaton 1971). This produces no functional instability so long as the accessory collateral ligament–volar plate unit is intact. The potential instability in flexion is more than adequately handled by the healing process. The volar pouch is re-established by a small elevator entering through the accessory collateral ligament area. A small amount of hydrocortisone may be then placed in the joint area (Howard et al 1953). The joint is positioned at 35–40° of flexion and then immobilized for 3–5 d. Active and active assistive motion is then begun under hand therapy supervision. The joint is splinted between exercise periods in a static splint at 40° of flexion. A transcutaneous nerve stimulator unit may be helpful to control pain in the early rehabilitation period. A minimum of two visits per week to the hand therapist is recommended. Every other day is desirable for the first 8–10 d. The patient must be followed weekly for 8–10 weeks.

FLEXION CONTRACTURE

This condition presents several considerations: 1. what caused it? Factors may include: volar skin contracture; fascial contracture (Dupuytren's); flexor sheath scarring following repair; flexor sheath disruption allowing flexor tendons to bowstring; contracted or scarred flexor tendons, flexor tenosynovitis, or congenital sheath–tendon stenosis; volar plate scarring or contracture; retinacular ligament adherence or scarring (pseudo-boutonnière) (McCue et al 1975); collateral ligament or accessory collateral ligament scarring or contracture; volar displacement of lateral bands and loss of extensor power by disruption or adherence (boutonnière) (see Ch. 6); intra-articular incongruity or fibrosis; or bony block or exostosis. 2. If the soft tissue release is successful, can the joint be expected to function? Situations in which the answer may be 'no' are those in which the articular surfaces or the tendons powering the joint are extensively damaged. If the joint itself is damaged, contracture release should be coupled with joint reconstruction or replacement. If the muscle–tendon units cannot be expected to function following tenolysis, then motor reconstruction should be planned. If both joint and tendon damage are present, contracture release, joint reconstruction and staged tendon reconstruction should be considered along with the alternative of arthrodesis. The technique which follows is recommended by the present author. Full credit is given to the pioneer writings of Curtis (1954, 1966) and others (Rhode & Jennings 1971, Sprague 1976, Harrison 1977, Young et al 1978, Watson et al 1979).

Technique

If general or regional anaesthesia is used, some plan for an 'extensor check' must be made to insure an adequate extensor tenolysis has been done. Full flexion of the wrist and metacarpophalangeal joints will put enough passive stress on the common extensor to bring the proximal interphalangeal joint to within 10° of full extension. Active participation from the patient and therefore local anaesthesia are preferred where possible. Where volar structures are clearly the problem (Dupuytren's contracture, flexor sheath or tendon problems, volar plate or accessory collateral ligament contracture), variations on the volar zig-zag incision are recommended. If skin contractures must be released, the volar approach through Z-plasty or flap recession with skin graft is used (Fig. 4.11). If there is any chance that dorsal repair or reconstruction will be needed, midlateral incisions are preferred. The flexor sheath is released in the area of the C-2 and C-3 portion of the sheath. Windowing techniques are satisfactory to release sheath contractures that are not the result of extensive sheath injury. Attempts are made to preserve the A-3 pulley. The increased flexor moment arm present with even mild bowstringing may cause a recurrent contracture. If needed, the sheath can be opened using a Z-technique and repaired later (Fig. 4.12a).

The flexor tendons are explored and their excursions assured. If the flexors are the major problem, tenolysis and/or tendon reconstruction is mandatory. Retraction of the flexor tendons will reveal the volar plate and its origins from the proximal phalanx. The A-3 pulley identifies the fibrous portion of the volar plate while a vincular stalk proximal to the joint locates the arch formed by the two proximal origins of the volar plate (Fig. 4.12b). Careful dissection in this arch and lateral to the sheath will demonstrate the proximal transverse digital artery feeding the vincular stalk (Fig. 4.12c). The proximal origins of the volar plate may then be safely released or excised. The lateral edges of the volar plate are then followed distally, leading to the accessory collateral ligament which, when excised, demonstrates the lower borders of the collateral ligament (Fig. 4.12d). A

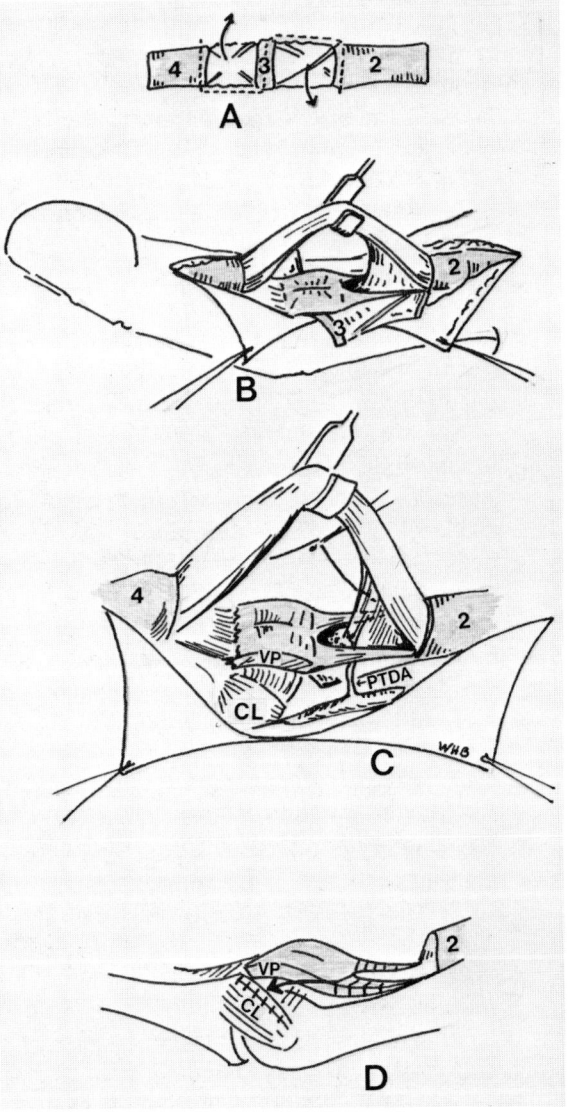

Fig. 4.12 A diagramatic view of the steps in exposure and release of a proximal interphalangeal joint flexion contracture. The numbers refer to the annular pulleys. VP—volar plate; CL—collateral ligament; PTDA—proximal transverse digital artery (see text).

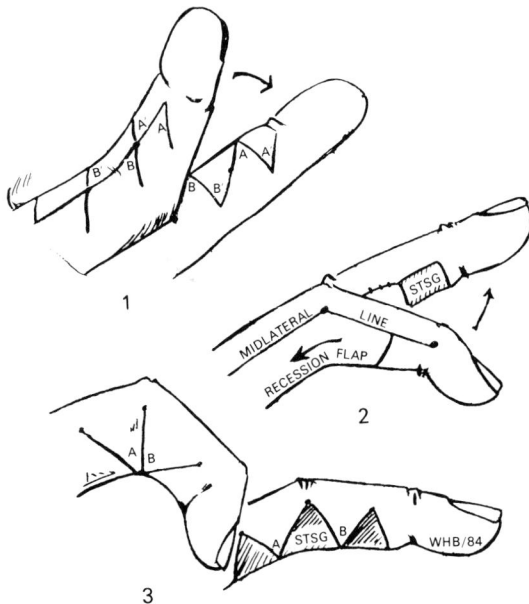

Fig. 4.11 While many flexion contractures can be released without formal release of the skin, these techniques are available when skin contributes significantly to the flexion contracture.

small elevator is used to release any collateral ligament adherence to the condyles. The transverse and oblique retinacular ligaments are excised and the lateral bands are elevated from the lateral collateral ligaments. Redundancy of the transverse fibres between the lateral bands and the central slip may be elliptically excised and the defect closed with one or two small sutures. The joint should, at this point, be passively extensible to 0° and the extensor check performed. The surgeon should persist in extensor tenolysis or reconstruction until full extension is possible. The joint is then transfixed with a small wire at 5–10° of flexion. This is removed in 5 d at which time active and active/assistive motion is begun with interval splinting in near full extension. The follow-up should be at intervals and for the duration noted for extension contracture.

CAPSULAR INSTABILITY

Post-traumatic volar capsular instability or laxity is the result of a volar plate injury. The site is most often at the distal plate–bone interface (Bowers et al 1980). A hyperextensible joint is often not a functional problem but yet an annoying one. The hyperextended proximal interphalangeal joint causes increased tension of the flexor profundus with subsequent flexion at the distal interphalangeal joint such that the digit resembles the swan-neck posture of the chronic mallet finger. This posture also places the line of initial pull of the flexor digitorum superficialis so near to the axis of motion of the proximal interphalangeal joint that temporary inhibition of flexion may occur causing the patient to complain of transient locking. If the tear in the volar capsule is sufficiently large, the condyles of the proximal phalanx may buttonhole through this defect into the flexor sheath causing subluxation or true dorsal dislocation (see Fig. 4.8). In these instances, finger function is noticeably impaired and treatment is sought. Repair of this instability is by either direct capsular repair (favoured by the present author) or by construction of a volar restraint using a tendon graft (Adams 1959, Thompson et al 1978) or the adjacent flexor superficialis (Swanson 1960, Curtis 1964, Wiley 1965).

Technique

A volar zig-zag approach is used. The exposure of the volar plate is identical to that for release of a flexion contracture (see Fig. 4.12). The tear in the volar plate is usually very obvious once the flexors are retracted. The condyles may buttonhole through the tear (see Fig. 4.8). The old insertion of the volar plate and the ineffective granulation at the distal margin of the torn volar plate are freshened. A curette is used to roughen the bone to which the volar plate is to be reattached. Drill holes are made in each volar lateral corner of the middle phalanx (Fig. 4.13). The drill holes exit dorsally in the area of the triangular ligament. A counter incision is made dorsally to view the exit of the drill holes. The triangular ligament may be excised. Using non-absorbable nylon type suture on small needles, a double pullout wire technique is used to secure each corner of the volar plate to the freshened metaphyseal bed of the base of the middle phalanx. The pullout sutures are brought dorsally through the drill holes, exit through the skin and are tied over a button. The joint is pinned under direct vision at 40° with a small wire. The joint is protected with a cast. The cast and pin are removed at 3 weeks and flexion is begun while extension is blocked with a splint. Pullout sutures are removed

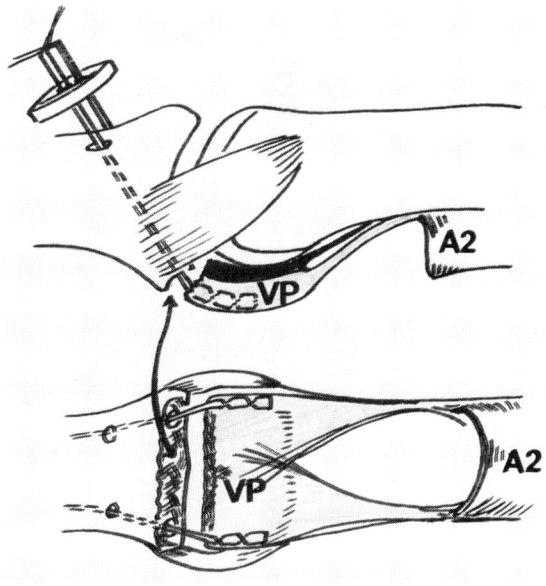

Fig. 4.13 The pull out wire techniques of repairing the volar plate.

at 4 weeks. Extension block splinting is continued for a full 8 weeks and thereafter no therapy is employed other than continued work on flexion. The joint should be buddy taped in re-injury situations. No attempt is made to treat the 20 or 30° flexion contracture remaining as it will resolve slowly over a period of time.

Chronic lateral instability

Chronic lateral instability is most often the result of an untreated or poorly treated grade III collateral ligament injury. The patient usually gives a history of injury followed by chronic swelling, pain and decreased motion. Examination will demonstrate the lateral instability and perhaps a permanently injured joint surface. If so, arthroplasty or arthrodesis is usually the best choice. If the joint contours are intact and some cartilage covers the midrange joint surface, ligament reconstruction may give a reasonable result. The patient should be made aware that pain relief and stability are primary goals and range of motion, albeit important, is a secondary goal.

Technique

Anaesthesia may be regional or general as no intraoperative patient cooperation is needed. The incision should be midlateral on the side of the instability. The early surgical goal is to redefine the original injury by careful scar excision. This is best accomplished with magnification by finding the normal volar margins of the lateral bands proximal and distal to the joint and carefully following these until the lateral side of the joint is defined. The scar over the collateral ligament may be removed and the injury site can be found. The central slip should be inspected and the lateral margin of the volar plate defined by removing the accessory collateral ligament. The volar recess is cleared of scar and the joint surfaces are inspected. If, at this point, the joint rests easily reduced and a full passive range of motion is possible, no further exploration is necessary. If reduction is difficult or a full passive range of motion is not possible, the contralateral ligament must be inspected. This ligament will usually be intact but may be either adherent to the condyle or contracted. If the volar plate and central slip are intact, a counter incision should be used to view the contralateral collateral ligament. If the central slip or volar plate are torn, the joint may be laterally displaced and the collateral ligament viewed. In either case, adherence or contracture must be released—usually by excision of the dorsal half of the collateral ligament. If necessary, repair of the central slip and volar plate are now carried out. It is the present author's preference to use a 4/0 non-absorbable suture anchored to bone through small diameter drill holes. Reconstruction of the completely disrupted collateral ligament is now carried out (Fig. 4.14). In order to achieve a semblance of normal collateral ligament function, the reconstructed ligament must be positioned on a line from the volar lateral corners of the middle phalanx to the natural recess on the side of the condyle of the proximal phalanx. The recess is deepened with a gouge and then two small drill holes are placed obliquely through the proximal phalanx.

The ipsilateral slip of the flexor digitorum superficialis is harvested by cutting it at its emergence from the A-2 pulley leaving it attached distally. A groove is fashioned by splitting the remnants of the attachments of the original collateral ligament at the volar lateral corner of the middle phalanx and the bone is roughened in this area. The flexor digitorum superficialis is swung

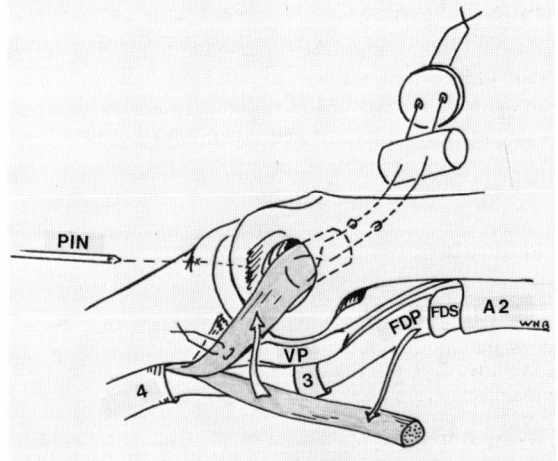

Fig. 4.14 Use of one limb of the flexor digitorum superficialis to reconstruct anatomically the collateral ligament. FDP—flexor digitorum profundus; FDS—flexor digitorum superficialis; VP—volar plate. Numbers refer to annular pulleys.

into this groove where a single horizontal mattress suture stabilizes it. A non-absorbable 4/0 suture is woven into the flexor digitorum superficialis and its two ends are passed through the drill holes in the proximal phalanx. The sutures are pulled tight and tied over the bone on the contralateral side. The position of 15° is selected for immobilization and a small wire is used to transfix the joint. Immobilization for 4 weeks is followed by careful mobilization using the techniques for collateral ligament injury. Both Lane (1978) and Palmer & Linscheid (1978) have illustrated similar techniques for collateral ligament reconstruction which include alternatives for reconstruction of the volar plate as well.

Ligament attenuation

Chronic attenuation of the collateral ligament of the interphalangeal joints producing painful instability is rare. This type lesion is the basis for the original communication regarding 'gamekeeper's thumb' (Campbell 1955). Although there are no references to this lesion occurring at the proximal interphalangeal joints, the present author's experience suggests that it does occur in young women of an asthenic habitus whose gracile digits are stressed by occupational or recreational activities which cause continuous stress on the collateral ligaments. Stresses which have been related to this disorder are typing, computer keyboard usage, or musical instrument fingering such as on the flute or the neck of a violin. The present author has managed three cases of chronic ligament attenuation at the proximal interphalangeal joint

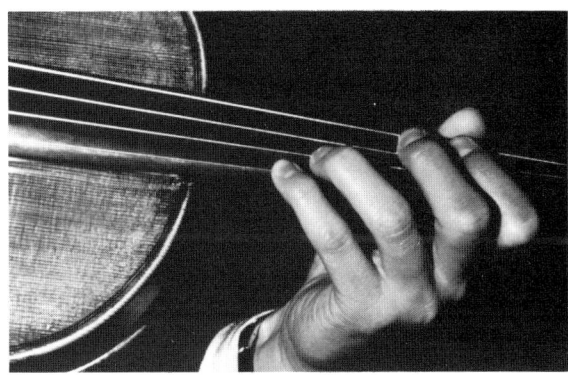

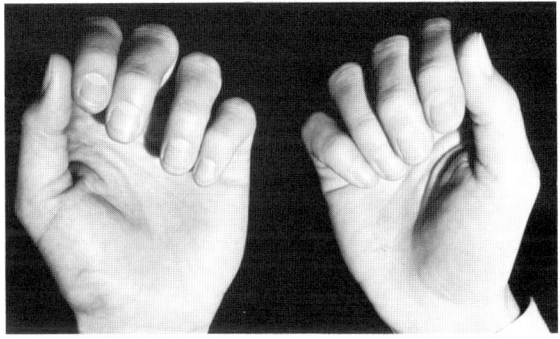

Fig. 4.15 Attenuation of the ulnar collateral ligament of the proximal interphalangeal joint of the left middle finger in a concert violinist.

(Fig. 4.15). Each occurred in individuals who pursued their particular activity for 6–8 h per day. Each responded to long-term custom splinting and to decreased practice time. The diagnosis was made by the typical history without evidence of injury and by physical examination suggesting a lax ligament at the proximal interphalangeal joint.

REFERENCES

Adams J P 1959 Correction of chronic dorsal subluxation of the proximal interphalangeal joint by means of a volar criss-cross graft. Journal of Bone and Joint Surgery 41A: 111

Ali M S 1984 Complete disruption of collateral mechanism of proximal interphalangeal joint of fingers. Journal of Hand Surgery 9B: 191–193

Bowers W H 1978 The post-traumatic swan-neck deformity—two common causes. North Carolina Medical Journal 39: 171–172

Bowers W H 1981 The proximal interphalangeal joint volar plate II: a clinical study of hyperextension injury. Journal of Hand Surgery 6: 77–81

Bowers W H, Wolf J W, Nehil J L, Bittinger S 1980 The proximal interphalangeal volar plate I: an anatomical and biochemical study. Journal of Hand Surgery 5: 79–88

Carroll R E 1973 Personal communication

Campbell C S 1955 Gamekeeper's thumb. Journal of Bone and Joint Surgery 37B: 148–149

Curtis R M 1954 Capsulectomy of the interphalangeal joints of the finger. Journal of Bone and Joint Surgery 36A: 1219–1232

Curtis R M 1964 Treatment of injuries of the proximal interphalangeal joint of the finger. Current Practice in Orthopedic Surgery 2: 125

Curtis R M 1966 Joints of the hand. In: Flynn J E (ed) Hand surgery, 1st edn. Williams & Wilkins, Baltimore, p 367

Eaton R G 1971 Joint injuries of the hand, 1st edn. Charles C Thomas, Springfield

Eaton R G, Dray G J 1982 Dislocations and ligament injuries in the digits. In: Green D P (ed) Operative hand surgery, 1st edn. Churchill Livingstone, New York, p 637

Garroway R Y, Hurst L C, Leppard J L, Dick H M 1984 Complex dislocations of the proximal interphalangeal joint. Orthopaedic Review 13:21–28

Green D P, Rowland S A 1975 Fractures and dislocations in the hand. In: Rockwood C A, Green D P (eds) Fractures, 1st edn. J B Lippencott, Philadelphia, p 310

Green S M, Posner M A 1985 Irreducible dorsal dislocations of the proximal interphalangeal joint. Journal of Hand Surgery 10A:85–87

Harris C, Riordan D C 1954 Intrinsic contracture in the hand and its treatment. Journal of Bone and Joint Surgery 36A:10

Harrison D H 1977 The stiff proximal interphalangeal joint. Hand 9:102–108

Howard L D, Pratt D R, Bunnell S 1953 The use of compound F (hydrocortisone) in operative and nonoperative conditions of the hand. Journal of Bone and Joint Surgery 35A:944–1002

Johnson F G, Greene M H 1966 Another cause of irreducible dislocations of the proximal interphalangeal joint of the finger. Journal of Bone and Joint Surgery 48A:542–544

Kilgore E D, Newmeyer W L, Brown L G 1976 Post-traumatic trapped dislocations of the proximal interphalangeal joint. Journal of Trauma 6:481–487

Lane C S 1978 Reconstructions of the unstable proximal interphalangeal joint: the double superficialis tenodesis. Journal of Hand Surgery 3:95–97

Lee S B 1982 Pseudoboutonnière deformity, its pathogenesis and treatment. Orthopedic Review 11:81–86

Littler J W, Eaton R G 1967 Redistribution of forces in the correction of the boutonnière deformity. Journal of Bone and Joint Surgery 49A:1267

McCue F C, Honner R, Gieck J H 1975 A pseudoboutonnière deformity. Hand 7:166–170

Meyer M A 1958 Irreducible volar dislocations of the proximal interphalangeal joint. Clinical Orthopedics 158:215–218

Murakami Y 1974 Irreducible volar dislocation of the proximal interphalangeal joint of the finger. Hand 6:87–90

Palmer A K, Linscheid R L 1978 Chronic recurrent dislocation of the proximal interphalangeal joint of the finger. Journal of Hand Surgery 3:95–97

Peimer C A, Sullivan D J, Wild D R 1984 Palmar dislocations of the proximal interphalangeal joint. Journal of Hand Surgery 9A:39–48

Posner M A, Wilenski M 1978 Irreducible volar dislocations of the proximal interphalangeal joint caused by interposition of an intact central slip. Journal of Bone and Joint Surgery 60A:133–134

Redler I, Williams J T 1967 Rupture of a collateral ligament of the proximal interphalangeal joint of the finger. Journal of Bone and Joint Surgery 49A:322–326

Rhode C M, Jennings W D Jr 1971 Operative treatment of the proximal interphalangeal joint. American Surgeon 37:44–59

Rodriguez A L 1973 Injuries to the collateral ligament of the proximal interphalangeal joints. Hand 5:55–57

Spinner M, Choi B Y 1970 Anterior dislocation of the proximal interphalangeal joint. Journal of Bone and Joint Surgery 52A:1329–1336

Sprague B L 1976 Proximal interphalangeal joint contractures and their treatment. Journal of Trauma 16:259–265

Stener B 1962 Displacement of a ruptured ulnar collateral ligament of the metacarpophalangeal joint of the thumb. Journal of Bone and Joint Surgery 44B:869–879

Stern P J 1981 Stener lesion after lateral dislocation of the proximal interphalangeal joint—indication for open reduction. Journal of Hand Surgery 6:602–604

Stern P J, Kiefhaber T R, Grood E S 1985 Lateral stability of the proximal interphalangeal joint—presented at annual meeting American Society for Surgery of the Hand, Las Vegas 1984. Journal of Hand Surgery 10A:429

Swanson A B 1960 Surgery of the hand in cerebral palsy and swan-neck deformity. Journal of Bone and Joint Surgery 42A:951

Thompson J S, Eaton R G 1977 Volar dislocation of the proximal interphalangeal joint. Journal of Hand Surgery 2:232

Thompson J S, Littler J W, Upton J 1978 The spiral oblique retinacular ligament (SORL). Journal of Hand Surgery 3:482–487

Watson H K, Light T R, Johnson T R 1979 Checkrein resection for flexion contracture of the middle joint. Journal of Hand Surgery 4:67–71

Wiley A M 1965 Chronic dislocation of the proximal interphalangeal joint: a method of surgical repair. Canadian Journal of Surgery 8:435

Young V L, Wray R C Jr, Weeks P M 1978 The surgical management of stiff joints of the hand. Plastic and Reconstructive Surgery 62:835–841

Zook E G, Van Beek A L, Wavak P 1979 Transverse volar skin laceration of the finger: sign of volar plate injury. Hand 11:213–216

N. J. Barton

5 Intra-articular fractures and fracture-dislocations

Fractures involving the interphalangeal (IP) joints may result in pain, stiffness or deformity. Of these three, the most common problem is stiffness, but there is a great difference in the *effect* of stiffness in the two IP joints of the fingers. At the distal interphalangeal (DIP) joint it produces relatively little disability, because the distance through which the tip of finger moves during full flexion of the DIP joint alone is only about 4 cm. In contrast, full flexion of the proximal interphalangeal (PIP) joint alone causes 8 cm of movement of the fingertip, because the lever arm of the finger distal to the joint is longer (Fig. 5.1). Restriction of this movement causes major disability in two ways: there is loss of flexion and thus gripping power in the finger, and the finger sticks out and gets in the way. Thus at the PIP joint the aim should always be to regain movement if possible, while at the DIP joint stiffness may be acceptable if the joint is stable and painless.

In practice, the situation is more complicated, because the two IP joints are interdependent. The drawings in Figure 5.1, although taken from tracings of the present author's finger, are misleading because they depict passive movements: actively the PIP joint cannot be flexed as much without also flexing the DIP joint slightly, and the DIP joint cannot be flexed at all without also flexing the PIP joint. This is presumably because, although flexion of each joint is by a separate tendon, extension is achieved (and flexion is controlled) by a common plexus of tendons serving both joints. This means that if, following a fracture, one interphalangeal joint becomes stiff, then there is nearly always some loss of movement of the other (uninjured) joint. This makes the problem of stiffness greater than one might have expected.

PROXIMAL INTERPHALANGEAL JOINT

Fractures of the head of the proximal phalanx

Avulsion fractures

These are comparatively uncommon on the proximal side of the joint, but occasionally a flake of

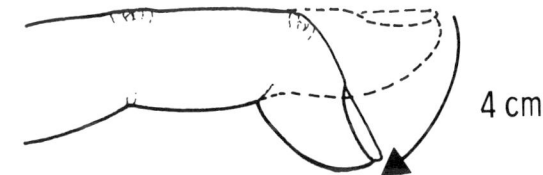

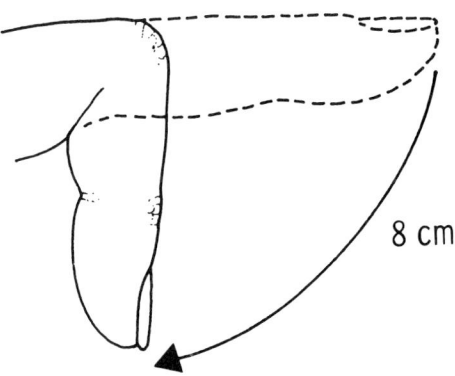

Fig. 5.1 Stiffness of the proximal interphalangeal joint causes much greater restriction of movement of the fingertip than does stiffness of the distal joint.

bone is pulled off from the insertion of one of the collateral ligaments. These can be regarded and treated as ligamentous injuries (see Ch. 4), but the doctor has the advantage of being able to see on the X-ray exactly where the detached piece lies. If it is in the joint, it must be removed (Rodriguez 1973).

Condylar fractures

London (1971) has classified these injuries into three types (Fig. 5.2). He found them to be most common in the little finger and least common in the middle finger, although that has not been the present author's experience.

London type I fractures may be stable and therefore not displace: treatment by early active movement is then appropriate.

Most condylar fractures are of the second type: oblique fractures in which the fragment tends to slide proximally, leaving a step in the articular surface. Occasionally, an oblique or spiral fracture in the distal half of the proximal phalanx runs into the joint, so that most of the joint surface is on the distal fragment, which then displaces proximally, leaving only a spike on the end of the proximal fragment projecting beyond the rest of the joint surface (London type IIb). From the functional viewpoint, it does not really matter whether the majority of the articular surface is on the displaced fragment or on the part which stays in place: either way, the joint surface is significantly disrupted.

Surprisingly little has been written about these fractures which, although not common, are among the most important type of phalangeal fracture, because ordinary conservative treatment usually produces a thoroughly bad result, due to pain, stiffness, *and* deformity.

It is possible to reduce such fractures by traction. This technique has fallen out of favour, but Ellis recommended simple skin traction as a satisfactory method. A narrow strip of non-elastic adhesive strapping is stuck to each side of the finger and to a notch in the distal end of an aluminium splint. The splint is then bent into a partially flexed position which, since the finger forms part of a larger circle than the splint, pulls the strapping tight and applies traction. (This technique is described for shaft fractures by Fitzgerald & Khan 1984). It is possible to achieve reduction of articular fractures in this way, but it is very difficult to maintain; moreover, it seems undesirable to *immobilize* a fracture of this type at all, especially in flexion. This method is suggested only for an undisplaced fracture.

It follows that operative treatment is indicated for displaced condylar fractures. It may be possible to reduce the fracture by manipulation and to hold it by a Kirschner wire introduced percutaneously, but since the purpose is to achieve very accurate reduction, open reduction (Jeffery 1966) is preferable.

McCue et al (1970) reported a series of 35 cases, a large number for an uncommon injury. All but two were men, and the injuries all occurred during sporting activities, usually ball games. (There are, of course, other causes, but this paper is on 'athletic injuries'.) They carried out open reduction of the fracture and joint surface, which was then held with Kirschner wires, usually two. The finger was immobilized on a volar metal splint with the PIP joint flexed 25° and the DIP joint 20°. After 3 weeks, active movements were begun, although for another 2 weeks the splint was still worn for protection at night and during heavy use or sport.

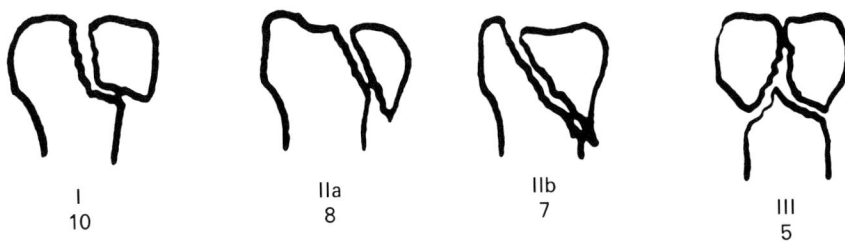

Fig. 5.2 Types of condylar fractures (reproduced with permission from 'Sprains and fractures involving the interphalangeal joints' by P S London 1971 The Hand 3:157) The figures below indicate the number of each type of fracture in London's series.

The figures obtained for the range of movement are very good: all but one patient regained 80° of flexion and even he had 70°. Some patients had a mild flexion contracture of 10–15°.

The present author prefers a semi-open technique (Barton 1984). The fracture is exposed proximally but the joint is not opened. If the visible part of the fracture is perfectly reduced, then the invisible part which runs through the articular surface will also be perfectly reduced. Fixation can be achieved with one or two Kirschner wires (Fig. 5.3), but the 2 mm screw from the AO small fragment set is better because, if it is introduced as a lag-screw, interfragmentary compression is applied and the fixation is thus more rigid (see Fig. 5.16**d**). Active movements are begun next day.

Type III, or T-shaped fractures, are rare; the present author has not encountered one in a finger (but see Fig. 5.17). Plate fixation is possible but, in the phalanges, invariably leads to adherence of the extensor tendon and consequent limitation of flexion. Therefore treatment of such a fracture by open reduction of the intercondylar element, fixing the two condyles together with a small screw or Kirschner wire is recommended; then, if possible, stabilize the transverse element with an oblique Kirschner wire, but if not, simply reduce it and immobilize it in extension for 3 weeks.

Sometimes patients with condylar fractures are not seen until a few weeks after the injury, or later still (Fig. 5.4). It is then very difficult to know what is the best thing to do. In the present author's experience, after 10–14 d the fracture has united and any attempt at open reduction is likely to involve so much damage to the joint that it will be even stiffer. If there is only a small depressed section of joint surface, it will probably cause little trouble and should be left alone. If *most* of the joint surface is depressed, considerable improvement can be achieved by trimming off the spike protruding from the proximal fragment which is impinging on the base of the middle phalanx and also

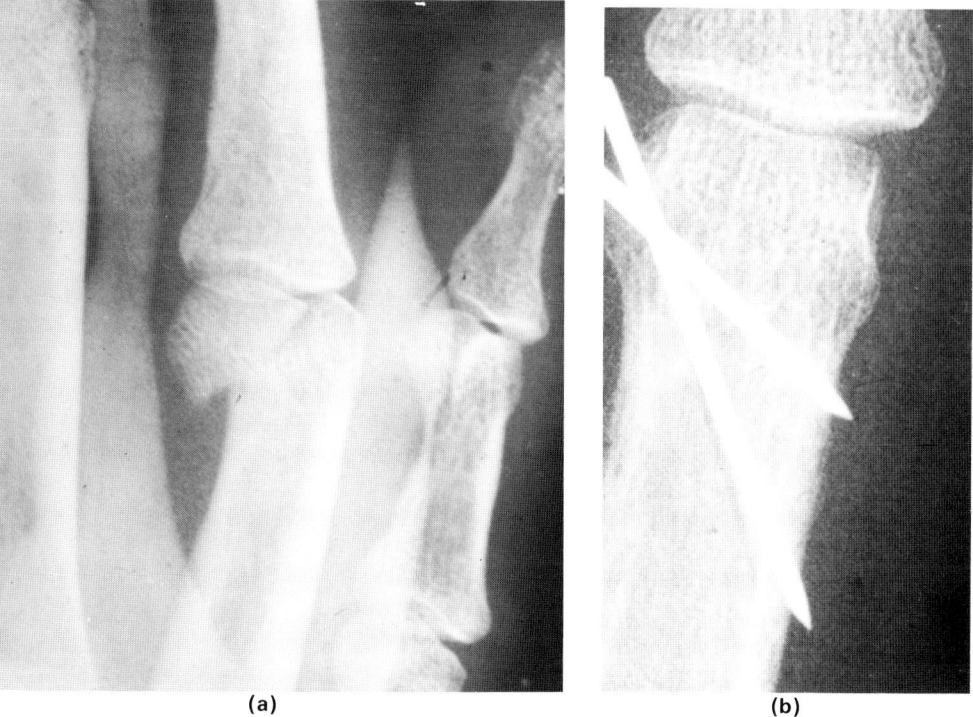

Fig. 5.3 (**a**) Oblique fracture (London type II) of condyle of proximal phalanx. The radiological view is also oblique: not usually helpful in the hand, but giving a good view of this particular type of fracture. (**b**) Same fracture, after open reduction and fixation with two Kirschner wires. The joint regained a range of movement from 5 to 95°.

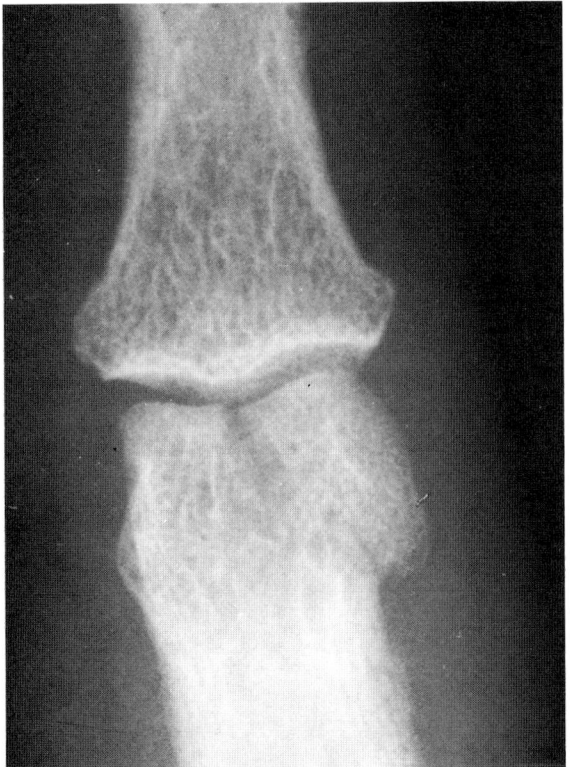

Fig. 5.4 This 48-year-old coal miner's right index finger was crushed by a fall of stone. He thought the injury was just a sprain and did not attend hospital until 16 d later, when it was decided to treat him by active movements. It is probably a London type I fracture, which is why it did not displace proximally. Remarkably, he went back to work only 9 d after that; when reviewed 8 weeks later, the PIP joint had a range from 0–90°, but DIP movement was limited to 0–45°. There was some ulnar deviation at the PIP joint but only occasional pain.

preventing the normal movement of the collateral ligament during flexion. This can be combined with a corrective angular osteotomy if necessary. When half the joint surface is depressed, there is no entirely satisfactory solution and the choice lies between accepting the situation, attempting to realign the joint surface by longitudinal or oblique osteotomy through it, prosthetic replacement, or arthrodesis. It is unwise to carry out any irreversible procedure too soon, as the pain does get less over a year or two although, of course, the stiffness and deformity remain. The patients may just stop complaining about them, but they do seem to become accustomed to the finger so that it causes less trouble than if it was arthrodesed (see Fig. 5.4).

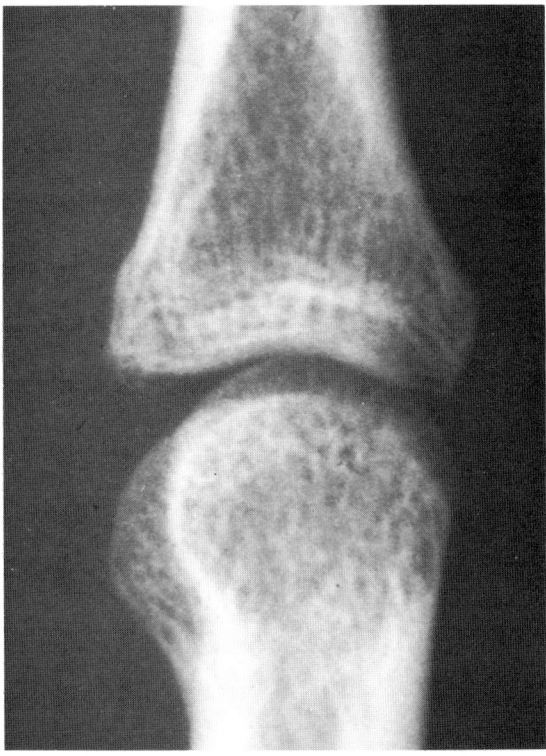

Fig. 5.5 Undisplaced fracture of a small fragment from the volar lip of the base of the middle phalanx, without subluxation. The patient was a medical student whose finger was hyperextended by a rugby football. These fractures usually do well whatever the treatment: this patient was treated by active mobilization and rapidly regained full movements.

Fractures of the base of the middle phalanx

Avulsion fractures of the dorsal lip

This is the bony version of the boutonnière injury, but fortunately the fracture draws attention to what has happened, in contrast to the purely tendinous avulsion of the central slip of the tendon which is so often overlooked.

If there is little or no displacement, the fracture can well be treated by simple immobilization. There are no published figures on which to base a recommendation of the duration of immobilization, but 6 weeks is suggested, followed by 4 weeks in a Capener lively splint. McCue et al (1970) treated five such patients by excision of the fracture fragment and reattachment of the central slip to the bony surface. This inevitably tightens up the central slip and alters the delicate balance of tension between central slip and lateral bands. It is therefore not surprising that although their patients regained an average of 80° of flexion at the PIP joint, the average range of flexion at the DIP joint was only 20° and one still had hyperextension.

O'Brien (1982) recommends accurate reduction if displacement is over 2 mm. The fragment may be held by a wire inserted percutaneously, but for accuracy it seems better to expose the fragment. When its exact size and shape are known, a decision can be made as to the most appropriate method of fixation: usually this will be one fine Kirschner wire.

Avulsion fractures of the volar lip

This is one of the more common injuries of the PIP joint. The finger is hyperextended, usually by a fall on the outstretched hand but sometimes after being struck by a ball, and the strong volar plate at the PIP joint pulls off its distal insertion from the front of the base of the middle phalanx (Fig. 5.5). Frequently there is little or no displacement, and Eaton (1971) suggests that in such cases only the central part of the insertion of the volar plate has pulled off, while each side of the insertion remains intact. It is hard to understand why the volar plate should give way at its thick distal end or insertion into bone instead of through the much thinner proximal part of the check-rein straps (aptly compared to a swallow's tail), but Bowers et al (1980) showed that it is in fact the distal attachment which provides most of the restraint to hyperextension (see Ch. 4). Whatever the mechanism, it seems to be generally agreed that this type of fracture nearly always makes a good recovery.

Benke & Stableforth (1979) reviewed 30 patients with this type of injury who had been treated conservatively, and found that 24 had an excellent result, 5 were good, and only 1 had a bad result. The method of conservative treatment was not stated, but it presumably varied, as the duration of immobilization was said not to influence the outcome. They concluded that since 95% of patients can expect an excellent or good result, regardless of the method of management, splintage is unnecessary and the patient should be encouraged to mobilize the joint immediately. Bowers (1981) agreed that these injuries 'do quite well with minimal splinting or even without treatment', but stressed that avulsion of the distal end of the volar plate *without fracture* is a different proposition, not only because it is more difficult to diagnose, but because it may fail to heal (perhaps due to poor blood-supply) which produces a hyperextension deformity.

Dorsal subluxation with volar fracture

This injury usually results from a blow on the end of the finger, the most common cause being a ball which was not caught correctly (Fig. 5.6). It occurs fairly often in games such as cricket, baseball, and

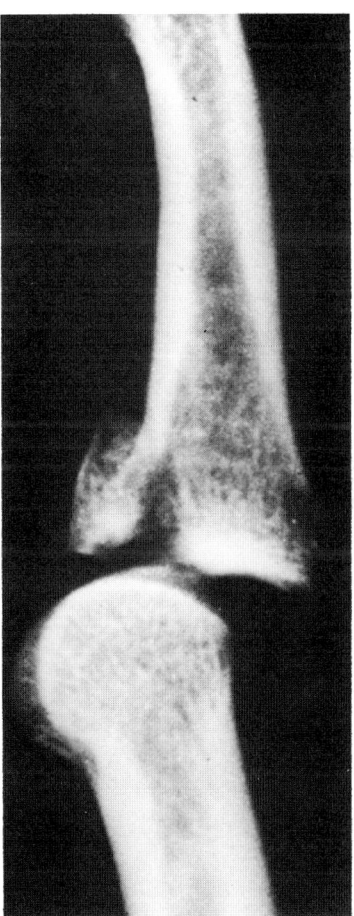

Fig. 5.6 Dorsal subluxation of PIP joint with a small volar fragment in a professional cricketer who misjudged a catch so that the ball hit the end of his finger. (Reproduced with permission from 'Fractures and joint injuries', 6th edn, J N Wilson (ed), Churchill Livingstone, 1982.)

Australian-rules football. The size of the volar lip fragment varies, but tends to be larger than in the simple avulsion fractures described above. The important part of the injury is the subluxation rather than the fracture, and in this it resembles Bennett's fracture-subluxation.

Treatment is essential: a dorsally subluxed PIP joint cannot be expected to work properly, and it never will. There is, however, a remarkable variety of methods of treatment and, although these injuries are not much commoner than condylar fractures, many papers have been published about them.

The subluxation can easily be reduced, and it will stay reduced if the joint is kept flexed; extension is the unstable position. However, it is well known that to immobilize the PIP joint in flexion is to invite a flexion contracture, especially if there was an injury directly involving that joint. Lee (1963) reviewed seven patients who had been treated by immobilization in flexion for an average of 18 days and found that, between 4 and 7 years after the injury, only three had a full range of movement, and six still experienced discomfort in cold weather. In one patient the dorsal subluxation had recurred: the finger was not painful but flexed only from 0–25°.

Robertson et al (1946) described treatment by transfixing the phalanx on each side of the fracture with a Kirschner wire and then applying elastic band traction to pull the proximal phalanx dorsally and the distal phalanx anteriorly, while a third, more distal, transfixing wire was used for longitudinal traction. Each band was fixed to the circumference of a large wire ring (which became known as a banjo splint), and active movements were begun straightaway. Traction was removed after 3 or 4 weeks. Details were given for seven patients of whom four regained full extension, two lacked only 5°, and one lacked 20°. The range of flexion was 70° in the worst cases and 90° in the best.

Agee (1978) devised a more compact but also more complicated dynamic external fixator, producing the same force-couple to maintain reduction of the subluxation, but dispensing with the need for longitudinal traction. Only two cases were described and the method seems not to have caught on, presumably because of its complexity and the fact that there are simpler and satisfactory alternatives. One of these is the ingenious extension-block splint, described by McElfresh et al (1972), which allows flexion but prevents extension. This is, however, rather cumbersome and has been simplified by Strong (1980) to achieve the same purpose of preventing extension, but leaving the front of the finger free (Fig. 5.7). Seventeen patients so treated were reported: 12 regained full extension, and another 3 lacked only 15°. One of the poor results was in a patient with 'mild compression of the rest of the articular surface', and the other was not treated until 4 weeks after the injury; this last patient was also one of the only two who failed to regain 90° of flexion.

If the volar fragment remains in its correct relationship to the head of the proximal phalanx, then reduction of the displaced main part of the middle phalanx onto the volar fragment will correct the subluxation, and if the fracture can then be internally fixed, the correction will be maintained. This method was recommended by Wilson & Rowland in 1966. They had treated 15 cases. The fracture was approached through a midlateral incision, and the distal ends of the collateral ligament and volar plate detached to reveal the joint and fracture. The fracture was then reduced and fixed by a small Kirschner wire on a power drill; the wire was passed right through and out of the back of the finger and then slowly withdrawn until its anterior end was flush with the cortical surface of the volar fragment, so that the wire did not prevent flexion of the joint. In comminuted fractures a pull-out wire was used which embraced the fragments with a loop and then passed out of the back of the finger where it was tied over a button. [Lister (1978) modified this method by twisting the wire loop on the back of the middle phalanx instead of bringing it out through the skin.] Even where a Kirschner wire was used, the reduction was judged unstable in some cases, and then a second Kirschner wire was passed across the joint to provide stability. The collateral ligament was repaired and the finger immobilized for 3 weeks, when exercises began. Any transarticular wire was removed at that stage and the osseous Kirschner wire 3 weeks later. The results were said to be satisfactory but not reported in detail: the least range of motion was 45° but only one finger regained a full range. However, none of these

INTRA-ARTICULAR FRACTURES AND FRACTURE-DISLOCATIONS 83

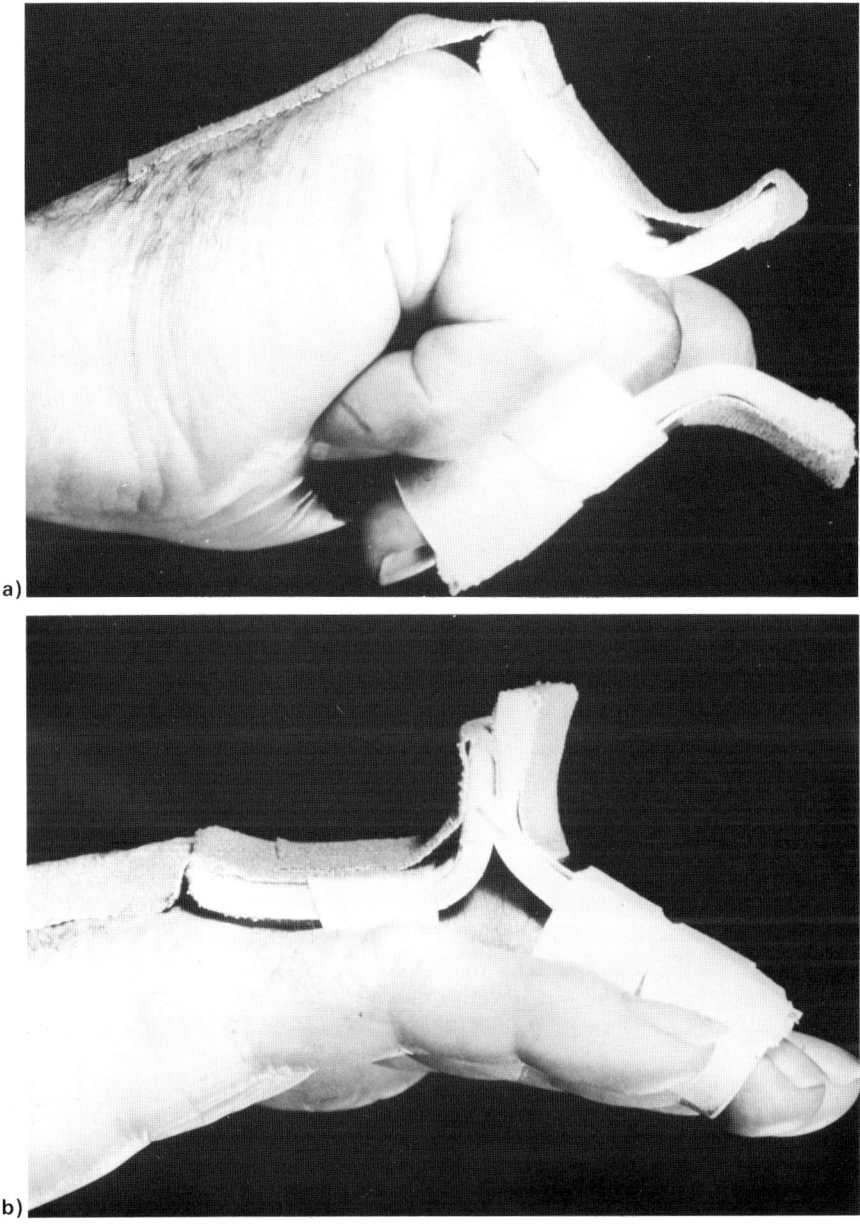

Fig. 5.7 Strong's method of extension block splintage. (**a**) In flexion, the two parts of the splint separate freely. (**b**) In extension, they come up against each other and limit the movement.

patients were operated on immediately after the accident, most having a delay of several weeks.

McCue et al (1970) used a very similar method in 21 cases, although they appear to have added the wire across the joint routinely. They obtained an average of 95° of flexion in cases with a large fracture fragment, 87° with a small fragment, and 82° with multiple small fragments. Glasgow & Lloyd (1981) reported a patient in whom they had succeeded in fixing the small volar fragment back to the rest of the middle phalanx by *percutaneous* Kirschner wiring, using a specially modified reduction forceps.

The problem of internal fixation of the volar

fragment is that there may also be damage of the central part of the articular surface (McElfresh et al 1972, Zemel et al 1981) and the fragments of cartilage-bearing cortex are so tiny that it is impossible to restore the normal anatomy. In these cases, a transfixing wire is necessary to maintain reduction and perhaps also distraction until some healing of the fracture has occurred. However, if it may be necessary to use a transarticular wire anyway, why not omit the difficult and uncertain exposure and fixation of the bony fragment? Reduction of the subluxation is always easy in fresh cases and can be done by simple manipulation; it can then be maintained by transfixing the PIP joint in some 30° of flexion by a Kirschner wire (Fig. 5.8). The principle is the same as in Wagner's method of treating Bennett's fractures. The wire is inserted through the bare triangular area of bone beyond the insertion of the central slip and before the lateral bands have come together. (Lister calls this the 'forgiving' area.) This method is attributed to Bunnell and is simple and satisfactory. It is suprising how quickly patients regain movement of the joint after removal of the wire 3 weeks later, but it is probably wise to protect the joint with an extension-block splint for another 3 weeks.

Another approach, also avoiding the difficulty of securely fixing back a tiny bony fragment, is to excise the fragment and suture the distal end of the volar plate into the defect, with the joint flexed about 35°. Eaton (1971) found that in recent cases this provided stable reduction and that it was rarely necessary to transfix the joint with a Kirschner wire. He used a pull-out wire suture which was removed at 3 weeks, after which active flexion, but not extension, was begun. Wiley (1970) reinforced this repair with one slip of the superficialis tendon.

Late cases are, of course, more difficult to treat. Donaldson & Millender (1978) reviewed the literature and concluded that operative procedures involving wide dissection and prolonged immobilization often resulted in limited motion. They obtained good results in four patients treated by an operation which was essentially an arthrolysis, open reduction and joint transfixion in flexion for 12 days, followed by extension block splinting for 4 weeks. Zemel et al (1981) prefer osteotomy, repositioning of the volar lip and a bone graft, again supported by temporary Kirschner wire

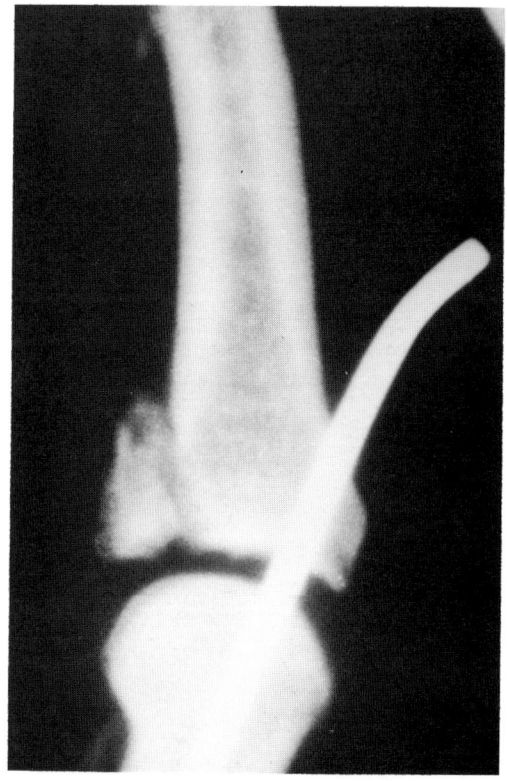

Fig. 5.8 Same patient as in Figure 5.6. The subluxation has been reduced by manipulation under anaesthetic and held by a Kirschner wire introduced percutaneously through the bare area near the base of the middle phalanx dorsally. Note the improvement in the position of the fracture, although this has not been exposed. (Reproduced with permission from Fractures and joint injuries, 6th edn, J N Wilson (ed), Churchill Livingstone, 1982.)

stabilization. They stress that 10 out of 14 patients had, in addition to the volar lip fracture, 'compression and/or crushing of a portion of the articular surface of the middle phalanx'. It seems likely that this is often the case but may not be appreciated at the time (Fig. 5.9), accounting for some bad results. The results of their procedure in 14 patients are described in detail: all but one gained more flexion and some gained as much as 60°. Three of the patients had been followed for as long as 10 years and had retained useful movement with no pain.

Volar subluxation with dorsal fracture

This is less common and very little has been written about it. Lee (1963) had only one example in his

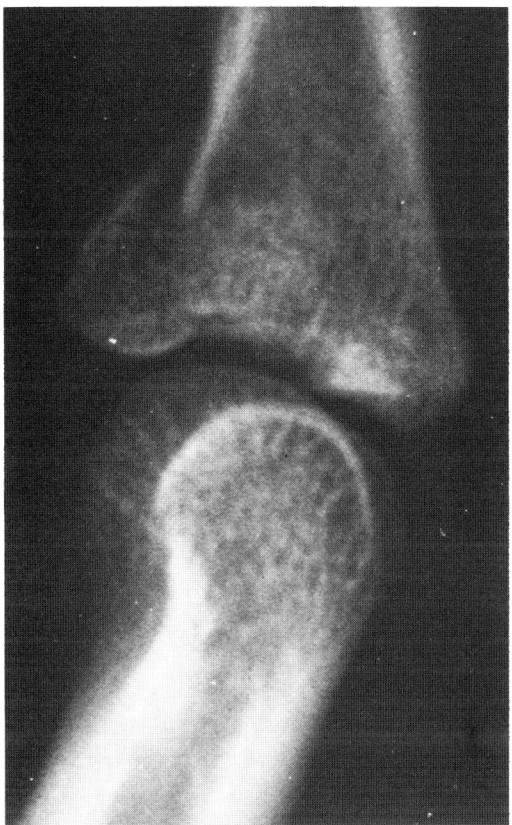

Fig. 5.9 This 21-year-old woman's finger was injured when her son fell on it. The X-ray was described as showing 'a very fine undisplaced fracture of the base of the middle phalanx, with only a very small fragment involved in the fracture'; it was not realized that the central part of the articular surface was also fractured and depressed.

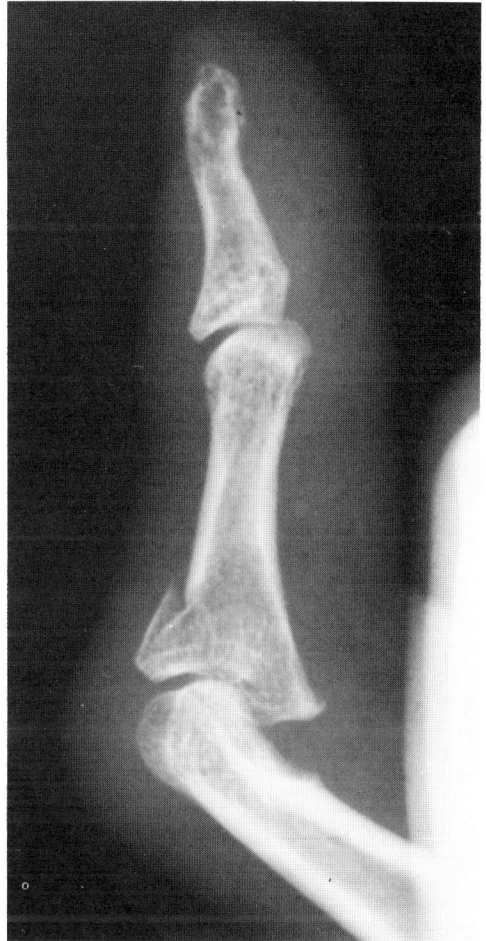

Fig. 5.10 This man sustained a volar subluxation of the PIP joint, with a dorsal fragment of middle phalanx remaining in its correct relationship to the proximal phalanx. The stable position for this unusual injury should be extension, but this patient had camptodactyly and had never been able to straighten the joint. The injury was therefore treated simply by early mobilization and he regained adequate movements.

series of articular fractures. Although the principles of treatment are the same, the fact that the injury is the other way round (Fig. 5.10) does affect the technique of treatment.

1. The stable position is extension, which makes it a more acceptable position in which to immobilize the joint
2. Surgical access to the fracture fragment is easier
3. The central slip of the extensor tendon is not a large structure and any attempt to advance it would alter the delicate balance of the extensor mechanism and might produce a swan-neck deformity. Excision of the fragment is, therefore, not advisable
4. Transfixion of the joint, although possible, is more difficult. The wire must not enter from the front of the finger, as that would compromise the flexor mechanism, and cannot enter from the back, as this is already fractured. It must therefore be introduced laterally and cross the joint obliquely

It seems reasonable to reduce the subluxation by manipulation and splint the finger in extension, but X-rays should be taken weekly for 3 weeks to detect any loss of reduction. Should this occur, a large fragment of bone should be fixed back in place; if the fragment is small, then Kirschner wire transfixion is probably the best answer.

Lateral compression fractures

The injury shown in Figure 5.11 is rare, but you may feel there is something familiar about it. Turn the picture upside down and you will see why. It is exactly comparable to an abduction fracture of the upper end of the tibia, the lateral rim and subjacent cortex of the bone being displaced outwards and the articular surface inside this depressed distally. In theory, one should treat this fracture in the same way as its tibial counterpart, i.e. by open reduction, restoration of the joint surface, internal fixation, and bone grafting to support the elevated central fragments. This particular patient was not seen until a later stage, but even soon after the fracture, it is doubtful whether good enough fixation of these very small fragments could have been achieved to have remained stable while the joint was being moved. Comminuted articular fractures are usually even more comminuted than one expects, and it may well be that the lateral cortex was not in fact in one piece as it appears on the X-ray.

An alternative method of treating tibial condyle fractures is by early mobilization of the joint in traction (Apley 1956) and this finger fracture (Fig. 5.11) was also treated by early active mobilization, although without traction, in an attempt to mould the fragments of the middle phalanx into approximately the right shape to fit the head of the proximal phalanx. The lateral angulation was accepted, the plan being to correct it later by osteotomy if it proved to be a problem to the patient.

Trojan (1972) considered it important to maintain good alignment by plaster splintage or percutaneous drill-wires.

Longitudinal fractures of the middle phalanx running into the PIP joint

This type of fracture (Fig. 5.12) is usually the result of a crushing injury, and the periosteal sleeve is intact or nearly so. The fractures are therefore stable and best treated by early mobilization.

Fractures involving both sides of the joint

These usually result from crushing injuries. The extensive fracturing, and the presence of some degree of skin damage, argue against internal fixation, and the prognosis for movement is poor. Active mobilization, as described above for fractures of the base of the middle phalanx, is not likely to be satisfactory, as there is no intact joint surface on the other side to act as a mould.

Generally, all one can do is to immobilize the joint in the best position (i.e. the position in which one would arthrodese it). This may be possible with simple splintage, but in unstable cases transfixion by a longitudinal Kirschner wire or some form of external fixation may be necessary. Weeks (1981) recommends traction on a hook glued to the fingernail, with the metacarpophalangeal (MP) joint flexed and the IP joints extended. Only exceptionally is primary arthrodesis appropriate, as the approach mentioned above leaves open three lines of later management:

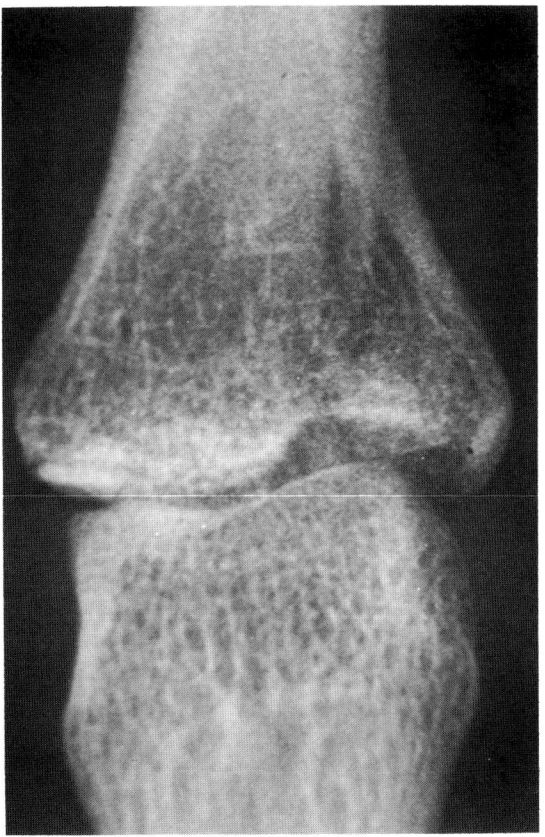

Fig. 5.11 Lateral compression fracture of the base of the middle phalanx (see text).

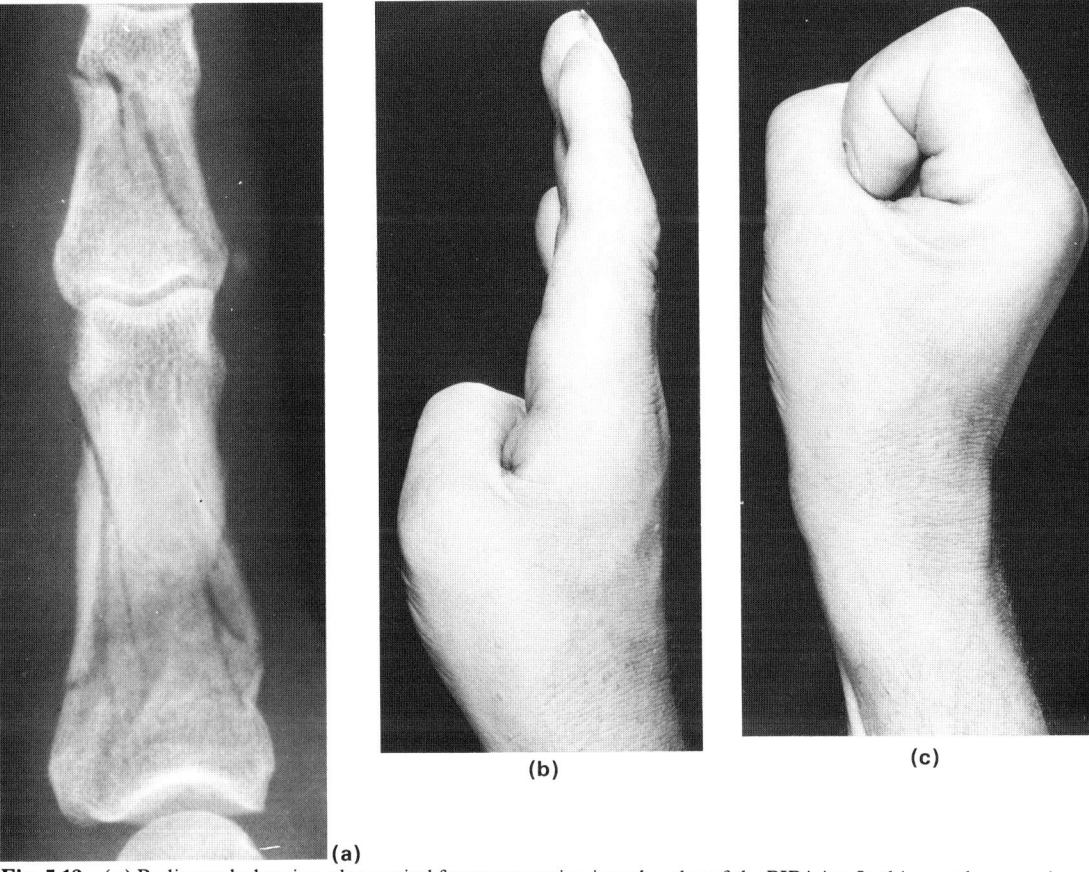

Fig. 5.12 (a) Radiograph showing a long spiral fracture running into the edge of the PIP joint. In this case there are also comminuted longitudinal fractures in the proximal phalanx, entering the MP joint. The finger had been crushed in a hydraulic press. The wounds were cleaned but not sutured, the hand was supported on a volar slab and active movements were begun 24 h later. (b) and (c) show the range of movements 3 months later.

1. The joint may fuse spontaneously or, more likely, regain a small amount of movement which is not always painful and may be useful to the patient. Either way, no further surgical treatment is needed.
2. Arthoplasty may be carried out later, usually requiring some sort of implant such as a Swanson's prosthesis. Although this will not give anything like a full range of movement, it is much preferred to arthrodesis.
3. Arthrodesis.

A single finger stiff at the PIP joint, in an otherwise normal hand, may be such a nuisance that the patient asks to have it amputated.

In severe crushing injuries, where other tissues are damaged beside the bone, primary amputation may be the best treatment. In these circumstances, the intact majority of the proximal phalanx should be retained, and in men who want a strong grip that is generally best anyway. In the border digits, the proximal phalanx and metacarpal head can be removed later if the patient does not like the appearance of the hand.

DISTAL INTERPHALANGEAL JOINT

Fractures of the head of the middle phalanx

In character, these are similar to fractures of the head of the proximal phalanx and they will, therefore, not be described in detail. The main difference is that the bone is appreciably smaller. Steel (1978) found that the small AO screws were too big for articular fractures of the DIP joint, and a Kirschner wire is probably better, but even this may cause problems (Fig. 5.13). Exact reduction is less important at the DIP joint, since both stiffness and deformity are less of a problem (30° of lateral angulation at the DIP joint produces much less lateral deviation of the fingertip than at the PIP joint because the lever is shorter), and in practice pain seems to be less of a problem too. Thus it may be reasonable at this joint to carry out closed percutaneous wiring, if the fragment is large enough.

Fractures of the base of the distal phalanx

Dorsal lip

There are two different mechanisms which may disrupt the insertion of the extensor tendon onto the base of the distal phalanx.

The first is when an actively extended finger is passively but forcibly flexed: this usually tears the tendon within its substance or avulses it from bone with a variably-sized piece of bone. This produces the well-known mallet finger.

The second is an end-on blow on the tip of the extended finger. This drives the concave base of the distal phalanx down onto the convex head of the middle phalanx (Stack 1969) which acts like an axe and chops through the distal phalanx causing what is sometimes called a mallet finger fracture (McMinn 1981). There may be no drooping of the tip and thus its designation as a 'mallet' fracture is undeserved. The resemblance to a mallet finger lies entirely on the general location of the bony injury in the distal phalanx. This is usually a sports injury, resulting from an imperfectly-judged attempt to catch a hard ball. In the USA it is therefore often referred to as a 'baseball finger', but it also occurs frequently in the more widely-played game of cricket, and in many other sports. The piece of bone which is broken off varies in size and may be quite large. In itself, the size is unimportant, but a large fragment allows subluxation of the remaining joint surfaces which does matter (Fig. 5.14).

The end-on blow may also cause contusion of the articular cartilage: this is a subject about which little is known, but it appears that chondrocytes can survive a lesser impact but may die after really violent blows (Mankin 1982). In practice, a good range of movement is usually regained and it seems unlikely that there is much lasting damage to the cartilage after this type of injury to the finger.

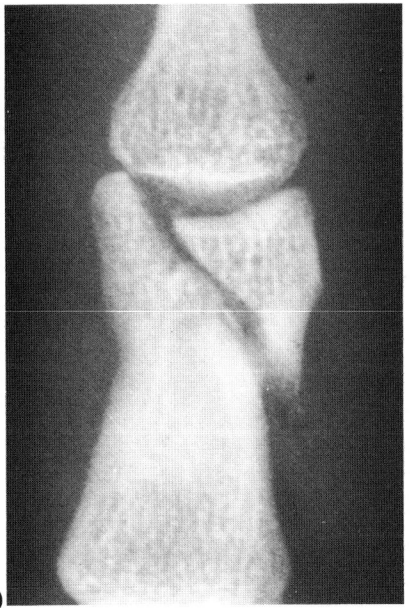 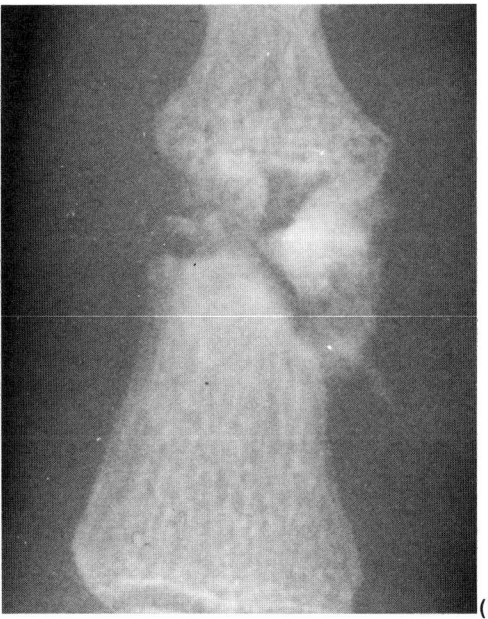

Fig. 5.13 (a) It was decided to treat this oblique condylar fracture by fixation with a Kirschner wire. (b) Unfortunately, this only broke the fragments into smaller pieces. The patient was seen later by the present author for a medico-legal report: the DIP joint was, of course, stiff but was not causing great problems.

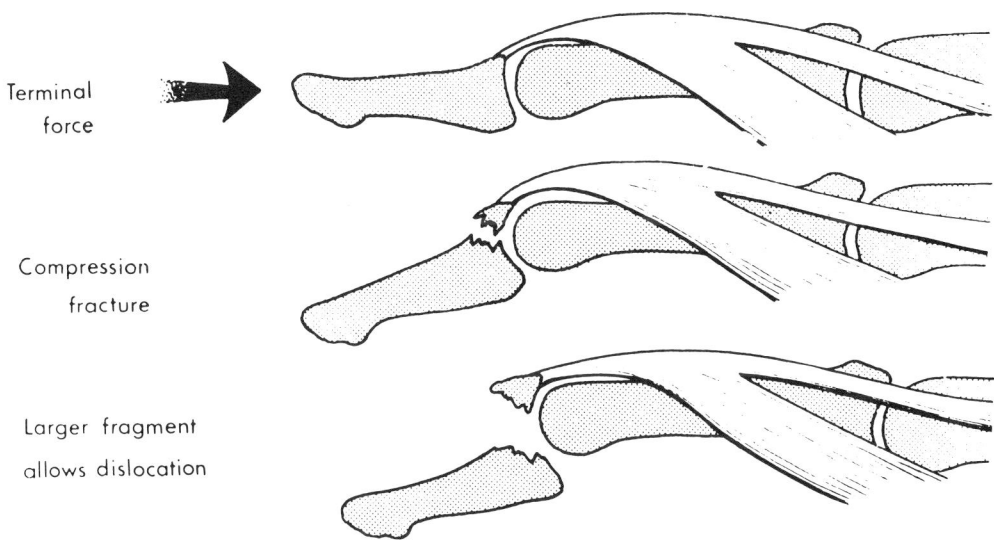

Fig. 5.14 Mallet finger fractures (Reproduced with permission from Mallet finger H G Stack 1969 The Hand 1:86.)

Small fractures, without any subluxation of the remaining joint surfaces, can be well treated conservatively, by splintage in a straight position until union has occurred: usually about 6 weeks. As long ago as 1963, Lee showed that even markedly displaced fragments would unite, although there was often some loss of movement at the DIP joint. Any splint which does the job and causes no complications is acceptable. The moulded polythene splint designed by Stack is the most satisfactory. (The splint is available in the UK from Pryor and Howard Ltd, Willow Lane, Mitcham, Surrey CR4 4US and in the USA from Link America Inc., East Hanover, New Jersey. A pirate version is also sold, shamelessly called the Stax splint.) It comes in five sizes which accommodate most fingers, but the dorsal transverse edge can be trimmed with a scalpel if necessary, or the splint can be split longitudinally along the dorsal midline to make it slightly larger. Crawford (1984) has reviewed 89 such fractures, comprising 20–50% of the joint surface, treated by the Stack splint with 'most satisfactory' results, provided that the splint was applied properly. With larger fragments and subluxation, some thought is required. Crawford has shown that these, too, can sometimes be controlled by a Stack splint, although it is important not to push the fingertip right into the end of the splint as this tends to hyperextend the distal phalanx and increase the palmar subluxation (Fig. 5.15).

If it is not possible to keep the subluxation reduced by external splintage, then some form of internal fixation is necessary. This was in fact probably the first type of phalangeal fracture of which internal fixation was reported (Pratt 1952). He used a longitudinal Kirschner wire, 0.045 inch (0.1 cm) in diameter, introduced through the tip of the distal phalanx and then on across the DIP joint. This can be done under a digital nerve block. Pratt actually used this for mallet finger fractures without subluxation, and he inserted the wire further proximally to hold the PIP joint in flexion: neither is necessary. An ordinary hollow needle, as used for injections, can be used instead of a Kirschner wire.

Other surgeons prefer to fix the small fractured fragment itself, by a very fine Kirschner wire or hypodermic needle, by a loop of malleable wire (Lister 1978), or even by a tiny screw. In the present author's experience, the fragment is seldom large enough to be fixed in this way and there is a fair chance of breaking it in to several even smaller fragments, in which case it will be necessary to use transarticular wire fixation anyway. The latter is therefore the first choice if splintage fails to maintain reduction of the subluxation. It is difficult to get the wire into the tip of the distal phalanx as

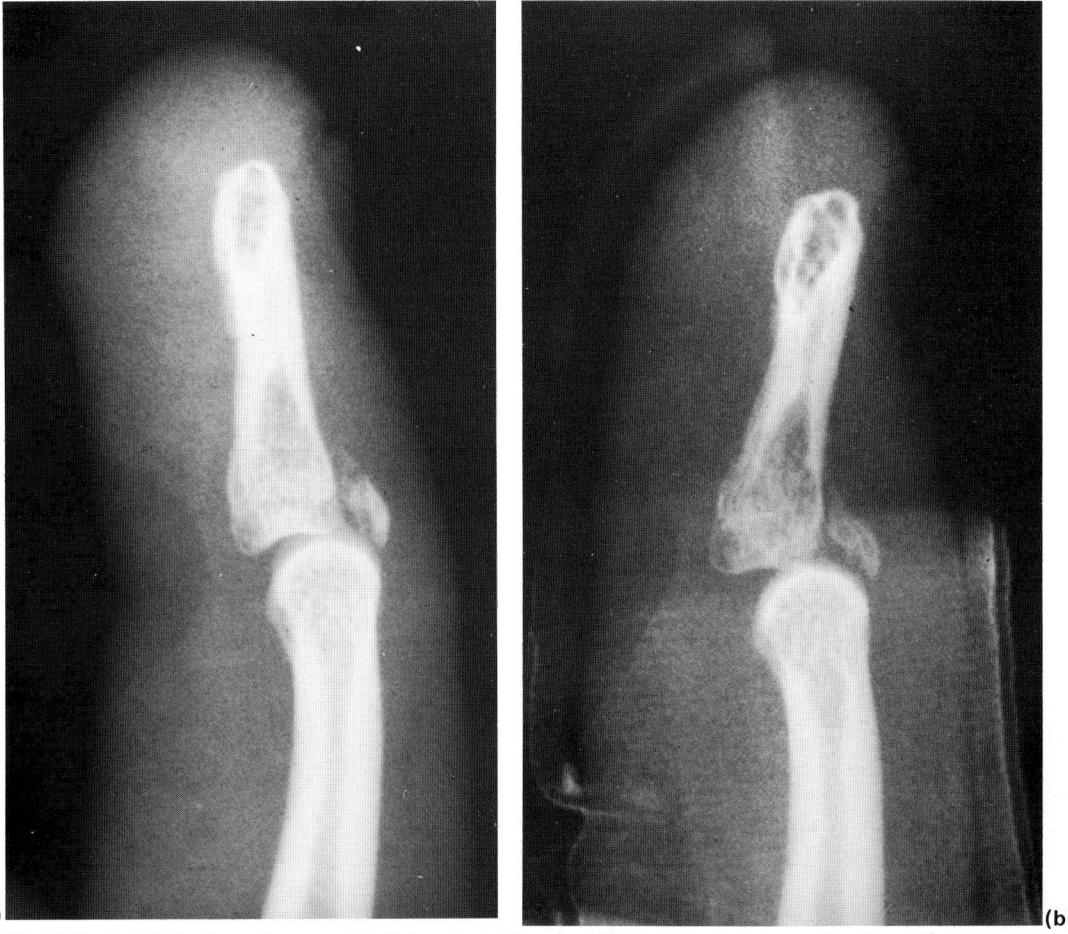

Fig. 5.15 (a) Mallet finger fracture with slight volar subluxation. (b) Incorrect treatment. The finger has been pushed too far into the splint, extending the distal phalanx and increasing the subluxation.

it tends to slip off the rounded end of the bone: a powered wire-introducer is helpful.

Volar lip

Hyperextension of the DIP joint may avulse the distal end of the volar plate with a tiny flake of bone. (Similar detached flakes, but obviously not recent injuries, are quite often seen as an incidental finding on X-rays taken for other purposes, and it is not really known whether they are a developmental abnormality or the result of an old injury.) It is doubtful whether hyperextension or a flexion contracture results, and it is unlikely that these need any treatment.

A larger fragment is likely to carry the insertion of the flexor digitorum profundus tendon and is a serious injury. Considerable violence is necessary to cause the injury, and the fragment is usually displaced, although the pulley over the middle phalanx (called A-4 by Doyle) prevents it from retracting far into the finger. One cannot be sure that the fragment indicates the site of the tendon end, because sometimes the tendon strips off the fragment without any ossific debris accompanying it (Robins & Dobyns 1975, Smith 1981). Exploration is required, and reattachment of the fragment (Leddy & Packer 1977).

Longitudinal fracture of the distal phalanx running into the DIP joint

As in the middle phalanx, these are due to crushing injuries. It is best to ignore the fracture altogether, and to treat the soft-tissue injury and mobilize the joint.

Fractures involving both sides of the joint

At the distal joint, arthrodesis is usually the most appropriate treatment, though if the skin has been damaged by crushing it may be wise simply to transfix the joint with a longitudinal wire to maintain length and then, if it proves necessary, carry out formal arthrodesis later.

SIMULTANEOUS FRACTURES OF BOTH INTERPHALANGEAL JOINTS

An end-on blow can produce fractures of both interphalangeal joints simultaneously. Small avulsion fractures should be treated by early active immobilization, as stiffening is obviously the enemy to be overcome.

If the fractures are unstable, it is unrealistic to expect to regain good movements of both joints. A more practical approach is to stabilize the DIP joint straightaway by transfixing it with a stout Kirschner wire. The efforts of the surgeon, therapist and patient are then concentrated on regaining as much movement as possible at the PIP joint, by whatever method is appropriate for the particular type of fracture, as described above.

INTERPHALANGEAL JOINT OF THE THUMB

This joint is functionally and anatomically intermediate between a proximal and a distal interphalangeal joint, but is closer to the latter. It is, however, much bigger than a DIP joint, so that internal fixation is more satisfactory. The normal range of movement varies considerably, having an inverse relationship to the range at the MP joint. Most people have more movement at their IP than MP joint, but even so, strength is more important than a full range at the IP joint of the thumb.

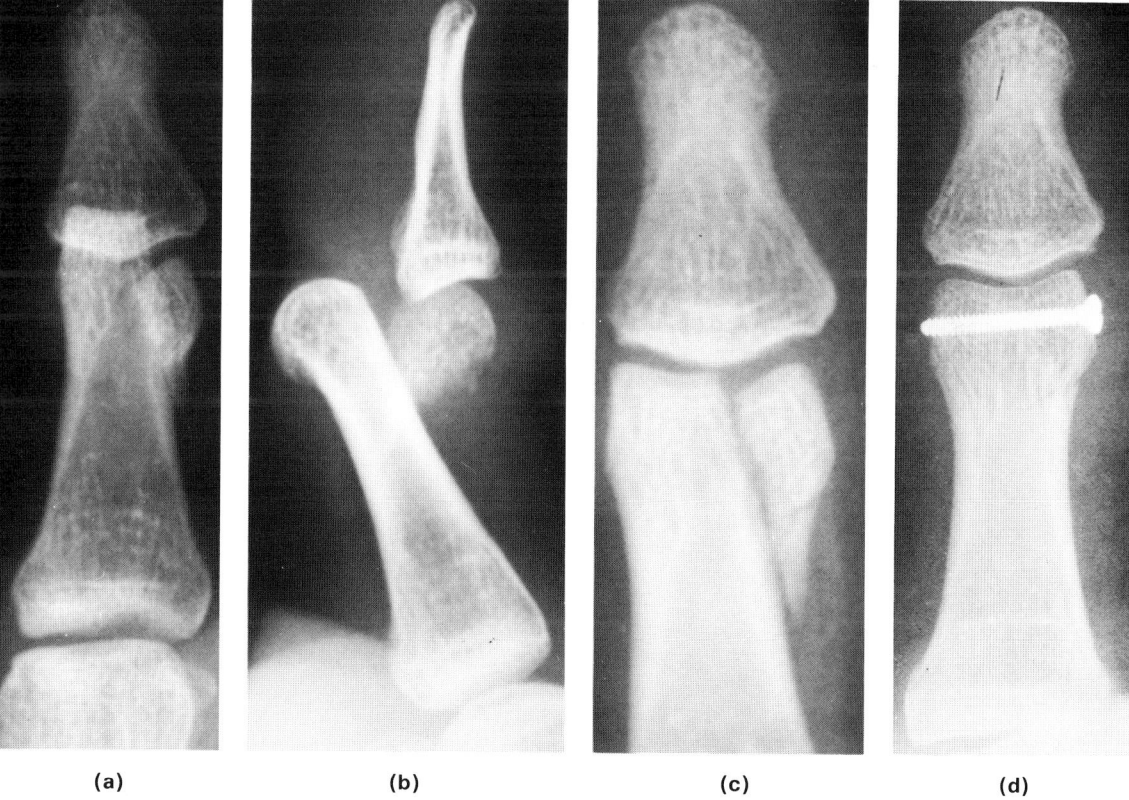

Fig. 5.16 (a) and (b) Fracture dislocation of the interphalangeal joint of the left thumb in a professional cricketer who was struck on the end of the thumb by the ball. (c) After closed reduction of the dislocation, there remains a considerable step in the joint surface. (d) After open reduction, the joint surface has been restored to normal and the fracture held with a small AO screw. The patient regained full movement of this joint.

Fractures of the head of the proximal phalanx

Small avulsion fractures should be treated by early mobilization. Large fractures, bearing a considerable articular surface, should be openly reduced and fixed (Fig. 5.16).

A T-shaped fracture of the head of the proximal phalanx of the thumb constitutes the only indication for the use of plates on the phalanges (Fig. 5.17).

Fractures of the base of the distal phalanx

Small avulsion fractures, without subluxation, should be treated as they are in the finger. If the largest Stack splint is not big enough, a simple straight splint of metal or wood can be used.

Fracture-subluxations are uncommon in the thumb. If the fragment is large, it can be fixed back: if the fragment is small, the joint should be temporarily transfixed. In large fractures of the

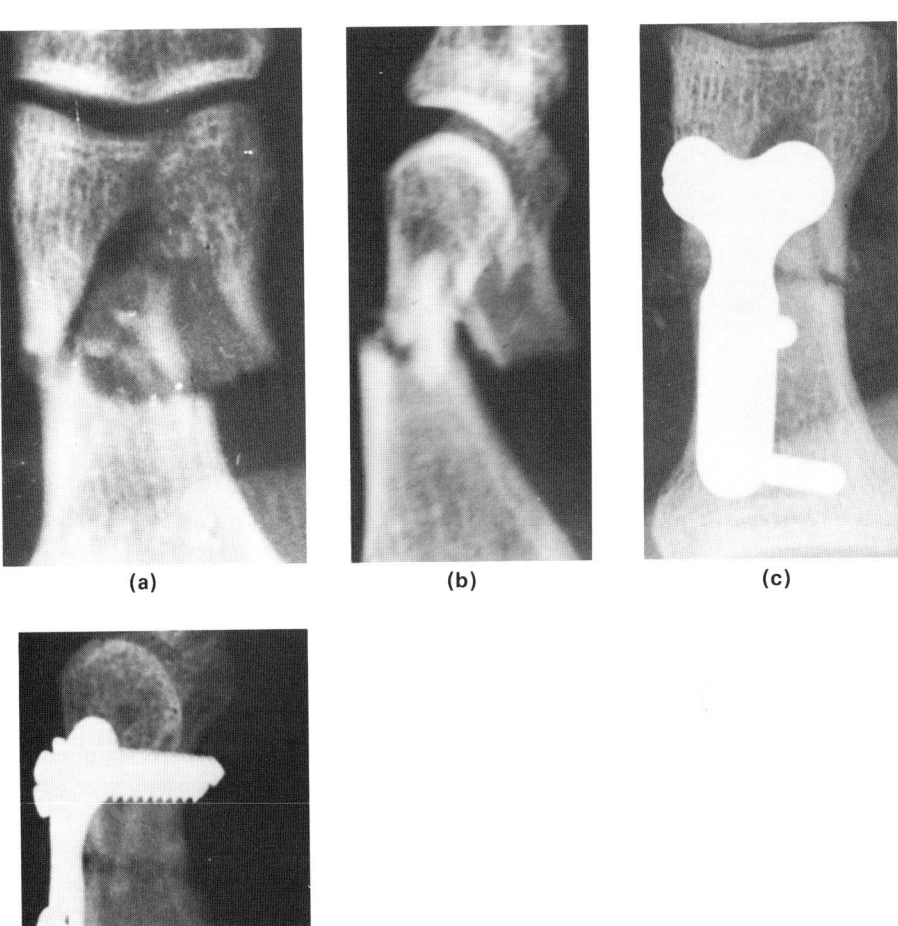

(a) (b) (c)

(d)

Fig. 5.17 (a) and (b) Compound T-shaped or intercondylar (London type III) fracture of the head of proximal phalanx of thumb. One condyle is extended and the other flexed. (c) and (d) After open reduction and fixation with the AO small T-shaped plate. Although the auteroposterior view still shows a tiny step in the joint surface, the lateral view shows restoration of the normal line of the front of the phalanx, allowing free movement of the flexor tendon. When the fracture had united, the plate was removed and tenolysis of the extensor tendon carried out; the patient regained 30° of flexion at the injured joint.

base of the distal phalanx, internal fixation should be considered. Often the fragment carries more of the articular surface than one would think, and open reduction and internal fixation is the only way to restore the joint to a reasonably normal condition.

REFERENCES

Agee J M 1978 Unstable fracture dislocations of the proximal interphalangeal joint of the fingers: a preliminary report of a new treatment technique. Journal of Hand Surgery 3: 386–389

Apley A G 1956 Fractures of the lateral tibial condyle treated by skeletal traction and early mobilisation. Journal of Bone and Joint Surgery 38B: 699–708

Barton N J 1984 Operative treatment of fractures of the Hand. In: Birch R, Brooks D (eds) Operative Surgery—The Hand, 4th edn. Butterworths, London pp 184–195

Benke G J, Stableforth P G 1979 Injuries of the proximal interphalangeal joint of the fingers. The Hand 11: 263–268

Bowers W H 1981 The proximal interphalangeal joint volar plate. II: A clinical study of hyperextension injury. Journal of Hand Surgery 6: 77–81

Bowers W H, Wolf J W, Nehil J L, Bittinger S 1980 The proximal interphalangeal joint volar plate. I: An anatomical and biomechanical study. Journal of Hand Surgery 5: 79–88

Crawford G P 1984 The molded polythene splint for mallet finger deformities. Journal of Hand Surgery 9A: 231–251

Donaldson W R, Millender L H 1978 Chronic fracture-subluxation of the proximal interphalangeal joint. Journal of Hand Surgery 3: 149–153

Eaton R G 1971 Joint injuries of the hand. C C Thomas Co. Springfield, Illinois

Fitzgerald J A W, Khan M A 1984 The conservative management of fractures of the shafts of the phalanges of the fingers by combined traction-splintage. Journal of Hand Surgery 9B: 303–306

Glasgow M, Lloyd G J 1981 The use of modified AO reduction forceps in percutaneous fracture fixation. The Hand 13: 214–216

Jeffery C C 1966 Peri-articular and intra-articular fractures. In: Stack H G, Bolton H (eds) 1975 The Proceedings of the Second Hand Club. The British Society for Surgery of the Hand, London p 382–383

Leddy J P, Packer J W 1977 Avulsion of the profundus tendon insertion in athletes. Journal of Hand Surgery 2: 66–69

Lee M L H 1963 Intra-articular and peri-articular fractures of the phalanges. Journal of Bone and Joint Surgery 45B: 103–109

Lister G 1978 Intraosseous wiring of the digital skeleton. Journal of Hand Surgery 3: 427–435

London P S 1971 Sprains and fractures involving the interphalangeal joints. The Hand 3: 155–158

McCue F, Honner R, Marriott C, Johnson J R, Gieck J H 1970 Athletic injuries of the proximal interphalangeal joint requiring surgical treatment. Journal of Bone and Joint Surgery 52A: 937–956

McElfresh E C, Dobyns J H, O'Brien E T 1972 Management of fracture-dislocation of the proximal interphalangeal joints by extension-block splinting. Journal of Bone and Joint Surgery 54A: 1705–1710

McMinn D J 1981 Mallet finger and fracture. Injury 12: 477–479

Mankin H J 1982 The response of articular cartilage to mechanical injury. Journal of Bone and Joint Surgery 64A: 460–466

O'Brien E T 1982 Fractures of the metacarpals and phalanges. In: Green D (ed) Operative Hand Surgery, Churchill Livingstone New York pp 583–635

Pratt D R 1952 Internal splint for closed and open treatment of injuries of the extensor tendon at the distal joint of the finger. Journal of Bone and Joint Surgery 34A: 785–788

Robertson R C, Cawley J T, Faris A M 1946 Treatment of fracture-dislocation of the interphalangeal joints of the hand. Journal of Bone and Joint Surgery 28: 68–70

Robins P R, Dobyns J H 1975 Avulsions of the insertion of the flexor digitorum profundus tendon associated with fracture of the distal phalanx. In: American Academy of Orthopaedic Surgeons Symposium on Tendon Surgery in the Hand, C V Mosby, St. Louis

Rodriguez A L 1973 Injuries to the collateral ligaments of the proximal interphalangeal joints. The Hand 5: 55–57

Smith J H 1981 Avulsion of a profundus tendon with simultaneous intra-articular fracture of the distal phalanx. Journal of Hand Surgery 6: 600–601

Stack H G 1969 Mallet finger. The Hand 1: 83–89

Steel W M 1978 The AO small fragment set in hand fractures. The Hand 10: 246–253

Strong M L 1980 A new method of extension-block splinting for the proximal interphalangeal joint. Preliminary report. Journal of Hand Surgery 5: 606–607

Trojan E 1972 Fracture-dislocation of the bases of the proximal and middle phalanges of the fingers. The Hand 4: 60–61

Weeks P M 1981 Acute bone and joint injuries of the hand and wrist: a clinical guide to management. C V Mosby Co, St. Louis

Wiley A M 1970 Instability of the proximal interphalangeal joint following dislocation and fracture dislocation: surgical repair. The Hand 2: 185–191

Wilson J N, Rowland S A 1966 Fracture-dislocation of the proximal interphalangeal joint of the finger. Treatment by open reduction and internal fixation. Journal of Bone and Joint Surgery 48A: 493–502

Zemel N P, Stark H H, Ashworth C R, Boyes J H 1981 Chronic fracture dislocation of the proximal interphalangeal joint. Treatment by osteotomy and bone graft. Journal of Hand Surgery 6: 447–455

6

Extensor surface injuries at the proximal interphalangeal joint

Disruption of tendons at the proximal interphalangeal joint initiates an imbalance with functional implications for the entire finger. Early recognition of the condition with an awareness of the pathomechanics permits early management with an improved prognosis.

Reversing proximal and distal interphalangeal joint deformity while retaining joint motion ranks among the most vexing problems which confront the reconstructive hand surgeon and hand therapist. This endeavour is intended to facilitate the recognition and management of the injured dorsal surface of the proximal interphalangeal joints of the fingers.

PERTINENT ANATOMY

The fibres of the extrinsic and intrinsic tendons interconnect over the proximal phalanx and about the proximal interphalangeal joint. The extrinsic extensor tendon trifurcates about the proximal interphalangeal joint: the broad, flat central slip inserts on the base of the middle phalanx; lateral slips supplement the intrinsic tendons to form the conjoined lateral bands. Each intrinsic tendon bifurcates: the medial slips attaching to the base of the middle phalanx adjacent to the central tendon; the parent tendons—each augmented by the lateral slip from the extrinsic extensor—continue distally as the conjoined lateral bands. The descent of the lateral bands with proximal interphalangeal flexion and ascent with extension are associated with an interplay of criss-crossing tendon fibres which move upon each other; the superficial layer from the extrinsic tendons overlaps the deeper layer from the intrinsic tendons (Schultz et al 1981).

Tension for extension of the fully flexed proximal interphalangeal joint is derived through the central fibres of the extrinsic central slip; the lateral bands pass through the axis of the joint in flexion and do not contribute to initiating extension. Tension is progressively transferred to the lateral bands as the joint extends; maximum tension in the more lateral fibres is reached in full extension (Micks & Reswick 1981).

Migration of the lateral bands is necessary for flexion of the distal interphalangeal joint, and for normal, synchronized extension of both interphalangeal joints. The normal 6 mm lengthening of the central tendon with proximal interphalangeal flexion is amplified 3–4 mm at the terminal tendon due to palmar shift of the lateral bands (Zancolli 1979). Forces transferred to the lateral bands by distal joint flexion do not result in any passive excursion of the extrinsic extensor tendons over the proximal phalanx if the proximal joint is unrestrained. These forces are dissipated by palmar migration of the lateral bands (Littler 1977). Passive flexion of the distal joint imparts 3–4 mm of transferred excursion to the central extrinsic tendon via the lateral bands if flexion of the proximal interphalangeal joint is blocked—an observation applied clinically when treating the boutonnière deformity. During active extension, the effective excursion of the terminal tendon at the distal joint is reduced to 3–4 mm because of the dorsomedial shift of the lateral bands.

Lateral band displacement with flexion and extension of the proximal interphalangeal joint is limited by the retinacular (retaining) ligaments. A broad band of fibres obliquely encircles the finger about the proximal interphalangeal joint, coursing from the flexor surface proximally in a dorsal-distal direction. The proximal fibres originate from and reinforce the distal annular (A2) segment of the flexor fibro-osseous sheath; the distal fibres originate from the palmar plate. The fibres palmar to the lateral bands—the transverse retinacular ligament—limit dorsal migration of the lateral bands during extension and assist lateral band descent during flexion. Dorsally these fibres connect the lateral bands: proximal fibres roof the insertions of the central tendon and medial slips of the intrinsic tendons; more distal fibres connect the converging conjoined lateral bands (triangular ligaments) (Fig. 6.1a, b). The transverse retinacular ligaments and continuous dorsal fibres are structurally analogous to the sagittal bands at the metacarpophalangeal joint. Retention of the transverse retinacular ligaments when surgically releasing the central tendon—described by Fowler for readjustment of mallet deformity (Milford 1971)—maintains active extension of the proximal interphalangeal joint without development of a boutonnière deformity (Rosenthal 1984). Resection of the transverse retinacular ligaments permits dorsal displacement and medial migration of the lateral bands which fosters development of a swan-neck deformity.

The oblique retinacular ligaments are variable structures which originate proximally from the lateral ridges of the proximal phalanx deep to the transverse retinacular ligament, palmar to the axis of the proximal interphalangeal joint. They course distally in the longitudinal axis of the finger and mix with fibres of the conjoined lateral bands over the middle phalanx, inserting on the distal phalanx dorsal to the axis of the joint. The oblique retinacular ligaments oppose hyperextension of the proximal interphalangeal joint. They contribute little to extension of the distal joint in the normal finger (Harris & Rutledge 1972, Zancolli 1979). These ligaments may participate in linked flexion of the normal finger. Normally, proximal interphalangeal joint flexion anticipates (exceeds) distal joint flexion, a reflection of tension transmitted through the oblique retinacular ligaments (Fig. 6.1c, d). Elimination of the oblique retinacular ligaments introduces an unnatural pattern of flexion: the distal joint initiates flexion, followed by the proximal interphalangeal joint in a rolling fashion (Zancolli 1979).

Contracture of the oblique retinacular ligament—termed intrinsic intrinsic tightness (Boyes 1971)—is tested by passively extending the proximal interphalangeal joint while passively flexing the distal interphalangeal joint. The test is not valid unless the proximal joint can be extended passively.

PATTERNS OF DEFORMITY

Boutonnière deformity

Boutonnière refers to 'buttonholed' herniation of the head of the proximal phalanx through the extensor tendons (Bingham & Jack 1937). Boutonnière deformity specifically conveys a flexion deformity of the proximal interphalangeal joint with an extension deformity of the distal interphalangeal joint; the metacarpophalangeal joint tends to hyperextend. Development of the deformity requires rupture of both the central extrinsic tendon and the dorsal retinacular fibres (Micks & Hager 1973). The retinacular fibres often survive the initial insult, tearing secondarily with progressing flexion of the proximal interphalangeal joint. Instigating injuries include forced flexion of the actively extended finger, direct trauma to the dorsum of the proximal interphalangeal joint and laceration. The early injury may only be associated with localized tenderness and swelling. X-rays are usually negative. Focal tenderness is the best single test for evaluating injured structures in the finger without early deformity (Wray et al 1984). Carducci (1981) performed arthrograms on injured proximal interphalangeal joints; a positive study revealed dye distal to the joint. His suggested examination, however, is reliable and more practical. Active extension of the proximal interphalangeal joint is assessed while the wrist and metacarpophalangeal joints are maintained in flexion. An extensor lag of greater than 15–20° is considered positive for a potential boutonnière deformity.

Lacerations are less deceiving, and the anatomical lesion is more apparent. Division of the central tendon and lateral bands will release both interphalangeal joints; no extension deformity of the distal joint develops.

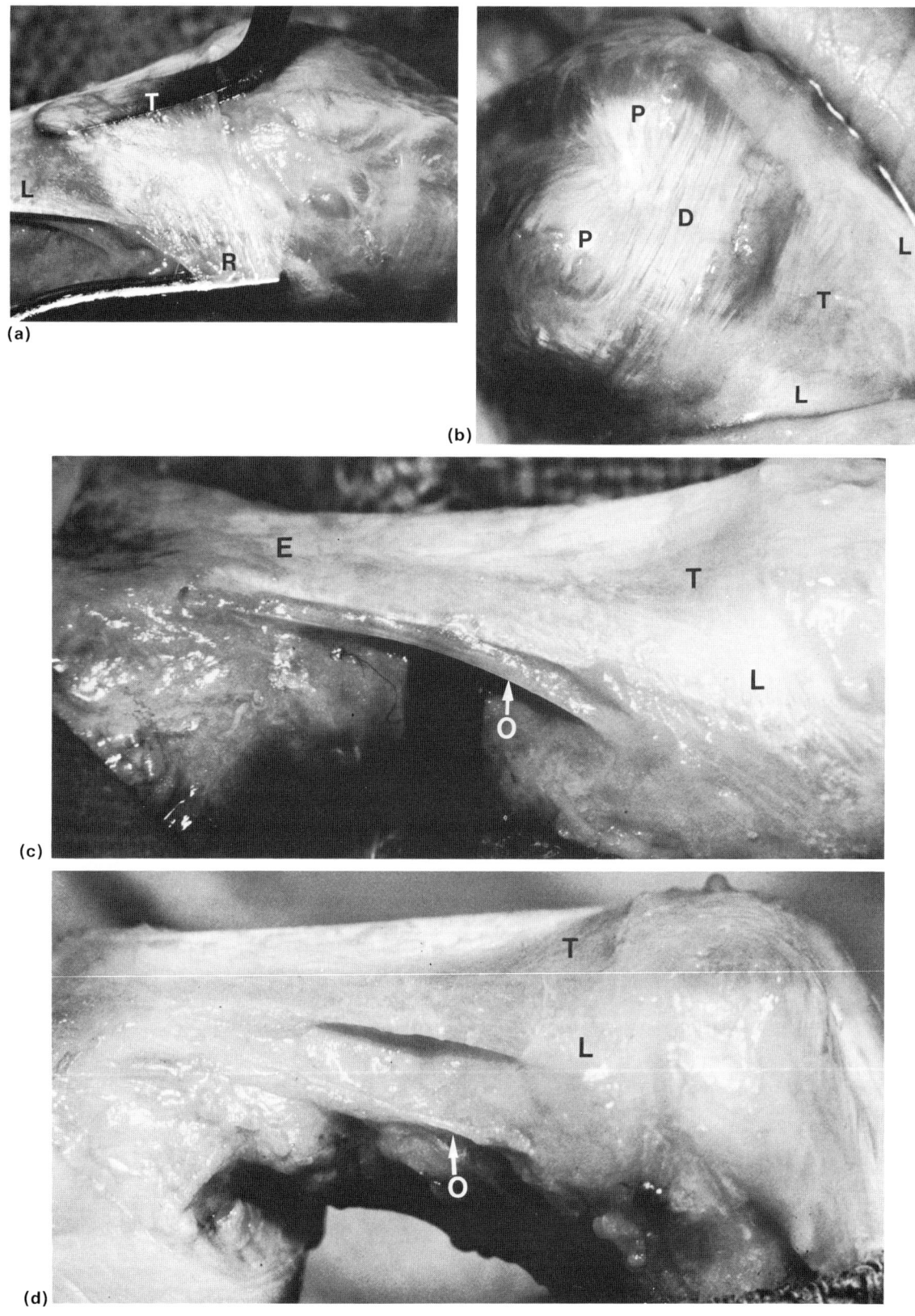

The stage of the lesion (Zancolli 1979) influences the prognosis and recommended treatment. Early recognition and treatment affect the prognosis favourably.

Stage 1

Rupture of the central tendon is associated with localized tenderness. Initially there may not be any flexion deformity. The unopposed flexor superficialis flexes the middle phalanx. The extrinsic extensor, released distally, concentrates forces at the metacarpophalangeal joint which tends to hyperextend. Increasing tension in the lumbrical muscle, the antagonist of the extrinsic extensor, reduces flexion of the distal phalanx by the profundus tendon (Stewart 1962). The proximal interphalangeal joint flexes; the distal joint extends principally from tension through the intrinsic muscles and lateral bands. The extrinsic tendon, tethered proximally by the sagittal bands, is prevented from influencing distal joint extension. Prevention of metacarpophalangeal hyperextension, however, permits the extrinsic extensors to effect extension of the interphalangeal joints (Fowler 1949). The dorsal retinacular ligaments stretch and rupture, allowing a palmar migration of the lateral bands. The proximal and distal joint deformities are passively correctable. Clinical tightness of the oblique retinacular ligament is not yet evident (Fig. 6.2**a**).

Stage 2

Flexion of the proximal joint and extension of the distal joint introduces laxity into the transverse and oblique retinacular ligaments. Lateral band descent progresses. The loose retinacular ligaments tighten, and the retinacular tightness test becomes positive. Passive correction of the proximal joint is possible since the lateral bands are not yet fixed palmar to the axis of the joint by adhesions or contracture of the transverse retinacular ligaments.

Proximal interphalangeal joint stiffness develops as the transverse retinacular ligaments shorten and the lateral bands become fixed in the palmar position (Fig. 6.2**b**).

Stage 3

Fixed deformity of proximal and distal interphalangeal joints becomes superimposed on tightness of the retinacular ligaments. Contractures of the palmar plate and accessory collateral ligaments evolve. The lateral bands become fixed palmar to the joint axis due to shortening of the loose retinacular ligaments, tightness of the intrinsic tendons and adhesions of the displaced lateral bands to the underlying joint capsule. Contracture of the lateral and palmar skin, tethered by cutaneous retinacular ligaments, add resistance to correction in the chronically deformed finger (Littler 1977). The flexed proximal and extended distal joint represent the fully developed boutonnière deformity (Fig. 6.2**c**).

Complex dislocations

This category includes dislocations which damage the extensor tendons and produce clinical deformity.

Semantic distinction between a complex injury—injury to multiple tissue systems—and a 'complexed' dislocation—articular interposition of tendon or ligament—has been suggested. When the proximal interphalangeal joint is flexed to 55° the lateral bands rest palmar to the joint axis. In this position the joint is more susceptible to torsional forces and more likely to incur a complex dislocation (Garroway et al 1984). A classification of five pathoanatomic types of complex dislocations of the proximal interphalangeal joints has been proposed; only the first two involve the extensor tendons.

Type 1: there is unilateral rupture of a collateral ligament with anterior intra-articular displace-

Fig. 6.1 Anatomy of the retinacular ligaments. (**a**) Vertical fibres about the proximal interphalangeal joint. These continuous fibres influence the descent and ascent of the lateral bands during flexion and extension. (**b**) Fibres bridging the lateral bands dorsally restrain palmar migration during flexion. (**c, d**) Oblique retinacular ligament. Orientated in the longitudinal axis of the finger, the proximal fibres pass beneath the transverse retinacular ligament palmar to the axis of the joint; distal fibres mix with the lateral bands and terminal tendon. D = dorsal fibres; E = terminal tendon; L = conjoined lateral band; O = oblique retinacular ligament; P = condyle proximal phalanx; R = transverse retinacular ligament; T = triangular ligament.

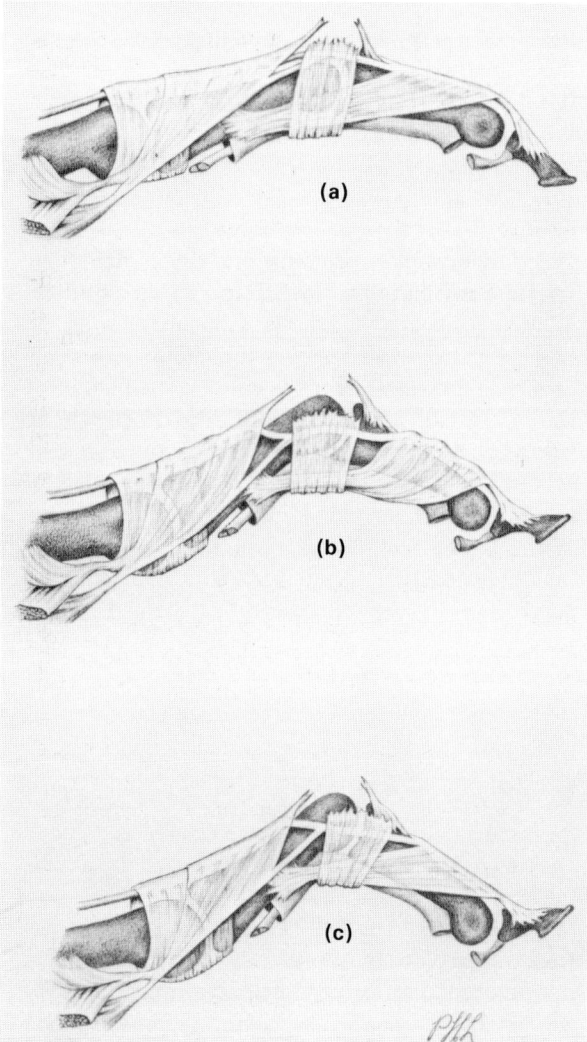

Fig. 6.2 Development of the boutonnière deformity. (**a**) Stage 1: the central tendon and triangular ligaments are torn. Unopposed flexion by the flexor superficialis initiates palmar migration of the lateral bands. (**b**) Stage 2: the lateral bands migrate palmar to the axis of the joint. Flexion of the proximal interphalangeal joint and extension of the distal joint progress. The retinacular ligaments are loose and the deformity is passively reversible. (**c**) Stage 3: contractures of the palmar plate and collateral ligaments of the proximal interphalangeal joint are superimposed upon contractures of the retinacular ligaments, tightness of the intrinsic muscles and fixation of the displaced lateral bands by adhesions. The deformity is fixed.

ment of the ipsilateral lateral band. The central tendon is preserved
Type 2: there is rupture of the central tendon in addition to the components of the type 1 injury

Rupture of the collateral ligament introduces axial instability. A flexion deformity of the proximal interphalangeal joint will develop if the central tendon and dorsal retinacular ligaments have also been ruptured. Anterior dislocation of the lateral band may block passive reduction of the deformity. The initial examination should include two-plane X-rays and axial stress views if instability is apparent.

Intrusion of the ruptured collateral ligament through the extensor tendons has been reported with dislocation of the proximal interphalangeal joint. Spinner & Choi (1970) described an anterior dislocation of the joint with rupture of the central tendon and palmar plate. The collateral ligament, avulsed from the proximal phalanx, was herniated between the oblique retinacular ligament and the lateral band. Stern (1981) reported a lateral dislocation with herniation of the avulsed collateral ligament between the central tendon and lateral band (a Stener-type lesion). A 15° extensor lag with axial instability was present clinically.

Pseudoboutonnière deformity

This deformity, described by McCue et al (1970), resembles the classical boutonnière deformity, but hyperextension of the distal joint is less severe than in the true boutonnière deformity (McCue et al 1975). The primary injury, however, is avulsion of the proximal attachments of the palmar plate from an oblique hyperextension injury. Early X-rays are normal and the implications of the injury may not be appreciated initially. Calcification appears at the site of the avulsed proximal attachment of the palmar plate 3–6 months following injury and may enlarge over the ensuing 6 months to form a spur; spurs were more commonly located on the radial side of the proximal phalanx than on the ulnar (oblique X-rays are recommended). Deformity ranges from 'mild' (<40°) to 'severe' (>45° and often progressive) flexion of the proximal interphalangeal joint. There is unilateral scarring of the lateral band on the side of the spur.

The deformity may be prevented by early active motion combined with supportive dynamic splinting (Lee 1982).

Attritional boutonnière deformity

Burkhalter & Carneiro (1979) referred to the deformity which results from attenuation of intact extensor tendons over the proximal interphalangeal joint as the attritional boutonnière deformity. Longstanding flexion of the joint causes pressure against the extensor tendons by the head of the proximal phalanx. The tendons are intact, but are functionally ineffective. The pathomechanics of the deformity are otherwise similar to those already described in the traumatic boutonnière deformity. Aetiologies include rheumatoid arthritis, Dupuytren's contracture, spasticity of the extrinsic extensor tendons, neurological diseases (amyotrophic lateral sclerosis, Charcot-Marie-Tooth disease), palmar skin contractures, intrinsic paralysis with claw deformity, ischaemic necrosis due to pressure (burns) and chronic dislocations. Deformities associated with rheumatoid arthritis are covered in Chapter 8.

Extensor tenodesis

The anatomical form, intimacy with the underlying periosteum, and complex excursion requirements of the extensor tendons about the proximal interphalangeal joint render them vulnerable to restraint from adhesions and physical alteration by scar. Restrained tendons tether flexion of more distal joints.

Reciprocal passive extension of the interphalangeal joints with metacarpophalangeal flexion is the extensor plus phenomenon. Dorsal restraint of the extensor tendons reduces active extension as well as active and passive flexion of the proximal interphalangeal joints; distal joint motion is also impaired. Compensatory increase in the proximal displacement of the extrinsic tendons is prevented by the sagittal bands which limit tendon excursion to 20 mm during flexion and extension of the metacarpophalangeal joint. The extensor tendon excursions associated with motion of the proximal and distal interphalangeal joints were discussed previously (see above). The reciprocal release of distal joints by passively extending more proximal joints is helpful in localizing adhesions (Rosenthal 1984).

TREATMENT OF TENDON INJURIES

The treatment of injuries to the extensor tendons is based on the type of injury and duration of deformity. Care of the acute open injury depends upon the extent of damage to the tendons, the findings on examination and the presence of fracture. Different methods have been described for tidy and avulsion wounds. Treatment of the chronic deformity depends on the extent of deformity, mobility, and aetiology. Treatment in all instances is tailored to the functional demands of the patient, and should reflect consideration of the patient's age, a realistic assessment of prognosis with treatment, and relevant infirmities. Littler's (1977) aphorism deserves emphasis: 'Despite the apparent logic of the procedure, the results are not entirely predictable.'

Closed injuries

The posture of the injured finger and location of swelling and tenderness are helpful in surmising the extent of tendon injury (Table 6.1). Testing active extension (see above: boutonnière deformity), passive extension and axial stability is essential. Routine X-rays should be augmented by oblique films following hyperextension injuries and when axial instability is present.

Localized findings, without loss of active or passive extension, axial instability or fracture, nevertheless imply a partial dorsal tendon injury which may progress unless the proximal interphalangeal joint is protected in extension by splinting. The metacarpophalangeal and distal interphalangeal joints are left free. Active distal joint motion is pursued. The injury is reassessed in 1 week. Absence of clinical findings with normal extensor function permits resumption of activities without further splinting. Continued tenderness indicates need for protective splinting for an additional 2 weeks.

Table 6.1 Treatment of closed injuries of the extensor tendons of the proximal interphalangeal (PIP) joint

• Suggestive examination • Active extension • Passive extension • No fracture	• Active extension loss • Passive extension • No fracture	• Active extension loss • Passive extension loss • ?Axial instability • ?Fracture
Splint PIP joint Reassess in 1 week	Splint PIP joint for 6 weeks ?Kirschner wire	Primary repair Open red fracture ?2nd stage tendon reconstruction

Inability to complete active extension of the proximal interphalangeal joint following injury is construed as a rupture of the central tendon. Associated interruption of the dorsal retinacular ligaments permits anterior displacement of the lateral bands with inability to initiate extension from the flexed position. In the absence of fracture, closed injuries are treated by uninterrupted splinting of the proximal interphalangeal joint for 6 weeks. Active metacarpophalangeal flexion shifts the extensor mechanism distally, opposing proximal retraction of the torn central tendon. Distal joint motion continues actively, and also opposes retraction of the central tendon by tension transferred through the lateral bands. Passive correction of the proximal interphalangeal joint with full active distal joint flexion indicates restoration of 'balance' between extrinsic and intrinsic tendon systems (Doyle 1982). Active motion is begun after 6 weeks, with interval splinting between active motion periods during the next 2 weeks. Splinting is only discontinued when there is no recurrence of deformity associated with unsupported active motion.

A Kirschner wire, inserted obliquely across the proximal interphalangeal joint, is a dependable substitute for splinting in patients who are not likely to comply with the demands of a splinting programme. Elliott (1971) recommended removal of the Kirschner wire after 5 weeks, followed by a week of uninterrupted splinting of the proximal interphalangeal joint, and night splinting for an additional week.

The duration of a deformity has become less significant in predicting success with splinting. Improved hand therapy has contributed to improved results even in longstanding cases. Boyes (1971) advocated splinting as late as 30 days following injury. McFarlane & Hampole (1973) reported that splinting offered a good prognosis in any case in which the proximal interphalangeal joint could be passively corrected, since this implied that the lateral bands were still mobile. Doyle (1982) endorsed splinting as late as 6 months following closed injuries. The parameter of time may be applied flexibly when determining treatment for chronic deformities.

Axial instability or unilateral widening of the proximal interphalangeal joint, indicating collateral ligament rupture, associated with loss of active or passive extension of this joint are indications for primary operative repair (Spinner & Choi 1970, Neviaser & Wilson 1972).

An avulsion fracture associated with functional interruption of the central tendon is also an indication for primary operative repair of a closed injury (Tubiana 1968; Boyes 1970). The position of the proximal interphalangeal joint following operative reconstruction of reducible larger articular fractures may be deleterious to concurrently repaired extensor tendons. Souter (1967, 1974) felt that these combined injuries implied a poor prognosis, and recommended staging the repairs. The fracture is repaired initially. Tendon reconstruction is deferred until the fracture has healed and passive joint mobility has been achieved.

The individual requirements of the patient should be considered when major joint damage is associated with extensor tendon injury. The selection of primary arthrodesis or primary tendon repair with secondary arthroplasty should reflect these considerations.

Open injuries

Open injuries present a gamut of challenges (Table 6.2). Tidy slicing injuries preserve the substance of the extensor tendons. Untidy injuries locally shred tissues, necessitating debridement and rendering secure repair uncertain. Reinforcement of the primary repair is often necessary. Dorsal avulsion

Table 6.2 Treatment of open injuries of the extensor tendons of the proximal interphalangeal (PIP) joint

Tidy	Untidy	Avulsion
Primary repair	Primary repair	Flap coverage
Kirschner wire	?Reinforcement	Local
	Snow (1973)	Russell
	Hellmann, Aiche	Joshi
	Littler (1964)	Remote
	Kirschner wire	Secondary tendon reconstruction
		Littler (1967)
		Salvi
		Joshi
		Snow (1976)
		Stack
		Fowler
		Nichols, Weeks
		Flatt

injuries indicate pedicle flap coverage with secondary reconstruction of the destroyed tendons.

Tidy injuries

Tidy injuries of the central tendon—clean lacerations without tendon destruction—should be repaired and the proximal interphalangeal joint stabilized in extension. A Kirschner wire may be removed after 3 weeks (McFarlane & Hampole 1973), but the proximal interphalangeal joint support continues for 5–6 weeks following repair (Doyle 1982). Splinting is discontinued only when there is no recurrent deformity with continued active motion without support. Following repair of the lateral bands in addition to the central tendon, the metacarpophalangeal joint and both interphalangeal joints are immobilized for 3 weeks following repair; this position protects the repair site from proximal retraction of the repaired tendon segments. Active motion of the metacarpophalangeal joint is then permitted but the proximal interphalangeal joint is supported for an additional 2 weeks, a total of 5 weeks' immobilization.

The specificity of the repair technique has received varying attention. Kaplan (1959) emphasized restoring the broad, flat insertion of the central tendon. Boyes (1970) supported a common figure-of-eight suture for tendon and skin. McFarlane & Hampole (1973) advocated a 'cluster' suture for the injured tendons. Doyle (1982) summed up reported sentiments when he wrote that any method for joining the tendon ends was satisfactory if the joint was supported following the repair. Considering the functional dynamics of the extensor tendons at the level of the proximal interphalangeal joint, however, it is meritorious to attempt an anatomic restoration which provides for repair of the extrinsic and intrinsic tendons individually. The central tendon and lateral bands are sutured separately, using a fine calibre, non-absorbable suture such as 5-0 white Mersilene® (Ethicon).

Suturing the lateral bands dorsal to the proximal interphalangeal joint, preventing their shift, permits flexion of the proximal joint but prevents concurrent flexion of the distal joint (Harris & Rutledge 1972, Zancolli 1979).

Untidy injuries

An untidy injury destroys tissue locally and requires debridement which may interfere with performing a secure tendon repair. Reinforcement of the repaired tendon is advisable when the suture line is tenuous or when loss of tendon segments prevents accurate approximation without tension. Transposed adjacent tissues provide reinforcement of the primary repair. A distally based medial segment of the extrinsic tendon, folded distally over the damaged central tendon, has been advocated by Snow (1973) (Fig. 6.3). When the remaining extrinsic tendon is deficient and cannot be utilized for reinforcement, the medial segments of both lateral bands may be mobilized and sutured centrally over the proximal interphalangeal joint (Hellmann 1964, Aiche et al 1970) (Fig. 6.3). One remaining lateral band, divided distally over the middle phalanx and reinserted into the base of the middle phalanx or remaining stump of the central tendon (Littler 1964) is an alternative for reinforcement of the primary repair (Fig. 6.3).

The proximal interphalangeal joint is pinned in extension with a Kirschner wire for 3 weeks, followed by continued support with splinting for an additional 2–3 weeks. The initial 3 weeks immobilization includes the wrist and metacarpophalangeal joint (Tubiana 1968, Zancolli 1979). Flexion of the metacarpophalangeal joint precludes proximal retraction of the extrinsic tendon and relaxes the repaired lateral bands (Stewart 1962).

Avulsion injuries

These injuries result in loss of dorsal skin with segments of the extensor tendons, precluding both repair and reinforcement using retained local tissue. A staged reconstruction is required, initially with a pedicle flap; tendon reconstruction is performed secondarily.

Pedicle flaps include local and remote flaps. A proximally-based local transposition flap is useful for smaller defects. Two local flap techniques, described for secondary reconstruction of the burned finger with poorly vascularized tissues over the proximal interphalangeal joint, have theoretical appeal for application in selected acute injuries. Russell et al (1981) designed a proximally based,

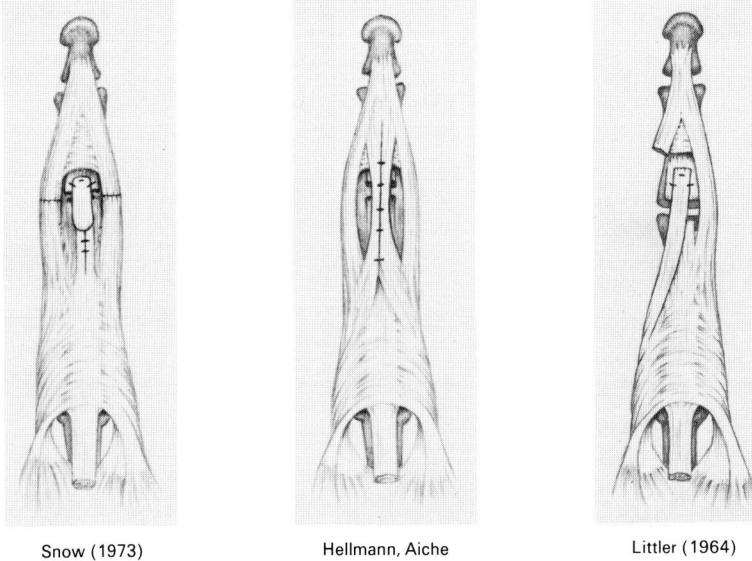

Fig. 6.3 Methods for reinforcement of extensor tendons in untidy dorsal surface injuries.

arterialized flap which was elevated from the side of the injured finger and rotated dorsally to cover the proximal interphalangeal joint. The digital nerve was not mobilized. Joshi (1982) described an arterialized tendo-cutaneous flap containing an uninjured lateral band which was rotated dorsally for reconstruction of the dorsum of the proximal interphalangeal joint. The more traditional cross finger flap is also applicable, and does not require as precise a dissection as an arterialized flap. Remote pedicle flaps, such as the groin pedicle, are also useful, particularly when multiple fingers are involved.

Selection of the method for secondary reconstruction of the avulsed extensor tendons is determined by the condition of the dorsal skin and remaining available extensor tendons (Van Der Meulen 1972). Littler & Eaton (1967) reefed both lateral bands dorsally over the proximal interphalangeal joint and remnant of the central tendon, preserving the lumbrical tendon and oblique retinacular ligaments to provide extension of the distal joint (Fig. 6.4). Salvi (1969) relocated the retained lateral bands dorsal to the axis of the joint with bi-axial dorsally-based flaps of the transverse retinacular ligaments ('capsular flaps') which were sutured dorsally as a surgical substitute for the dorsal retinacular ligaments (Fig. 6.4). Joshi's (1982) tendo-cutaneous flap has already been mentioned (Fig. 6.4).

Snow (1976) described a method for reconstructing congenitally deficient finger extensor tendons using the interosseous muscle–tendon unit from an adjacent digit (Fig. 6.4). He has used this method successfully for late reconstruction of traumatic deformities in four cases (Snow 1984).

Stack (1971) bridged the defect in the extrinsic extensor using the flexor superficialis, which he divided proximally, passed dorsally through the middle phalanx and sutured to the distal remnant of the central tendon (Fig. 6.4).

Free tendon grafting for reconstruction of the damaged extensor surface of the finger provides an alternative in selected patients. With a discrete lesion of the extrinsic tendon, without significant scarring of the lateral bands, free tendon grafting of the central tendon to the middle phalanx restores an independent extensor to the proximal inter-

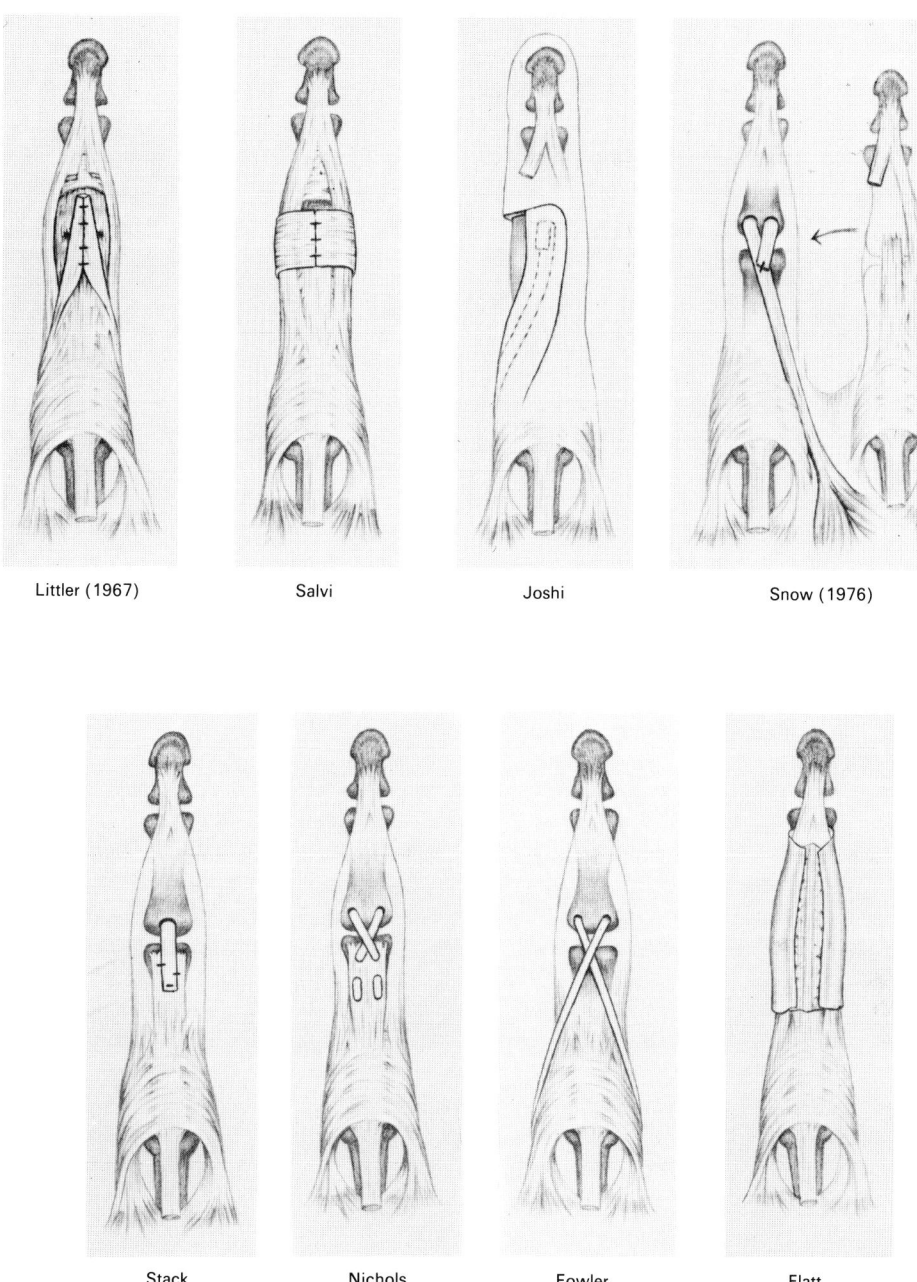

Fig. 6.4 Methods for replacement of extensor tendons in avulsion dorsal surface injuries.

phalangeal joint (Nichols 1951) (Fig. 6.4). Weeks (1967) modified this method by weaving the tendon graft into the lateral bands as well as the extrinsic tendon remnant, functionally replacing the dorsal retinacular ligaments. Fowler (Boyes 1970) described tendon graft reconstruction using the intrinsic muscles at the base of the finger for the motors (Fig. 6.4). His method has application when the central tendon as well as the lateral bands are not available, or when dorsal skin does not permit dissection, as in the burn boutonnière deformity (Larson et al 1970). Flatt (1983) has successfully replaced major dorsal defects of the finger extensor tendons with the palmaris longus tendon and contiguous deep fascia. The deep fascia provides a trough for the lateral bands, restoring extension forces to both interphalangeal joints while providing restraint to palmar displacement of the lateral bands (Fig. 6.4). This procedure has merit in extensive defects, with application in cases as late as 18 months following injury (Suzuki 1973). Time appears to be less relevant to prognosis than is passive correction of the deformity preoperatively. Free tendon grafting is exacting. Flatt (1983) poignantly reflected that 'adequate tension' was 'impossible to define but essential to success.'

Infected injuries

A wound infection interferes with conventional guidelines for treatment and poses a dilemma which is not easily solved. The risk of sepsis destroying a surgical effort designed to shorten treatment and improve function is weighed against the cautious but more lengthy pursuit of non-operative methods. Selecting the most propitious course becomes judgmental. The septic tidy laceration precludes repair. Exposed articular cartilage is vulnerable to the infection as well as to dessication. Supportive culture-specific antibiotics and protective moist dressings cover the unfavourable phase until repair can be accomplished in the presence of a surgically clean wound with negative cultures. Tendon repair and Kirschner wire stabilization of the proximal interphalangeal joint is then reasonable. Persistence of the sepsis remands the case to continued non-operative care with splinting and wound care. The implications for functional restoration in the non-operative course are guarded and presume diligent and prolonged supervision. A functional plateau may not be reached for prolonged periods in such cases (Rosenthal 1984).

Chronic deformities

The established deformity from a boutonnière lesion or tenodesed extensor tendons should be symptomatic and present a functional impairment or treatment is not indicated. Mild flexion deformity of the proximal interphalangeal joint, 20–30°, may be of little clinical consequence if comfortable active flexion of both interphalangeal joints is retained (Boyes 1971). The cumbersome stiff finger which is subject to repeated trauma, unsightly and unable to flex at the distal joint, however, deserves attention. No determination of a surgical scheme can be made until maximum improvement has been gained through splinting and supervised hand therapy, continued unabated as long as progress is continuous. The longer a deformity exists, the more difficult reversal becomes (Pardini et al 1979). Nevertheless, there is no definite time beyond which a trial of corrective splinting and therapy should be discounted as futile when initially approaching treatment of a deformity (Table 6.3).

Mobile boutonnière deformity

Deformities responsive to corrective splinting of the proximal interphalangeal joint with concurrent mobilization of the distal joint fall within stage 1 and 2 of boutonnière pathogenesis (see above: Patterns of deformity). Prognosis is more favourable with passive correction of the proximal interphalangeal joint (McFarlane & Hampole 1973). Active distal joint flexion is essential for maintaining correction of the proximal interphalangeal joint; lack of distal flexion predisposes to a recurrent deformity (Zancolli 1979). Static splinting of the distal joint in flexion retards recurrence of proximal deformity in resistant cases (Stewart 1962, Zancolli 1979). Preoperative therapy must be pursued until passive extension of the proximal interphalangeal joint has levelled off at a 'best

Table 6.3 Treatment of chronic deformity of the proximal interphalangeal joint due to extensor tendon injury

Boutonnière mobile deformity	Boutonnière fixed deformity	Extensor tenodesis
?Accept deformity	Distal tenotomy	Tendolysis
Splint PIP +	(Fowler,	Serial tenotomy
mobilize DIP	Dolphin)	(Kilgore 1975)
Staged tendolysis	Joint release +	Resection extrinsic
(Curtis)	tendon repair	tendon (Littler
Repair	(?staged)	1964)
Elliott	PIP arthroplasty	
Littler (1967)	PIP arthrodesis +	
Matev	distal tenotomy	

PIP: proximal interphalangeal
DIP: distal interphalangeal

effort' level. *Active* postoperative extension rarely exceeds *passive* preoperative extension following extensor tendon reconstruction unless a major joint release accompanies the tendon reconstruction (Elliott 1971, Curtis et al 1983) (Fig. 6.5).

Curtis et al (1983) promulgated a staged technique for reconstruction of the chronic traumatic boutonnière deformity which surgically releases the deformity while carefully recognizing the functional anatomy of the extensor tendons. Preoperative passive correction is required. The procedure is begun under digital block anaesthesia; wrist block is avoided because of intrinsic paralysis. Stage 1 is a meticulous tendolysis of the extrinsic tendons, transverse retinacular ligaments and lateral bands. Failure to achieve full active extension is followed by stage 2, release of the transverse retinacular ligaments. Loss of 20° or less of active extension following stage 2 is followed by stage 3, a distal tenotomy of the lateral bands over the middle phalanx as described by Fowler (Littler 1964, Dolphin 1965). Lack of more than 20° active extension after stage 2 indicates the need for extensor tendon reconstruction, stage 4. Curtis et al advocate the method of Elliott (1970) (Fig. 6.7).

Elliott's anatomical reconstruction involves a tendolysis with surgical definition of the central tendon and both lateral bands. The scarred segment of the central tendon is resected, the central tendon is reapproximated at its insertion and the lateral bands are retained dorsally with sutures (Fig. 6.7). Littler & Eaton's (1967) method folds both lateral bands dorsally over the remnant of the central tendon to effect extension of the proximal interphalangeal joint. The lumbrical tendon and oblique retinacular ligaments remain to extend the distal joint (Fig. 6.7). With tightness of the oblique retinacular ligament, release of the distal joint can be achieved with a triangular resection of the oblique retinacular ligaments and inferior borders of the lateral bands at the base of the middle phalanx on both sides—an intrinsic intrinsic release (Zancolli 1979). Matev's (1964) reconstruction involves more extensive dissection with mobilization of the lateral bands to their insertions, but permits restoration of a balanced, independent extensor tendon for both proximal and distal interphalangeal joints. His technique also releases the extension deformity of the distal interphalangeal joint (Matev 1969) (Fig. 6.7).

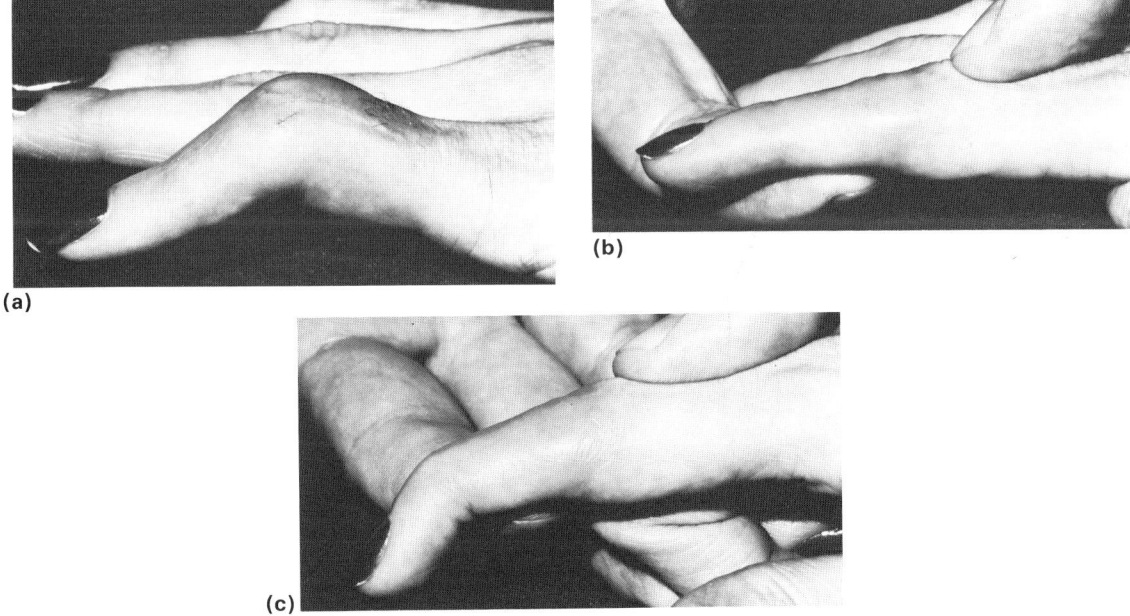

Fig. 6.5 Progressive reversal of the established boutonnière deformity with dynamic splinting and supervised hand therapy. (**a**) The deformity. (**b**) Passive extension of the proximal interphalangeal joint obtained by splinting. (**c**) Recovery of distal joint flexion is essential for restoration of balance as well as for preventing recurrence of deformity after splinting is discontinued. (Reprinted with permission from Rosenthal, 1984.)

106 THE INTERPHALANGEAL JOINTS

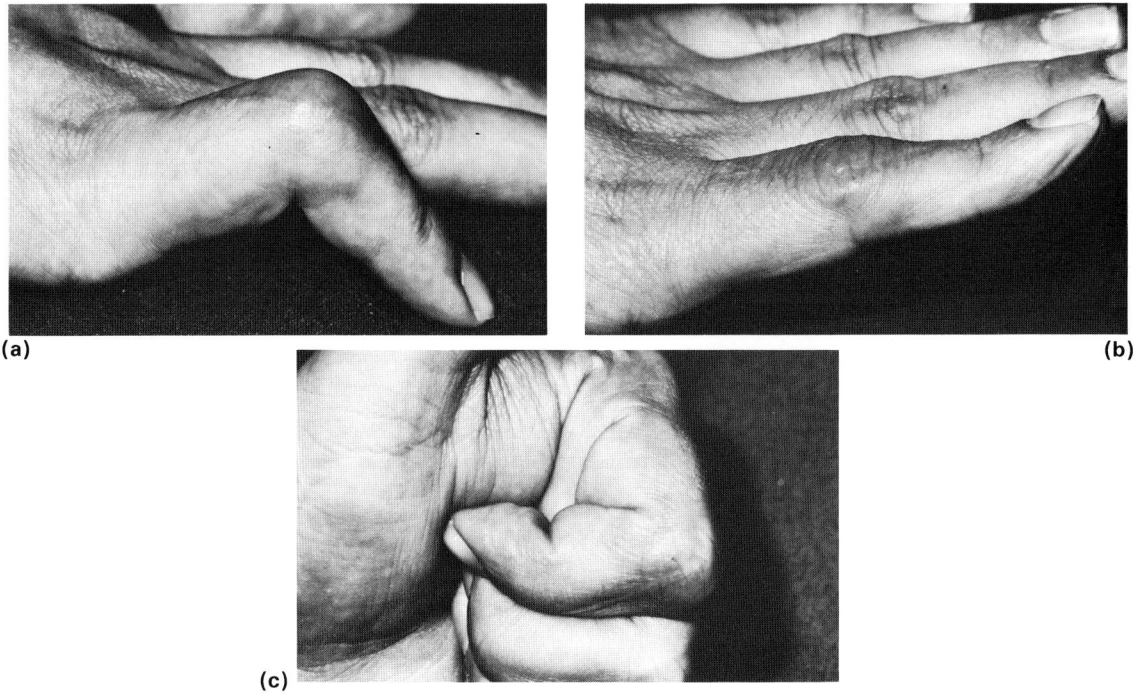

Fig. 6.6 Successful tendolysis for chronic deformity in a 25-year-old man. (**a**) Active extension when first seen 7 months after attempted reconstruction of boutonnière deformity with reefing of the lateral bands over the proximal interphalangeal joint. Passive extension was achieved with splinting. (**b**) Active extension 6 months after tendolysis with dorsal capsulotomy of proximal interphalangeal joint. (**c**) Active flexion.

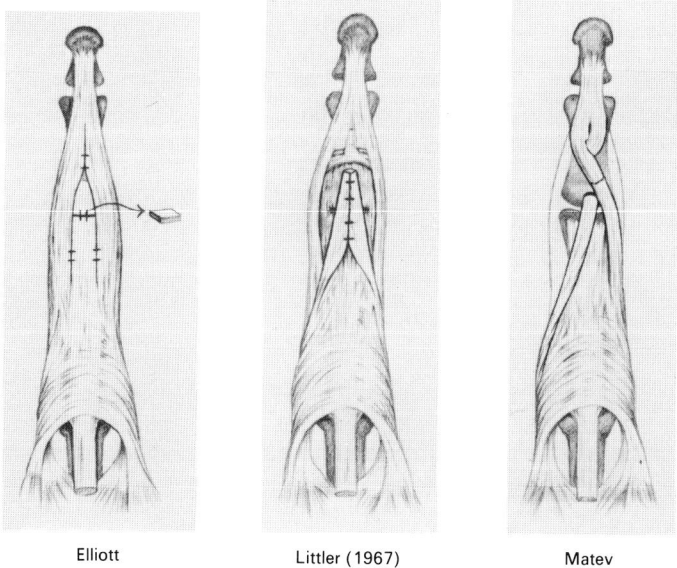

Elliott   Littler (1967)   Matev

Fig 6.7 Methods for reconstruction of the chronic boutonnière deformity.

Selection of the most appropriate method for reconstruction involves consideration of the active and passive motion of both joints and the configuration of the injured tendons at the time of surgery. Elliott's anatomical reconstruction requires the central tendon and both lateral bands. His restoration of the normal extensor tendon relationships is fundamentally appealing. Littler & Eaton's (1967) reconstruction which restores extension to the proximal interphalangeal joint may be used when the central tendon is deficient. Distal joint tightness may not be corrected, however, without an intrinsic intrinsic tenotomy or distal extensor tenotomy. Matev's method, feasible without a central tendon, involves a relatively complicated readjustment of the lateral bands, but permits rebalancing of both proximal and distal interphalangeal joint deformities. Each method has merit in specific situations.

Attritional boutonnière with intrinsic paralysis. Burkhalter & Carneiro (1979) released the transverse retinacular ligaments and sewed the lateral bands in the midline over the proximal phalanx in the chronic attritional boutonnière deformity associated with high ulnar nerve lesions. This static tenodesis by the paralysed intrinsic muscles reversed the claw deformity at the metacarpophalangeal joint. A distal tenotomy was performed if the distal interphalangeal joint was tight in extension. They cautioned that this procedure should only be performed when there is little prospect for recovery of the intrinsic muscles.

Fixed boutonnière deformity

The deformity which is resistant to passive correction by splinting is, by definition, a stage 3 deformity. Tendolysis and reconstruction of the extensor tendons cannot be expected to improve upon the passive correction of joint deformities achieved preoperatively. Release of the proximal joint contracture must precede extensor tendon restoration, usually as the first of staged operative procedures (Burton 1982, Curtis et al 1983). Inability to correct surgically the capsular stiffness of the proximal interphalangeal joint is an indication for an implant arthroplasty (Burton 1982, Curtis et al 1983), or arthrodesis of the joint with distal tenotomy (Elliott 1971).

Distal tenotomy—already discussed as stage 3 in Curtis' technique—cannot be expected to augment active extension of the proximal interphalangeal joint by more than 20° even with liberation of the extensor tendons by lysis and sectioning of the transverse retinacular ligaments. Distal tenotomy does, however, significantly release the extension contracture of the distal joint, improving flexion and finger function (Dolphin 1965).

Burn boutonnière

The extensor tendons are at risk from direct damage by heat, secondary ischaemia from compression beneath eschar and thinning due to pressure from the underlying proximal phalangeal head of the flexed joint (Maisels 1965). Prophylactic splinting of the metacarpophalangeal joints in flexion and the interphalangeal joints in extension, with skeletal traction pins if necessary, avoided the development of a single boutonnière deformity in 200 children with hand burns (Larson et al 1970). Treatment of the established deformity is delicate. Resurfacing with vascularized flaps has been discussed (Russell et al 1981). McCormack (1971) required 30° of passive motion of the proximal interphalangeal joint, implying a relative lack of intra-articular adhesions, as a prerequisite for considering reconstruction of the burned boutonnière deformity. The mobile deformity may be reconstructed with free tendon grafts as described by Fowler (Boyes 1970), using small axial incisions remote from the precarious dorsal skin (Larson et al 1970). Stiff deformities are best treated by arthrodesis of either the proximal or distal interphalangeal joint, or both (Maisels 1965, Larson et al 1970, Elliott 1971, McCormack 1971).

Extensor tenodesis

Scar blockage of the extensor tendons limits active and passive motion of the extensor tendons over the proximal phalanx, and can mimic intrinsic tightness by restraint of the dorsal apparatus more proximally (Rosenthal 1978). Maximum improvement with preoperative therapy and splinting is assumed (Fig. 6.6). Joint assessment by examination and X-rays precedes surgery. Surgery is

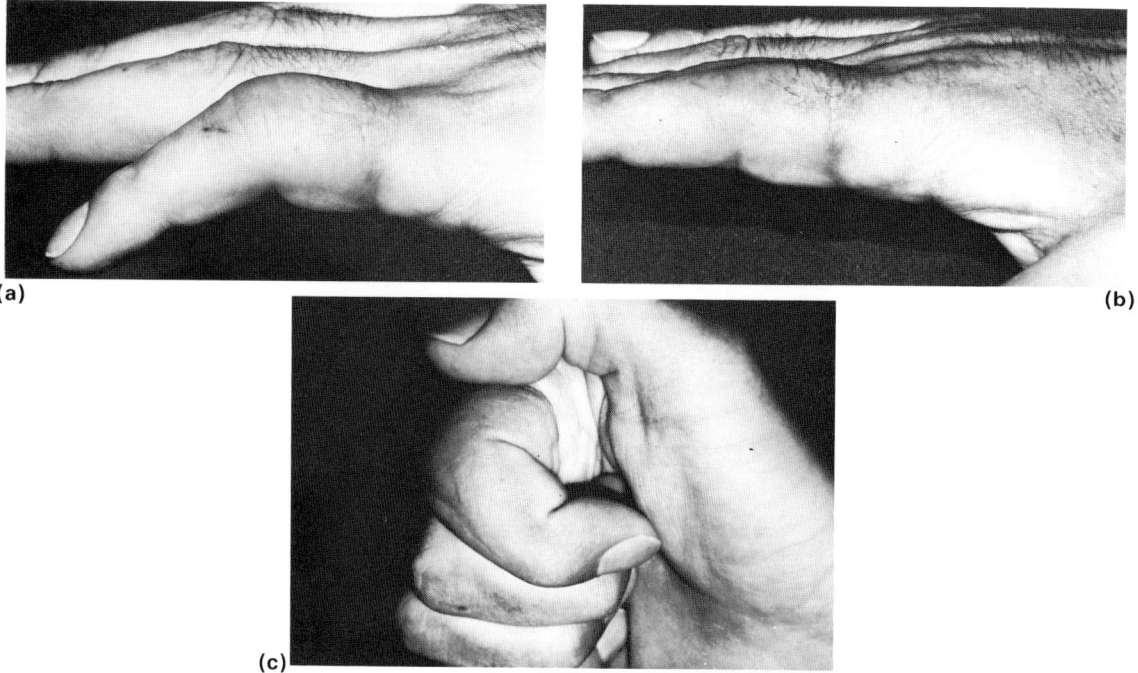

Fig. 6.8 Extensor tenodesis 8 months after laceration of extensor tendons with an open fracture of the proximal phalanx. (**a**) Preoperative active extension. Passive extension was complete. (**b**) Active extension 5 weeks after tendolysis. (**c**) Active flexion which equalled the passive potential recorded at surgery.

performed under block at the metacarpal neck level. Tendolysis implies release of all restraining adhesions, plus unyielding retinacular ligaments, and restores passive descent of the lateral bands with proximal interphalangeal joint flexion (Fig. 6.8). Persistence of a tenodesis effect following an adequate lysis infers structural alteration of the extrinsic tendon. The extrinsic tendon may then be lengthened with a serial tenotomy (Kilgore et al 1975), a segmental resection (Littler 1964), or an insertional reattachment. Kilgore et al released the distal fibres of the radial sagittal bands—clearing migration of the sagittal bands over the radial tubercle of the metacarpal head—if serial tenotomy did not relieve the extensor-plus tenodesis. The distal fibres of the ulnar sagittal band were then released if tightness persisted. Littler segmentally resected the scarred extrinsic tendon, preserving the intrinsic tendons and dorsal retinacular ligaments for extension of the interphalangeal joints. A third option is reattachment of the surgically lengthened central tendon more proximally on the middle phalanx, effecting a lengthening tenorrhaphy. This releases the proximal restraint of the scarred extrinsic tendon and preserves both extrinsic and intrinsic tendons.

REFERENCES

Aiche A, Barsky A J, Weine D L 1970 Prevention of boutonnière deformity. Plastic and Reconstructive Surgery 46:164–167

Bingham D L C, Jack E A 1937 'Buttonholed' extensor expansion. British Medical Journal 2:701–702

Boyes J H 1970 Bunnell's surgery of the hand, 5th edn. J B Lippincott, Philadelphia p 439–442, 475–477

Boyes J H 1971 Boutonnière deformity (discussion) In: Cramer L M, Chase R A (eds) Symposium on the hand, vol. 3. C V Mosby, St Louis p 56

Burkhalter W E, Carneiro R S 1979 Correction of the attritional boutonnière deformity in high ulnar nerve paralysis. Journal of Bone and Joint Surgery 61A:131–134

Burton R I 1982 Extensor tendons—late reconstruction. In: Green D P (ed) Operative hand surgery. Churchill Livingstone, New York Ch. 44, p 1480–1482, 1489–1499

Carducci A T 1981 Potential boutonnière deformity. Its recognition and treatment. Orthopaedic Review 10:121–123

Curtis R M, Reid R L, Provost J M 1983 A staged technique for the repair of the traumatic boutonnière deformity. Journal of Hand Surgery 8:167–171

Dolphin J A 1965 Extensor tenotomy for chronic boutonnière deformity of the finger. Journal of Bone and Joint Surgery 47A:161–164

Doyle J R 1982 Extensor tendons—acute injuries. In: Green D P (ed) Operative hand surgery. Churchill Livingstone, New York. Ch 43, p 1449–1454

Elliott R A 1970 Injuries to the extensor mechanism of the hand. Orthopedic Clinics of North America 1:335–354

Elliott R A 1971 Boutonnière deformity. In: Cramer L M, Chase R A (eds) Symposium on the hand, vol 3. C V Mosby, St Louis p 42–54, 56

Flatt A E 1983 Care of the arthritic hand, 4th edn. C V Mosby, St Louis p 146–147

Fowler S B 1949 Extensor apparatus of the digits. Journal of Bone and Joint Surgery 31B:477

Gama C 1979 Results of the Matev operation for correction of boutonnière deformity. Plastic and Reconstructive Surgery 64:319–324

Garroway R Y, Hurst L C, Leppard J, Dick H M 1984 Complex dislocations of the proximal interphalangeal joint. Orthopaedic Review 13:21–28

Harris C, Rutledge G L Jr 1972 The functional anatomy of the extensor mechanism of the finger. Journal of Bone and Joint Surgery 54A:713–726

Hellmann K (1964) Die Wiederherstellung der Strecksehnen im Berich der Fingermittelgelenke. Langenbeck's Archiv für Klinische Chirurgie 309:36–38

Joshi B B 1982 A salvage procedure in the treatment of the boutonnière deformity caused by contact burn and friction injury. The Hand 14:33–37

Kaplan E 1959 Anatomy, injuries and treatment of the extensor apparatus. Clinical Orthopaedics 13:24–41

Kilgore E S, Graham W P, Newmeyer W L, Brown L G 1975 The extensor plus finger. The Hand 7:159–165

Larson D L, Wofford B H, Evans E B, Lewis S R 1970 Repair of the boutonnière deformity of the burned hand. Journal of Trauma 10:481–487

Lee B S 1982 Pseudo-boutonnière deformity, its pathogenesis and treatment. Orthopaedic Review 11:81–86

Littler J W 1964 Principles of reconstructive surgery of the hand. In: Converse J M (ed) Reconstructive Plastic Surgery. W B Saunders, Philadelphia p 1624–1631

Littler J W 1977 The digital extensor-flexor system. In: Converse J M (ed) Reconstructive Plastic Surgery. Vol 6 2nd edn. W B Saunders, Philadelphia. Ch 75, p 3166–3175

Littler J W, Eaton R G 1967 Redistribution of forces in the correction of the boutonnière deformity. Journal of Bone and Joint Surgery 49A:1267–1274

McCormack R M 1971 Principles of treatment and reconstruction of the burned hand and finger. In: Cramer L M, Chase R A (eds) Symposium on the hand, vol 3. C V Mosby, St Louis Ch 8, p 66–72

McCue F C, Honner R, Johnson M C, Gieck J H 1970 Athletic injuries of the proximal interphalangeal joint requiring surgical treatment. Journal of Bone and Joint Surgery 52A:937–955

McCue F C, Honner R, Gieck J H, Andrews J, Makala M 1975 A pseudo-boutonnière deformity. The Hand 7:166–170

McFarlane R M, Hampole M K 1973 Treatment of extensor injuries of the hand. Canadian Journal of Surgery 16:366–375

Maisels D O 1965 The middle slip or boutonnière deformity in burned hands. British Journal of Plastic Surgery 18:117–129

Matev I 1964 Transposition of the lateral slips of the aponeurosis in treatment of longstanding 'boutonnière deformity' of the fingers. British Journal of Plastic Surgery 17:281–286

Matev I 1969 The boutonnière deformity. The Hand 1:90–95

Micks J E, Hager D 1973 Role of the controversial parts of the extensor of the finger. Journal of Bone and Joint Surgery 55A:884

Micks J E, Reswick J B 1981 Confirmation of differential loading of lateral and central fibers of the extensor tendon. Journal of Hand Surgery 6:462–467

Milford L 1971 The hand. C V Mosby, St Louis, p 105

Neviaser R J, Wilson J N 1972 Interposition of the extensor tendon resulting in persistent subluxation of the proximal interphalangeal joint. Clinical Orthopaedics 83:118–120

Nichols H M 1951 Repair of extensor tendon insertions in the fingers. Journal of Bone and Joint Surgery 33A:836–841

Pardini A G, Costa R D, Morais M S 1979 Surgical repair of the boutonnière deformity of the fingers. The Hand 11:87–92

Rosenthal E A 1978 Tenolysis. AAOS Sound Slide program no. 719

Rosenthal E A 1984 The extensor tendons. In: Hunter J M, Schneider L H, Mackin E J, Callahan A D (eds) Rehabilitation of the hand, 2nd edn. C V Mosby, St Louis Ch 29, p 324–352

Russell R C, Van Beek A L, Wavak P, Zook E G 1981 Alternative hand flaps for amputations and digital defects. Journal of Hand Surgery 6:399–405

Salvi V 1969 Technique for the buttonhole deformity. The Hand 1:96–97

Schultz R J, Furlong J, Storace A 1981 Detailed anatomy of the extensor mechanism at the proximal aspect of the finger. Journal of Hand Surgery 6:493–498

Snow J W 1973 Use of a retrograde tendon flap in repairing a severed extensor tendon in the PIP joint area. Plastic and Reconstructive Surgery 51:555–558

Snow J W 1976 A method for the reconstruction of the central slip of the extensor tendon of a finger. Plastic and Reconstructive Surgery 57:455–459

Snow J W 1984 Personal communication

Souter W A 1967 The boutonnière deformity. A review of 101 patients with division of the central slip of the extensor expansion of the fingers. Journal of Bone and Joint Surgery 49B:710–721

Souter W A 1974 The problem of boutonnière deformity. Clinical Orthopaedics 104:116–133

Spinner M, Choi B Y 1970 Anterior dislocation of the proximal interphalangeal joint, a cause of rupture of the central slip of the extensor mechanism. Journal of Bone and Joint Surgery 52A:1329–1336

Stack H G 1971 Buttonhole deformity. The Hand 3:152–154

Stern P J 1981 Stener lesion after lateral dislocation of the proximal interphalangeal joint—indication for open reduction. Journal of Hand Surgery 6:602–604

Stewart I M 1962 Boutonnière finger. Clinical Orthopaedics 23:220–222

Suzuki K 1973 Reconstruction of post-traumatic boutonnière deformity. The Hand 5:145–148

Tubiana R 1968 Surgical repair of the extensor apparatus of the finger. Surgical Clinics of North America 48:1015–1031

Van Der Meulen J C 1972 The treatment of prolapse and collapse of the proximal interphalangeal joint. The Hand 4:154–162

Weeks P M 1967 The chronic boutonnière deformity. A method of repair. Plastic and Reconstructive Surgery 40:248–251

Wray R C, Young V L, Holtmann B 1984 Proximal interphalangeal joint sprains. Plastic and Reconstructive Surgery 74:101–107

Zancolli E A 1979 Structural and dynamic basis of hand surgery, 2nd edn. J B Lippincott, Philadelphia pp 23–37, 46–59, 79–92

R. Honner

7. Acute and chronic flexor and extensor mechanism injuries at the distal joint

ACUTE FLEXOR TENDON INJURIES AT THE DISTAL JOINT

Flexor tendon injuries associated with open wounds

Lacerations at the anterior aspect of the distal interphalangeal joint often divide the flexor tendon. In simple wounds, the soft tissue attachments and vincula often prevent the profundus tendon from retracting far and, under these circumstances, if the wound is satisfactory, a direct repair of the tendon can be carried out. In cooperative patients, a Kessler (1973) type of suture is used, using 5/0 monofilament suture material, with a 6/0 monofilament suture running circumferentially around the tendon. The early passive movement programme with elastic band traction popularized by Kleinert et al (1973) and Lister et al (1977) has given acceptable results. In less satisfactory circumstances, where it is considered that the patient may not be able to cooperate with this type of early passive movement, good results can still be obtained by keeping the digit completely still for 3 weeks with a dorsal plaster cast and then starting gentle active motion with a therapist.

Where the injury is more severe, and particularly when the injury is close to the insertion of the flexor tendon, an advancement of the cut end of the tendon is a more satisfactory technique than an attempt at direct suture. A 4/0 monofilament suture is used to make an interweaving suture in the distal end of the tendon. This suture is passed through a hole drilled into the base of the distal phalanx and tied over a button on the nail, embedding the cut end of the tendon into the shaft of the distal phalanx (Figs. 7.1, 7.2 and 7.3). This suture is removed 6 weeks later by simply cutting one side of the stitch and removing the stitch and button.

Skilled postoperative therapy is required; in addition to the progressive mobilization and strengthening of the repaired flexor digitorum profundus, early isolation and control of the flexor superficialis movement and power, with avoidance of proximal interphalangeal joint contracture, is also important.

Closed ruptures of the tendon

Occasionally closed rupture of the flexor profundus tendon can occur at its distal attachment. Before

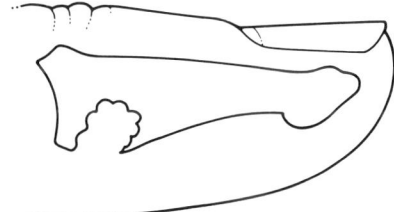

Fig. 7.1 Lateral diagram of the distal phalanx showing hole fashioned by narrow chisels and gauges.

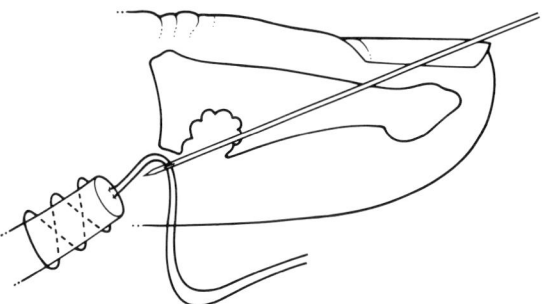

Fig. 7.2 An interweaving suture in tendon end in eye of needle passed through distal phalanx and distal portion of nail with a power drill.

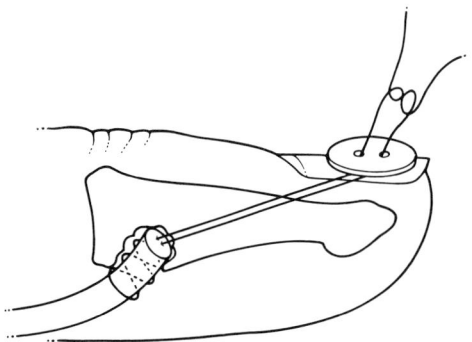

Fig. 7.3 The tendon suture is pulled through the distal phalanx by the needle and tied over a button, ensuring the tendon end passes into the distal phalanx.

considering the management of these injuries, the acute condition is defined as presenting within the first 2 weeks from injury, as in these cases it is often possible to carry out a direct repair of the damaged tendon.

These injuries commonly occur in otherwise healthy young people often engaged in vigorous sport (Honner 1975, Lunn & Lamb 1984). They may occur in any age group with forceful extension of the flexing digit. It occurs much more commonly in the ring finger. This may be for anatomical reasons, relating to the size of the ring finger ray (Bynum et al 1985), the tethering of the extensor tendon system, or anatomical arrangements in the flexor profundus muscle and the lumbricals and the distal attachment of the tendon (Carroll & Match 1970, Fahrer 1981, Lunn & Lamb 1984). The management selected for this injury depends on the age of the lesion at presentation, the functional needs of the patient for that particular finger, the general health and cooperation of the patient, and the degree of retraction of the avulsed tendon. Some patients may not have sufficient functional impairment to warrant reconstructive surgery. The finger with a ruptured profundus and intact superficialis has about 80% of normal function. Any treatment selected should have little chance of interfering with the intact superficialis function in that digit.

These acute injuries of the flexor tendon should all have radiographic examination; sometimes, small fragments of bone are avulsed (Leddy & Packer 1977), rarely, large fragments disrupting the distal joint are found (Smith 1981), and there have been reports of pathological avulsion fractures (Ogunro 1983, Fromison & Shall 1984). Occasionally, a fracture here *does not* mean avulsion of the tendon but instead a volar plate injury. This, of course, is not an operative lesion and can be distinguished by careful evaluation (Bowers & Fajenbaum 1979).

Small avulsion fractures help to localize the end of the ruptured tendon, but do not alter the reconstruction required. The larger fragments and pathological lesions require their own specific treatment as well as tendon reconstruction. The patient presents with a history of injury in the previous few days, there is active control and good power in flexion of the proximal interphalangeal joint, but no active movement at the distal joint of the damaged digit. This is most apparent when the patient attempts to make a fist. In some patients, the ruptured end of the profundus tendon can be palpated just anterior to the proximal phalanx, indicating that it has not retracted proximally through the superficialis decussation, and therefore can be easier to advance and repair. Occasionally, the tendon may be trapped *in* the decussation and interfere with superficialis function. Exploration through a zig-zag anterior incision is recommended. The limiting factor to repair is collapse and fibrosis affecting the A-4 pulley (Doyle & Blythe 1975). Depending on factors such as the degree of local trauma and the age of the patient, it is usually possible to dilate the distal pulley and advance a ruptured profundus tendon within the first 2 weeks after injury. If the profundus tendon cannot be palpated anterior to the proximal interphalangeal joint, it can generally be felt as a tender mass, often associated with some deep bruising, in the palm. This represents a more serious injury to the tendon sheath system. Before exploration, the various options must be discussed with the patient as this degree of injury causes bleeding throughout the whole of the sheath. The pulleys (A-1 and A-2) over the proximal phalanx tend to contract more firmly and more quickly than the distal pulley (A-4). In the first week after injury, it is usually possible to advance the profundus tendon through the proximal portion of the sheath, through or around the decussation of the superficialis and through the A-4 pulley. This is variable and needs to be approached with caution, as it is possible to create adhesions within the proximal sheath destroying the superficialis function. If it is not possible to advance the ruptured profundus tendon, then the surgeon will have to make a decision about alternative techniques: simple excision of the profundus, staged reconstruction, or fusion of the distal joint, which will be discussed in the management of the chronic lesions.

CHRONIC FLEXOR TENDON INJURIES AT THE DISTAL JOINT

When the opportunity for early management of these injuries is missed, each patient requires careful assessment with treatment selected on the basis of the functional requirement for that digit and the ability demonstrated by the patient to cooperate in a postoperative exercise programme.

A review of 44 successive cases (Honner 1975) showed that approximately one-third of the patients needed no surgical reconstruction, one-third were helped by an arthrodesis of the distal joint of the finger and one-third by flexor tendon grafting through an intact superficialis. Before any surgery is contemplated, full passive motion of the distal joint and normal proximal interphalangeal joint function have to be established, and the various options and requirements discussed with the patient.

Arthrodesis of the distal joint in 20–30° of flexion is useful for some patients. It improves the stability of grip and overcomes the tendency to hyperextension at the distal joint due to the unopposed action of the extensor system. When arthrodesis of the distal joint is selected, removal of the ruptured profundus tendon from the palm avoids the tenderness that develops in the palm with heavy work. This is due to the presence of the physical mass of the ruptured tendon and the surrounding synovial tissue proliferation. Arthrodesis has been found more satisfactory than tenodesis to improve the stability at the distal joint. The method recommended has been described by Anderson (1970), a modification of Robertson (1964), and more recently described by Lister (1978), and Hoge & Jensen (1982). It requires a dorsal H-shaped incision, cutting directly down to bone through tendon. The joint articular cartilage is excised to leave flat opposing surfaces. The position of 20–30° of flexion is recommended. Fixation is by a central Kirschner wire passed longitudinally through the distal phalanx and then retrograde into the middle phalanx, reinforced with a horizontal wire cerclage suture through transverse drill holes in the adjacent phalanges. This secure fixation allows early motion at the proximal interphalangeal joint. (Figs. 7.4, 7.5 and 7.6).

There is a small number of patients who present late where there is a definite functional need for active flexion at the distal joint. One-stage tendon grafts through the intact superficialis have been utilized by some surgeons. Since Pulvertaft's initial report in 1960, others have reported large series, all with some failures (Jaffe & Weckesser 1967, Goldner & Coonrad 1969, Stark et al 1977, McClinton et al 1982), although the recent report by Lunn & Lamb (1984) described good results and no failures in nine cases.

Because these patients have some 80% of normal function, the surgical technique selected must have the least possible chance of interfering with the function of the proximal interphalangeal joint. For

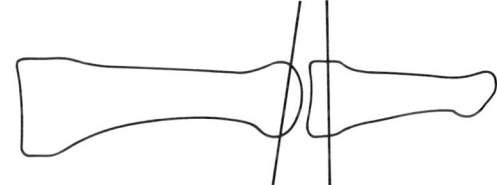

Fig. 7.4 A lateral view of the distal interphalangeal joints showing planes of bone and articular cartilage resection.

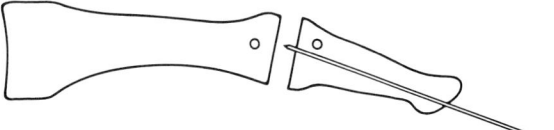

Fig. 7.5 A lateral view showing Kirschner wire in distal phalanx and the two holes transversely in the adjacent bones prepared for the circumferential wire suture.

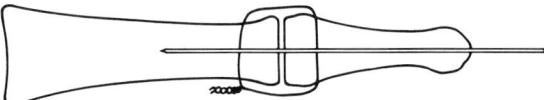

Fig. 7.6 A dorsal view of the distal joint, showing the circumferential wire suture tightened and the Kirschner wire passed across the joint.

this reason the two-stage technique described by Hunter & Salisbury (1971) has been used (Wilson et al 1980) and is the recommended surgical technique. A recent review (Honner 1984) describes 35 successive cases in which this technique was used. There were no problems with return of superficialis function or proximal interphalangeal joint contractures and the average range of motion at the distal joint was 41°. In the first stage, exploration of the finger through an anterior zig-zag incision is performed, with a separate transverse incision in the palm used to remove the profundus tendon. A silastic tendon spacer is then inserted and attached distally at the base of the distal phalanx, passing through or around the superficialis decussation through the proximal flexor sheath, the palm, and into the distal forearm, where the proximal end lies free in the space between the flexor superficialis and the flexor profundus. Postoperatively, active exercises are commenced to regain full proximal interphalangeal joint function and careful passive mobilization of the distal joint is performed.

Some 2 months later, when full function has been returned to the joints, the second stage is performed. The ends of the silastic tendon are exposed through small incisions and a plantaris tendon graft from the leg is used to replace the silastic tendon. This is fixed distally to the distal phalanx and sutured to the profundus tendon mass in the distal forearm by an interweaving suture. The forearm, wrist and hand are immobilized in flexion for 3 weeks. During this time, active and passive motion of the proximal interphalangeal joint can be achieved and, 3 weeks postoperatively, the active movement at the distal interphalangeal joint is commenced.

ACUTE EXTENSOR TENDON INJURIES AT THE DISTAL JOINT

Open lacerations

Frequently, patients present with a transverse laceration at or just proximal to the distal joint, with complete division of the extensor tendon, the digit usually falling into some 50° of flexion at the distal joint. This may be accompanied by a hyperextension deformity at the proximal interphalangeal joint. Where the general condition of the patient permits, the best treatment is exploration of the wound and repair of the extensor tendon as soon as is practicably possible. In patients where radiographic examination shows no underlying bone damage, simple wound cleansing and exploration establishes the diagnosis. The free ends of the extensor tendon can usually be approximated with two or three fine horizontal mattress sutures. The repair of this thin tendon is protected with a Kirschner wire passed longitudinally from the distal phalanx across the distal joint into the middle phalanx, holding the joint in slight hyperextension. The wire is left protruding from the pulp of the distal phalanx.

Postoperative comfort requires support of the injured finger for 5 days, then active exercises at the proximal interphalangeal joint are begun, protecting the wound with a small dressing. Three weeks after the initial surgery, the Kirschner wire can be removed and the distal joint protected with a small metal splint on the volar surface, holding the joint in slight hyperextension. Slight flexion and active extension at the distal joint can be gradually commenced 4 weeks after the operation. Some protective splinting will be needed for a total of 6–8 weeks after the surgery, depending on the progress of joint mobilization. Open wounds with fractures require appropriate internal fixation of the fragments, which may or may not have the extensor tendon attached to them. The fractures may be associated with significant disruption of the joint articular surfaces. Intraosseous wiring or sutures are used to restore the bony attachment of the extensor tendon and reconstitute the articular surface, and then a longitudinal Kirschner wire is passed across the reconstituted joint, to hold the distal joint in extension for 4 weeks after the reparative surgery (see Ch. 5).

Four weeks after the injury, the Kirschner wire is removed and the patient commences a gentle flexion and extension programme, supporting the distal joint in slight hyperextension with a volar metal splint when not exercising. The splint may be discontinued at 8 weeks.

Closed injuries

Closed rupture of the extensor tendon at the distal joint is a common injury in the middle-aged patient, can occur with minimal trauma, and is usually called a mallet finger. These closed injuries may be classified according to the requirements for treatment and their different prognoses.

Type I. A partial disruption of the extensor tendon at the distal joint due to attrition in the elderly. There is an extensor lag of 20–30°, with normal X-rays.

Type II. A complete avulsion of the extensor mechanism, in which the extensor lag is between 30 and 60°. Full passive flexion is present and there is often significant redness and swelling over the dorsum of the joint. The X-rays are normal.

Type III. A small avulsion fracture represents avulsion of the attachment of the extensor tendon, similar in clinical appearance to type II.

Type IV. Often occurring in the younger age group, this type results from a direct blow on the end of the finger, breaking off a significant portion of the articular surface at the base of the distal phalanx. The articular fragment that has the extensor tendon attached to it displaces dorsally and is sometimes quite rotated.

Type V. This is similar to type IV, often with a larger dorsal fragment. On the lateral X-ray the distal phalanx is seen to be subluxed volarward in relation to the alignment of the middle phalanx.

Management of the closed extensor tendon injuries

Type I is a partial rupture of the extensor and will heal satisfactorily if the distal joint is held in slight hyperextension with a simple volar metal splint (Fig. 7.7) for a period of 4 weeks.

Type II represents complete avulsion of the extensor tendon system, but the joint does not fall into 90° of flexion presumably because the oblique ligaments at the side of the extensor tendon (Landsmeer 1949, Stack 1969) support some

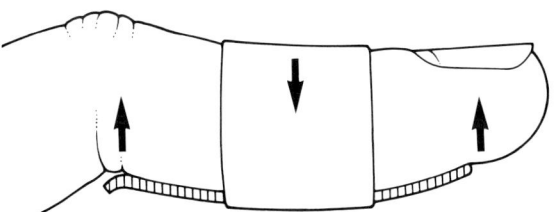

Fig. 7.7 A lateral view of the curved volar metal splint with single central adhesive strapping holding the distal joint in 20–30° hyperextension.

extension. The oblique retinacular ligaments do not appear to be present in all human fingers (Shrewsbury & Johnson 1977) and it would appear that some of the support preventing a severe flexion deformity in these patients is due to a tightness of the dorsal part of the collateral ligaments at the distal interphalangeal joint (Shrewsbury & Johnson 1980). The clinical management of type II and type III is the same. Good results have been achieved with prolonged splinting (Robb 1959, Hallberg & Lindholm 1960, Stark et al 1962, Abouna & Brown 1968, Auchincloss 1982, Moss & Steingold 1983) even when begun at prolonged intervals after injury. Some authors have recommended percutaneous Kirschner wire fixation of the distal joint in hyperextension for types II and III following the suggestions of Pratt (1952), but it seems that this form of internal splinting is best reserved for those patients who are unable to cope with the splinting programme.

The details of the splinting programme and the careful supervision of progress are essential to achieving a good result in this condition. A simple volar metal splint is recommended, shaped so that it applies a two-point pressure over the volar surface of the digit, with a single piece of elastic strapping over the dorsum of the distal interphalangeal joint, so that a mild three-point pressure system is instituted, holding the joint in some extension (see Fig. 7.7). In the first week some patients with marked swelling and tenderness at the distal joint find this too uncomfortable. For the first week they should be treated simply with a longer volar metal splint holding both interphalangeal joints in extension, until the local symptoms settle down and the distal joint splint can be applied.

The duration of splinting is important. The distal joint needs to be held in hyperextension for at *least* 4 weeks. If there is no lag present at that stage, then cautious flexion of some 30° can be allowed, with active extension and hyperextension being regularly exercised. In this interval, when the patient is not exercising, the volar supporting splint should be worn for a further 4 weeks, so that some form of splinting, particularly at night, continues for at least 8 weeks. Most patients regain good flexion and retain active extension 8 weeks after injury, but a few need a further period of exercise and protective splinting. It helps to emphasize that full active *flexion* of the joint is to be avoided for several months.

The management of type III injuries has been varied, but the majority of reports suggest that careful conservative treatment gives acceptable results. This can also be achieved by surgical repair, but the complication rates in surgical treatment are higher (Stark et al 1962, Auchincloss 1982, Moss & Steingold 1983, Wehbé & Schneider 1984). It would seem that open reduction of the type IV fracture should be reserved for the occasional case in the young person with good skin cover and a fragment one-third or larger of the articular surface, which has been significantly displaced and does not reduce with an attempt at splintage.

Type V injuries most often occur in the younger patient, usually with high velocity. Because the results of conservative treatment are poor (significant stiffness and discomfort) open reduction of the volar subluxation is recommended. The large fragment can be replaced and held in position with intraosseous wiring or sutures, and then a separate Kirschner wire is passed to hold the joint in hyperextension for some 4 weeks before its removal and the commencement of a careful splinting and exercise programme (Hamas et al 1978).

CHRONIC EXTENSOR TENDON INJURIES AT THE DISTAL JOINT

It is common for the elderly patient with type I and II injuries to present late, 3–6 weeks after the initial injury. Even at this late stage, a significant improvement in the position of the finger and the local symptoms due to the flexed distal joint can be achieved by a prolonged splinting programme. This usually consists of some 6 weeks' constant extension splinting—maintaining proximal interphalangeal joint function. This is followed by a further period of splinting of the distal joint, with cautious exercise. In the few patients with normal X-rays, who have disabling symptoms from failure of splinting programmes, surgical treatment may be considered. Stack (1969) has described the use of a plication stitch to shorten the extensor tendon in these patients. Iselin et al (1977) have described the technique of tenodermadesis, which appears to be more useful in the younger age group, and this has been confirmed by Kon & Bloem (1982). This technique can be carried out under local anaesthesia. Skin, tendon scar and sometimes part of the dorsal capsule are resected from the distal interphalangeal joint and the defect closed with interrupted sutures. The repair is protected with volar splinting for some 5 weeks and a progressive exercise programme, with intermittent splinting. Other procedures which are occasionally indicated are Fowler's central slip release (Bowers & Hurst 1978) and, occasionally, in the thick labouring hand with disabling symptoms due to the fixed flexion contracture at the distal joint, an arthrodesis of the distal joint in the position best suited to the patient's functional needs is worthwhile. The compression arthrodesis technique described in the section on avulsion of the flexor tendon at the distal joint is recommended (Anderson 1970).

REFERENCES

Abouna J M, Brown H 1968 The treatment of mallet finger. The results of 148 consecutive cases and a review of the literature. British Journal of Surgery 55:653–667

Anderson G R 1970 Arthrodesis of the distal interphalangeal joints, proceedings. Journal of Bone and Joint Surgery 52B:800

Auchincloss J M 1982 Mallet finger injuries; a prospective controlled trial of internal and external splintage. The Hand 14:168–173

Bowers W H, Fajgenbaum D M 1979 Closed rupture of the volar plate of the distal interphalangeal joint. Journal of Bone and Joint Surgery:146

Bowers W H, Hurst L C 1978 Chronic mallet finger; the use of Fowler's central slip release. Journal of Hand Surgery 3:373–376

Bynum D K, Gilbert J A, Wainer R A 1985 Avulsion of the flexor digitorum: an anatomic and biomechanical note. Journal of Hand Surgery 10A:433

Carroll R E, Match R M 1970 Avulsion of the flexor profundus tendon insertion. Journal of Trauma 10:1109–1118

Doyle J R, Blythe W F 1975 The finger flexor tendon sheath and pulleys. AAOS Symposium on Tendon Surgery in the Hand. C V Mosby Company, St. Louis, p 81–87

Fahrer M 1981 Interdependent and dependent actions of the fingers. In: Tubiana R (ed) The Hand, W B Saunders Company, Philadelphia, ch 40, p 402

Fromison A I, Shall L 1984 Flexor digitorum profundus avulsion through enchondroma. Journal of Hand Surgery 9B:343–344

Goldner J L, Coonrad R W 1969 Tendon grafting of the flexor

profundus in the presence of a completely or partially intact flexor sublimis. Journal of Bone and Joint Surgery 51A: 527–532

Hallberg D, Lindholm A 1960 Subcutaneous rupture of the extensor tendon of the distal phalanx of the finger, 'mallet finger'. Brief review of the literature and report on 127 cases treated conservatively. Acta Chirugica Scandinavica 119: 260–267

Hamas R S, Horrell E D, Pierret G P 1978 The treatment of mallet finger due to intra-articular fracture of the distal phalanx. Journal of Hand Surgery 3: 361–363

Hoge J, Jensen P Ø 1982 Compression arthrodesis of finger joints using Kirschner wires and cerclage. The Hand 14: 149–152

Honner R 1975 The late management of the isolated lesion of the flexor digitorum profundus. The Hand 7: 171–174

Honner R 1984 Treatment for isolated profundus injuries. Symposium on tendon surgery in the hand: another decade, March 1984. C V Mosby Company, St Louis (in press)

Hunter J M, Salisbury R E 1871 Flexor tendon reconstruction in severely damaged hands; a two-stage procedure using a silicone decron reinforced gliding prosthesis prior to tendon grafting. Journal of Bone and Joint Surgery 53A: 829–858

Iselin F, Levame J, Godoy J 1977 A simplified technique for treating maller fingers: tenodermadesis. Journal of Hand Surgery 5: 214–216

Jaffe S, Weckesser E 1967 Profundus tendon grafting with the sublimis intact. Journal of Bone and Joint Surgery 49A: 1298–1308

Kessler I 1973 The grasping technique for tendon repair. The Hand 5: 253–255

Kleinert H E, Kutz J E, Atasoy E, Stormo A 1973 Primary repair of flexor tendons. Orthopedic Clinics of North America 4: 865–876

Kon M, Bloem J J A M 1982 Treatment of mallet fingers by tenodermadesis. The Hand 14: 174–176

Landsmeer J M F 1949 The anatomy of the dorsal aponeurosis of the human finger and its functional significance. Anatomical Record 104: 31

Leddy J P, Packer J W 1977 Avulsion of the profundus tendon insertion in athletes. Journal of Hand Surgery 2: 66–69

Lister G 1978 Intraosseous wiring of the digital skeleton. Journal of Hand Surgery 3: 427–435

Lister G D, Kleinert H E, Kutz J E, Atasoy E 1977 Primary flexor tendon repair followed by immediate controlled mobilization. Journal of Hand Surgery 2: 441–451

Lunn P G, Lamb D W 1984 'Rugby finger' avulsion of profundus of ring finger. Journal of Hand Surgery 9: 69–71

McClinton M A, Curtis R M, Shaw Wilgis E F 1982 One hundred tendon grafts for isolated flexor digitorum profundus injury. Journal of Hand Surgery 7: 224–229

Moss J G, Steingold R F 1983 The long-term results of mallet finger injury; a retrospective study of one hundred cases. The Hand 15: 151–154

Ogunro O 1983 Avulsion of flexor profundus secondary to enchondroma of the distal phalanx. Journal of Hand Surgery 8: 315–316

Pratt D R 1952 Internal splint for closed and open treatment of injuries of the extensor tendon at the distal joint of the finger. Journal of Bone and Joint Surgery 34A: 785–788

Pulvertaft R G 1960 The treatment of profundus division by free tendon graft. Journal of Bone and Joint Surgery 42A: 1363–1371

Robb W A T 1959 The results of treatment of mallet finger. Journal of Bone and Joint Surgery 41B: 546–549

Robertson D C 1964 The fusion of interphalangeal joints. Canadian Journal of Surgery 7: 433–437

Shrewsbury M M, Johnson R K 1977 A systematic study of the oblique retinacular ligament of the human finger: its structure and function. Journal of Hand Surgery 2: 194–199

Shrewsbury M M, Johnson R K 1980 Ligaments of the distal interphalangeal joint and the mallet position. Journal of Hand Surgery 5: 214–216

Smith J H 1981 Avulsion of a profundus tendon with simultaneous intra-articular fracture of the distal phalanx. Journal of Hand Surgery 6: 600–601

Stack H G 1969 Mallet finger. The Hand 1: 83–89

Stark H H, Boyes J H, Wilson J N 1962 Mallet finger. Journal of Bone and Joint Surgery 44A: 1061–1068

Stark H H, Zemel N P, Boyes J H, Ashworth C R 1977 Flexor tendon grafting through intact superficialis tendons. Journal of Hand Surgery 2: 456–461

Wehbé M A, Schneider L H 1984 Mallet Fractures. Journal of Bone and Joint Surgery 66A: 658–669

Wilson R L, Carter M S, Haldeman V A, Lovett W L 1980 Flexor profundus injuries treated with delayed two-stage tendon grafting. Journal of Hand Surgery 5: 74–78

SECTION 3

Arthritis and Arthrosis: Reconstruction

J. E. Imbriglia

Rheumatoid and related arthritides of the interphalangeal joints

RHEUMATOID ARTHRITIS

Introduction

In managing rheumatoid conditions of the proximal interphalangeal (PIP) joint, the physician must first assess the entire hand, wrist and forearm. Pathology at the metacarpophalangeal (MCP) joint and the distal interphalangeal (DIP) joint will have major influences on the PIP joint. Tendon imbalance and ruptures proximal or distal to the PIP joint will alter the position and motion of the joint. For these reasons, reconstruction of the PIP cannot be an isolated event.

The function of the PIP joint is very important in determining the prognosis of future hand function. Normally, the PIP joint contributes 110° to a total digital arc of motion of 270°. This motion allows a finger with a fusion of the DIP joint to have nearly normal function. A 110° arc of motion at the PIP joint allows a finger with an MCP silicone replacement joint to be brought into the palm. Ray Curtis has called the PIP joint the 'epicentre' of hand surgery. This is certainly true in rheumatoid arthritis.

Conversely, if the PIP joint is destroyed, reconstructive procedures are relatively inadequate in duplicating PIP function. Arthrodesis may relieve pain and provide stability, but the loss of motion is quite disabling in itself. Current arthroplasty techniques may restore 50% of motion under the best conditions, and as reported by both Beckenbaugh (1977) and Flatt (1983c), stability remains a problem. If the MCP joint requires arthroplasty, then reconstructive efforts to repair the PIP joint are even further compromised. Most patients with joint destruction of both the MCP and PIP joints are best treated by an MCP arthroplasty and PIP arthrodesis, although dual joint replacement can occasionally succeed.

These comments make a critical implication in management of the PIP joint. Prior to articular surface destruction, synovitis and tendon imbalance about the PIP joint results in obvious loss of motion. It is at this stage that soft tissue procedures (e.g. intrinsic release, synovectomy) may restore motion and function, and perhaps more importantly retard the destruction in the joint. Compared to later efforts at both the MCP and DIP joints, soft tissue reconstructive procedures at the PIP joint provide great opportunities for functional gain. Millender et al (Millender & Nalebuff 1975d, Millender et al 1982) have put great effort into both classification and treatment of the disorders of the PIP joint for this reason.

Conclusions

1. PIP joint motion and stability are critical factors in determining a course of treatment in the arthritic hand, and in attempting to give a prognosis for future hand function
2. The treatment of the PIP joint should be undertaken only after careful evaluation of the MCP and DIP joints
3. Arthrodesis and arthroplasty of the PIP joint are salvage procedures. Soft tissue reconstruction prior to joint destruction may offer great gains both in motion and function

Extrinsic factors affecting PIP joint motion

The extrinsic factors affecting PIP motion in rheumatoid arthritis are:

1. Intrinsic tightness secondary to MCP joint involvement
2. Stretching or rupture of the terminal extensor tendon at the DIP joint
3. Flexor tenosynovitis and occasionally tendon rupture
4. Secondary skin contracture, especially in long-standing swan-neck deformities.

These extrinsic factors must be considered prior to performing a procedure directly on the joint. In Helal's (1975) series of 174 stiff proximal interphalangeal joints in rheumatoid arthritis, only three had articular surface destruction which was the main cause of the lost motion. The majority of stiff joints in his series were due to intrinsic imbalance and tightness. Metacarpophalangeal joint ulnar deviation and palmar subluxation often result in intrinsic tightness with loss of both active and passive motion of the PIP joint (Fig. 8.1). Intrinsic tightness can be tested by passively extending and radially deviating the MCP joint. If the PIP joint loses passive flexion then the intrinsic mechanism is tight. Intrinsic tightness may eventually contribute to the formation of a swan-neck deformity (Flatt 1983a). Obviously, it would be an error to attempt correction of the PIP joint without simultaneously correcting the primary problem at the MCP level.

Rupture or attenuation of the terminal extensor tendon over the distal joint may also cause tendon imbalance resulting in a swan-neck deformity. This situation may also occur if synovitis has weakened the palmar plate of the PIP joint resulting in secondary laxity. The treatment of a swan-neck deformity secondary to rupture of the terminal extensor tendon must include correction of deformity of the distal joint.

Flexor tenosynovitis can result in loss of both active and passive motion at the PIP joint. Backhouse et al (1971) reported that nodular tendonitis occurred in 50% of patients with rheumatoid arthritis. A nodule distal to the A-2 pulley may cause the finger to lock in extension; the passive range of motion of the PIP joint thus will be greater than the active. Left untreated, tendon rupture may occur. Nodularity of the flexor tendons in the palm may also cause restriction of active flexion. Wissinger (1971) has described this

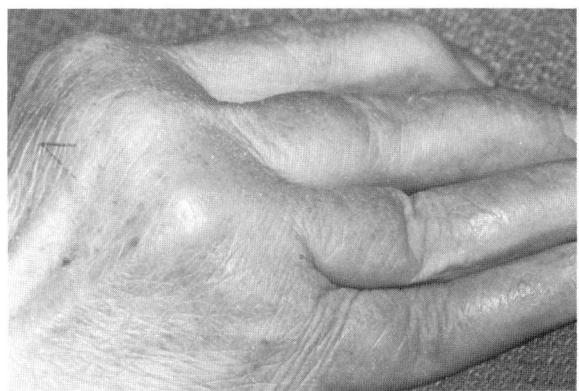

Fig. 8.1 MCP joint ulnar deviation and intrinsic tightness resulting in deformity at the PIP joint. Active and passive flexion is decreased.

as digital flexor lag. Generalized tenosynovitis will cause the finger to swell and the sheer bulk of the tenosynovium interferes with normal passage of the flexor tendons below the pulley system. Active *and* passive motion of the PIP joint will be decreased. In this case, a tenosynovectomy may be necessary to regain motion.

Intrinsic tightness, attenuation of the terminal extensor tendon, and flexor tenosynovitis may all co-exist in a given finger that has lost motion. Each must be corrected in attempts to regain function of the PIP joint.

Pathogenesis of boutonnière and swan-neck deformity

Invasive synovitis is the genesis of the boutonnière lesion. It causes attenuation and destruction of the ligaments, joint capsule, and tendons. Initially, synovitis interferes with motion simply due to the bulk in the joint. If the process continues, the central slip becomes attenuated and the lateral band fibres separate from the central slip. The lateral bands migrate palmar to the mid-axis of the joint and full active extension at the PIP joint is lost. The PIP joint gradually becomes fixed in flexion while the distal joints' flexion is limited. Continued synovitis, and decreased motion contribute to the final destruction of the joint surfaces. The final boutonnière deformity consists of hyperextension of the distal joint, fixed flexion contracture of the PIP joint and secondary hyperextension of the MCP joint (Fig. 8.2).

Swan-neck deformity may be secondary to

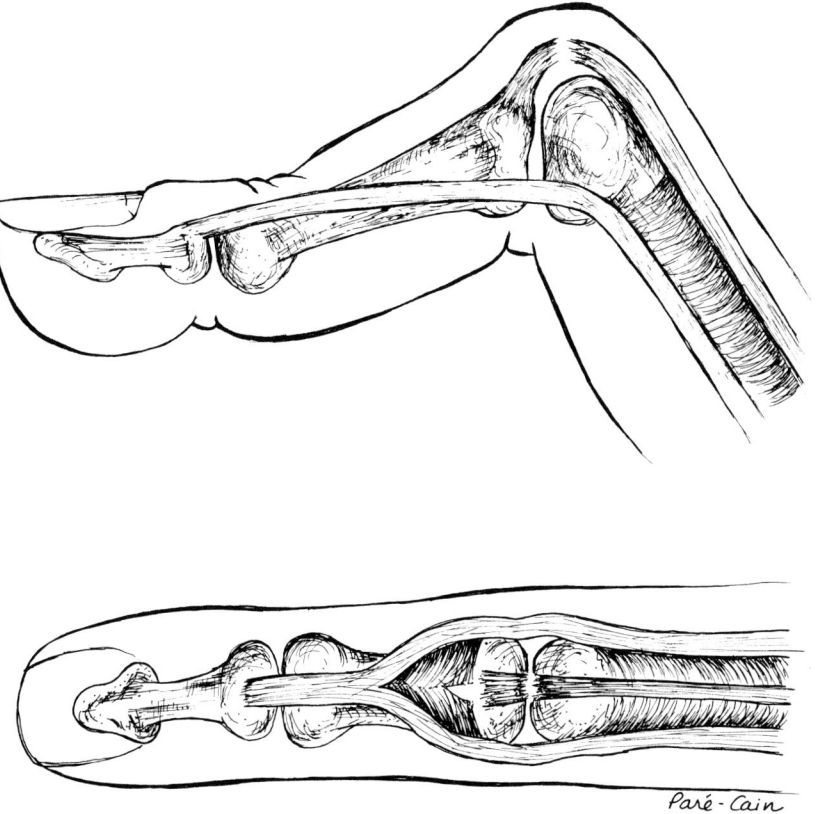

Fig. 8.2 Attenuative rupture of the central slip and palmar migration of the lateral bands resulting in a boutonnière deformity.

tendon imbalance proximal or distal to the PIP joint. Flatt (1983c) states that the usual cause is intrinsic muscle tightness with the head and the neck of the swan formed by secondary flexion of the DIP joint. Millender and Nalebuff (1975) have developed a classification of swan-neck deformities based on the mobility of the PIP joint and the condition of the joint surfaces.

Type I	PIP joint flexible in all positions
Type II	PIP joint flexion limited in certain positions
Type III	limited PIP joint motion in all positions
Type IV	stiff PIP joint with poor X-ray appearance

The cause of the type I deformity may be attenuation of the terminal extensor mechanism over the distal joint with secondary tendon imbalance and extensor overpull at the PIP joint. Primary PIP joint synovitis with stretching of the palmar plate may also be causative (Fig. 8.3).

When the PIP joint has limited flexion in certain positions (type II), the cause of the deformity may be intrinsic tightness. In type II, the amount of flexion at the PIP joint is influenced by the position of the proximal phalanx in relation to the metacarpal. If the PIP joint flexion decreases when the MCP joint is brought into extension and radial deviation, then the tight ulnar intrinsics are contributing to the deformity.

It is often a combination of these three problems (terminal extensor tendon rupture, palmar plate weakness, intrinsic tightness) that contributes to the final deformity. A given finger in an arthritic hand may progress through phases, i.e. the deformity may begin with a problem in the distal joint, but 6 months later, the degree of deformity may be increased by progressive intrinsic tightness at the level of the MCP joint. As the deformity worsens,

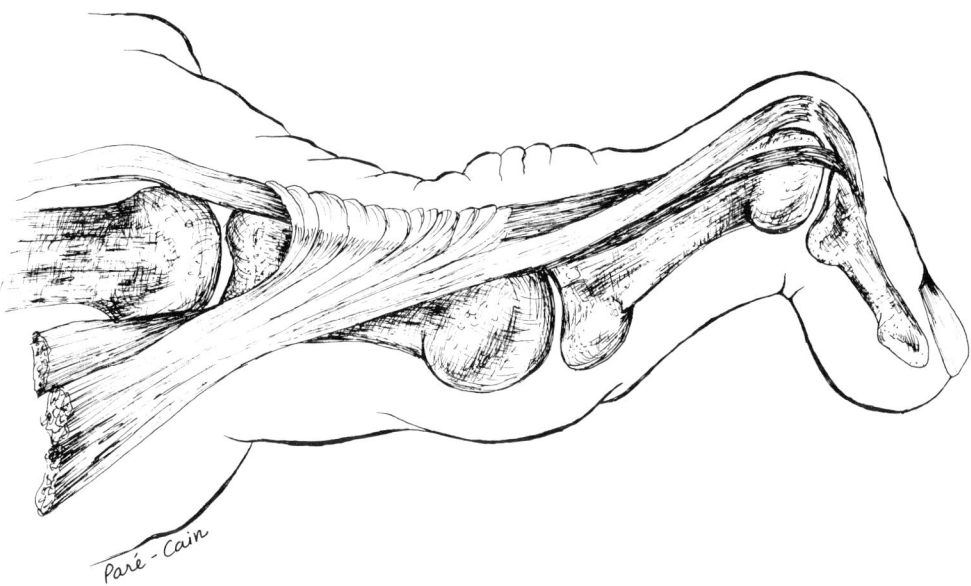

Fig. 8.3 A swan-neck deformity with attenuation of the terminal extensor tendon and hyperextension of the PIP joint.

soft tissues may contract, and the PIP joint loses active and passive motion in all positions (type III). The skin, tendons and peri-articular tissues have now contracted around the PIP joint so that attempts to relieve intrinsic tightness by positioning are of no help. The patient now has a severe disability (Fig. 8.4). The loss of both active and passive motion interferes with normal joint nutrition, and possibly hastens destruction of the joint surface (type IV). The time taken for a finger to go through these phases is variable and unpredictable. Careful observation is necessary since correction in the early phases is so much more beneficial than salvage in the final stages.

It is intriguing that a swan-neck deformity may co-exist with a boutonnière deformity in a given hand. The answer may lie in the differential degree of synovitis which can occur at various joints. If the synovitis is most aggressive at the PIP joint, a boutonnière deformity is likely to develop. If MCP joint synovitis predominates resulting in ulnar drift and MCP joint subluxation, a swan-neck may develop at the PIP joint level. This is more likely if the PIP joint has lost palmar stability.

Treatment: synovitis

Synovectomy in patients with rheumatoid arthritis is an established procedure with a long history of recorded clinic results as summarized by Gschwend (1985). MCP joint synovectomy and tendon re-alignment in rheumatoid arthritis is rarely indicated, as experience has shown that motion is lost and deformity recurs. In addition, the relatively good alternative of MCP joint arthroplasty is available.

The results of PIP joint synovectomies are more encouraging when one considers the alternatives.

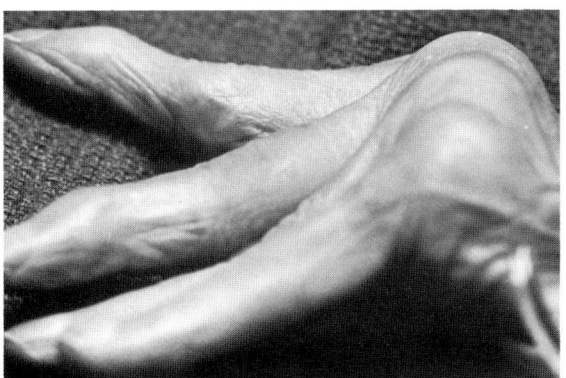

Fig. 8.4 Fixed swan-neck deformities with contractures of the periarticular soft tissues.

Like Gschwend (1985), the present author feels that the indication for synovectomy exists when the inflammation continues between the flare-up phases and in spite of basic therapy, because then the fear of basic joint destruction is justified. The question arises, what is basic therapy and for how long should it be carried out before synovectomy is performed? Basic therapy should consist of a course of gold salts, antimalarial drugs or salicylates. Immunosupressive drugs may be used instead of gold salts. Cortisone preparations are not considered basic therapy because a recession of swelling does not indicate any actual healing.

Local injection of cortisone combined with splinting may decrease swelling and thereby help the joint mechanically for a period of a few months. Intra-articular cortisone injections do not heal the synovitic process and recurrent synovitis is inevitable if there is a flare-up of the disease. Spontaneous remission of synovitis of the PIP joint may occur, and therefore the surgeon must allow for a certain period of observation before proceeding with surgery. Lipscomb (1971) suggested a period of at least 6 months. Millender et al (1982) implied that they wait a period of 9–12 months. Flatt (1983b) states that in certain hands, a period of 6 months is too long and the destructive process may have progressed to the point where synovectomy may not be useful. The time element alone does not provide the surgeon with an adequate guide for decision to perform a synovectomy.

The purposes of the surgical synovectomy are to relieve pain; to halt the destructive process; and to prevent and correct mechanical imbalance (i.e. boutonnière deformity). When the surgeon feels that the prognosis for the joint without surgery is poor, then surgical synovectomy is indicated in an attempt to achieve the above goals. The indications for synovectomy are both *immunological* and *biomechanical*. The synovectomy should be performed before severe erosion and joint space narrowing occur (immunological), and before biomechanical imbalance interferes with joint motion. The biomechanical indications are often overlooked. If progressive synovitis is causing a boutonnière deformity, synovectomy should be performed in an attempt to prevent further deformity. The results of boutonnière reconstruction in rheumatoid arthritis are poor, and the prevention of deformities is much preferred to late reconstruction. The biomechanical indication is present when proliferative synovial swelling leads to plugging of the joint, stretching or attenuation of the extensor mechanism, and loss of mobility (Fig. 8.5). The immunological indication is uncontrolled synovitis leading to cartilage deterioration and joint destruction. Synovectomy is contraindicated in a very sick individual who cannot withstand an anaesthetic or cannot cooperate with a postsurgical therapy programme. Activity of the disease does not represent an absolute contraindication, although one would prefer the patient to be as comfortable as possible in the postoperative period. The most common local contraindication would be radiographic destruction of the joint surface, in which case arthrodesis or arthroplasty is preferred.

Technique. The purpose of synovectomy is to remove as much of the synovium as possible without disturbing the mechanical stability of the joint. It is agreed that no synovectomy can be complete. Surgeons should strive to remove 80–90% of the synovium. Flatt (1983c) states that removing less than 70% of the synovium will probably yield an unsatisfactory result. The obvious bulging synovium should be removed, and the recesses deep to the collateral ligaments and palmar plate should be cleaned of all synovial tissue. Abnormal tissue on the osteocartilaginous border should be excised.

The joint is approached through a dorsal curvilinear incision. The plane between the tendons and subcutaneous tissues is developed preserving veins where possible. The synovium usually

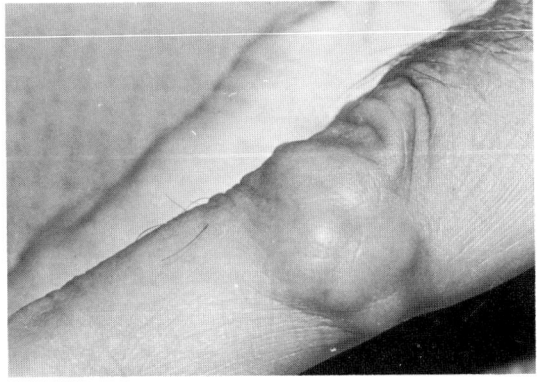

Fig. 8.5 Bulging synovium which mechanically interferes with joint motion.

bulges between the central slip and lateral band (Fig. 8.6). A longitudinal incision is made in the area of the bulge, the tendon is retracted and the dorsal synovium is removed. The present author always attempts to leave the central slip intact for fear of weakening the structure. If the synovium is bulging palmar to the lateral bands, then longitudinal incisions can be made through the transverse retinacular ligaments allowing dorsal retraction of the lateral bands. The transverse retinacular ligament incision can be made on either side of the joint. The collateral ligament recesses on the proximal phalanx are cleaned with a small curette. A longitudinal incision is made between the accessory collateral ligament and the palmar plate. The palmar pouch is cleared of any synovium. Incisions in the extensor mechanism are repaired with fine interrupted, absorbable sutures. The skin is closed. Gschwend (1985) recommends detaching the collateral ligament and simply sutures the

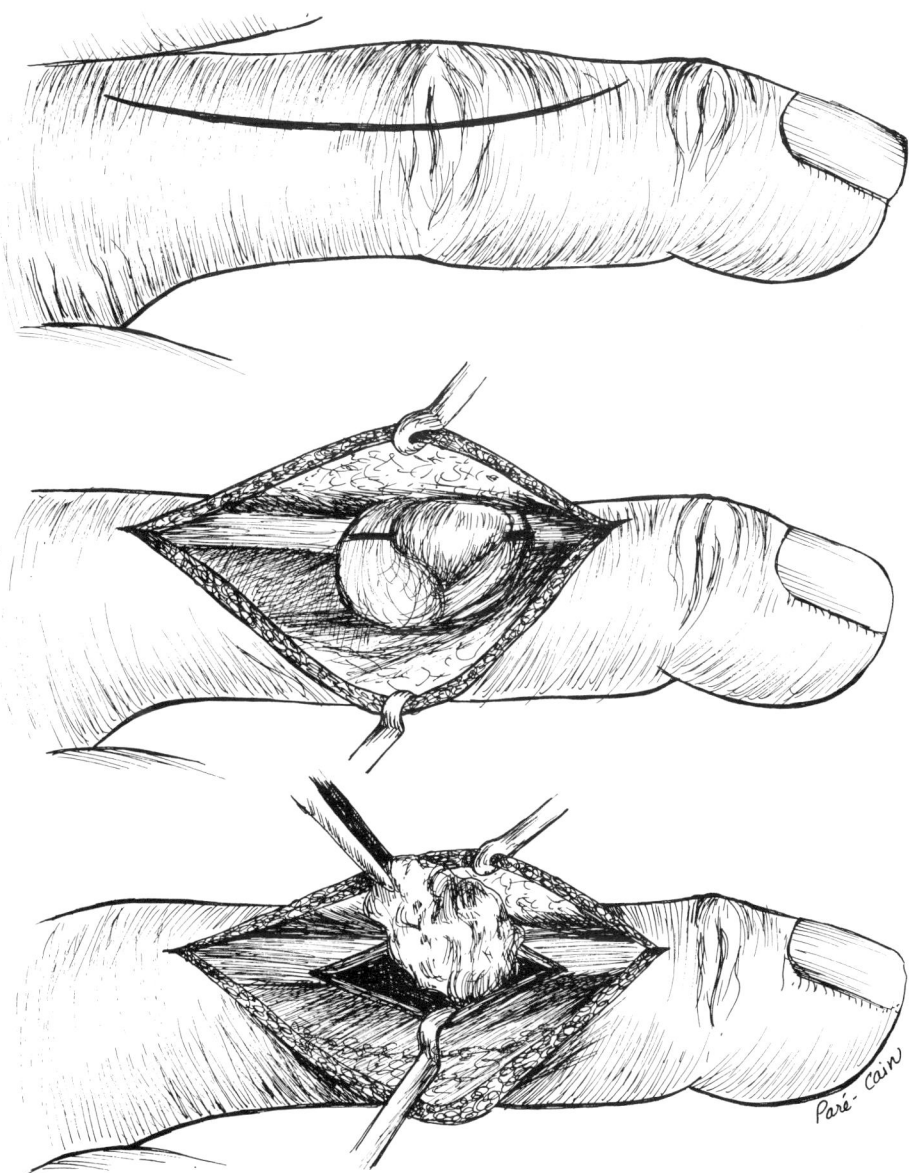

Fig. 8.6 The synovium of the PIP joint bulging through a tear in the extensor mechanism.

ligament back to its origin. Following the procedure, the joint is splinted in extension. Active and passive motion are started 4 d postoperatively. Night splinting in extension is continued for 3 weeks. A supervised therapy programme should be continued until the preoperative range of motion has been regained.

Results. Flatt (1983c), Ansell (1970), Raunio (1977), and Wilde (1974) have attempted to evaluate the results of PIP joint synovectomy. The common parameters have been (1) pain relief; (2) recurrent synovitis; (3) range of motion; and (4) the development of boutonnière deformities. The results are summarized in Table 8.1.

From these studies, certain trends are evident. Lasting pain relief can be expected in over 50% of patients. This pain relief should have a beneficial effect on function. Range of motion is not appreciably affected and there may be a decrease in range of motion with time. Synovitis will recur in a large percentage of patients (25–60%) with a concomitant deterioration of clinical results. A surprisingly low number of boutonnière deformities developed in these patients, and this may be the most beneficial effect of the operation.

Treatment: boutonnière deformity

Uncontrolled synovitis results in attenuation of the extensor mechanism over the PIP joint and the insidious development of a boutonnière deformity. The hyperextension deformity of the distal joint and the MCP joint are secondary to the tendon imbalance. The treatment, therefore, is directed to the PIP joint. Millender et al (1982) have classified boutonnière deformities in rheumatoid arthritis as mild, moderate and severe. Classification is based on the active and passive range of motion of the joint, and the X-ray evaluation.

Mild. At this stage, the PIP joint lacks 10–15° of full active extension. Passively, the PIP joint can be fully extended. The distal joint is usually hyperextended, but is able to flex as the PIP joint flexes. The patient, therefore, can make a fist. The PIP joint is usually swollen secondary to active synovitis. In this stage, the surgeon can attempt to regain motion at both the distal and proximal interphalangeal joints. He may also prevent the deformity from progressing rapidly to the next stage. To restore distal joint motion, an extensor tendon tenotomy should be performed. A transverse tenotomy is performed over the midportion of the middle phalanx. This allows easier flexion of the distal joint without the development of mallet finger due to support of the oblique retinacular fibres. Flatt (1983a) recommends a more distal tenotomy, but this may be at the risk of a mallet deformity. In addition to the extensor tenotomy, a PIP joint synovectomy should be performed at this stage if the joint is swollen. A reefing of the extensor mechanism can be performed as part of the synovectomy. The reefing of the extensor mechanism should allow better active extension of the PIP joint. Following tenotomy and synovectomy, active motion is started. Dynamic splints are used to assist PIP extension. At night, the PIP joint is splinted in extension for 3–4 weeks.

Moderate. As the extensor mechanism over the PIP joint becomes more attenuated, the flexion deformity increases. The lateral bands continue to displace in a palmar direction (see Fig. 8.4). The joint now lies in 50° of flexion and the hyperextension of the distal joint is more pronounced and does not fully correct with flexion of the PIP joint. The MCP joint hyperextends to compensate for the flexed PIP. If left in this condition, the boutonnière deformity may become fixed and soft tissue reconstruction may no longer be possible.

Table 8.1 Summary of the results of proximal interphalangeal (PIP) joint synovectomy

	Flatt (1983) (79 joints)	Ansell et al (1970) (115 joints)	Raunio (1977)	Wilde (1974) (98 joints)
Pain relief	50%	60%	60%	60%
Recurrent synovitis	24%	41%	50%	60%
Range of motion	−22°	No change	Slightly improved	−4°
Boutonnière deformity	4	5	?	1

Certain criteria should be met if the surgeon is undertaking a soft tissue reconstruction at this stage:

1. X-rays show an adequate joint space
2. Passive correction of the PIP joint deformity is possible
3. The flexor tendons are intact and functioning

Several techniques have been described. All have three basic components:

1. Reconstruction of the central slip
2. Positioning of the lateral bands such that their pull is once more dorsal to the mid-axis of the PIP joint
3. Tenotomy of the terminal extensor tendon to allow flexion of the distal joint

The dorsal incision is curvilinear and long enough to allow mobilization of the lateral bands and central slip. The central slip will be stretched out and there will be an abnormal separation between the lateral bands and the central slip through the oblique fibres. A transverse incision is made in the central slip 3–4 mm from the insertion on the middle phalanx. Longitudinal incisions are then made on either side of the central slip for approximately 1.5 cm and the central slip is mobilized. The transverse retinacular ligaments are incised allowing the lateral bands to be brought dorsally. While the PIP joint is held in full extension, the cut ends of the central slip are overlapped and repaired with non-absorbable sutures. The overlapped area is usually 3–4 mm. Instead of overlapping the ends, a portion of the central slip may be excised (3–4 mm), but because of the thinness of the tissue, the present author most often overlaps the tendon to gain the necessary tension in the tendon repair. The lateral bands are then sutured to the central slip under some tension, effectively placing more of their power at the PIP joint and attempting to remove some of the pull at the distal joint (Fig. 8.7). Passive flexion of the PIP joint is then checked. The joint should flex passively to 60°. After measuring the passive flexion, a Kirschner wire is placed across the joint holding it in an extended position. A tenotomy of the terminal

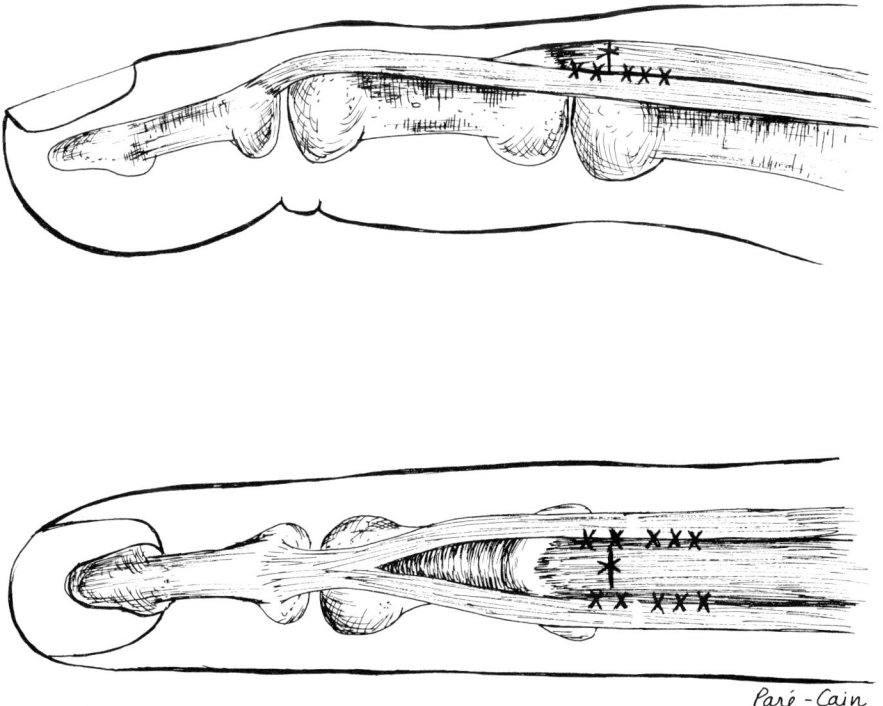

Fig. 8.7 Surgical reconstruction of a boutonnière deformity. The central slip must be repaired, and the lateral bands must be sutured back to the central slip dorsal to the mid-axis of the joint.

extensor tendon is then performed over the middle phalanx. The wound is closed with interrupted sutures. Distal joint motion is encouraged immediately. It is recommended to leave the Kirschner wire in for 2 weeks and then use external splints for another 4 weeks before beginning active flexion exercises.

Flatt (1983a) has described the use of a free tendon graft—palmaris longus—in reconstruction of the central slip in rheumatoid arthritis. Various techniques have been described in which one or both of the lateral bands are used to substitute for the central slip (see Ch. 6). These procedures increase the tension of the lateral bands and may result in secondary problems with active motion. The more 'anatomical' reconstruction is preferred and it is not necessary to use the other methods.

Severe. If the flexion deformity becomes fixed, surgical reconstruction to restore extension becomes increasingly difficult. If the flexion contracture is 30–40°, dynamic splinting may help. Alternatively, the surgeon could consider a PIP joint release combined with reconstruction of the extensor mechanism *if* the joint surface is congruous. The results of boutonnière reconstruction when there is a fixed flexion contracture are unpredictable and the procedure is not often indicated (Fig. 8.8). The patient with a 40° fixed flexion contracture, a further arc of motion to 90° and little pain is probably best left alone (except perhaps for an isolated terminal extensor tenotomy), as no soft tissue procedures can reliably restore extension and the 50° arc of motion is more functional than an arthrodesis or most arthroplasties. If further motion is lost and the contracture is in the range of 70–80° or if the joint surface is destroyed, arthrodesis or arthroplasty become the only choices for treatment. In choosing one of these procedures, the surgeon has certain guidelines: (1) in the index finger, arthrodesis is the procedure of choice because of the necessity for stability; (2) if MCP arthroplasty is going to be necessary in a given finger, arthrodesis at the PIP joint is again the procedure of choice as consistent results with silicone arthroplasties at both levels in one finger have not been obtainable. Silicone arthroplasty can be considered in the middle, ring and little fingers in patients who may not require MCP arthroplasties.

Arthrodesis

In the index finger, the position of fusion should be 30–35°. The angle increases as one proceeds to the ulnar side of the hand. The position of PIP fusion in the little finger should be 45–50°.

Technique. The fusion is performed through a dorsal incision splitting the extensor mechanism. Any remaining cartilage is removed. In boutonnière deformities with severe fixed contractures, some shortening of the proximal phalanx may be required to obtain the proper position. Two Kirschner wires are inserted in retrograde fashion across the fusion site. The present author cuts off the pins below the skin in most cases for two reasons: pins can be left in as long as necessary with less chance of pin tract infection than if the pins are exposed (Fig. 8.9). Once early healing has started, the finger is more functional without external pins. The biggest disadvantage to buried pins is the necessity for removal with local anaesthetic. Bone grafting is not necessary in most cases. The fusion rate using pinning techniques should be high (Carroll & Hill 1969). Granowitz & Vainio (1966) reported eight non-unions in 122 arthrodeses. Moberg (1960) has described a technique of fusion using an intramedullary bone peg for stability. The present author has no experience with this technique, but from the description, the

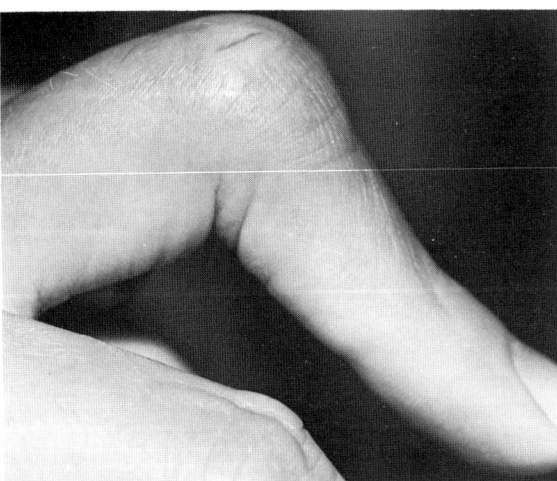

Fig. 8.8 A severe boutonnière deformity with a fixed contracture of 70°. Surgical reconstruction to restore active motion is very difficult.

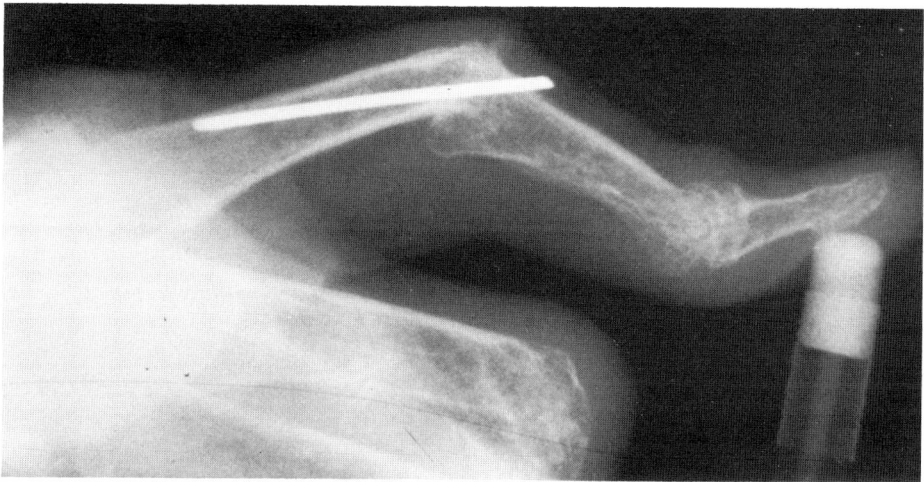

Fig. 8.9 Arthrodesis of the PIP joint with pin fixation.

technique is demanding and time consuming, and it would appear to be impractical to attempt multiple fusions in one sitting using the described method.

Arthroplasty

A number of different types of arthroplasties have been attempted at the PIP joint in rheumatoid arthritis. An inadequate number of long-term clinical studies makes it difficult to determine how good or bad the results really are. The metal prosthesis designed by Flatt (1983c) was not used in boutonnière deformities. Beckenbaugh (1977) reviewed the Mayo clinic's experience using cemented prostheses. The results were unsatisfactory due to loosening, periosteal bone formation and recurrence of deformity. Proximal interphalangeal joint arthroplasties using cemented prostheses have been abandoned. Swanson (1973b) did evaluate the use of silicone prostheses in 54 boutonnière deformities. The average arc of motion postoperatively was 67°. Sixteen patients had a persistent extensor lag postoperatively of approximately 10°.

Technique. The joint is approached through a dorsal incision. The central slip will appear to be very attenuated and the lateral bands will be displaced palmarward. The central slip is detached leaving a small stump of tissue on the phalanx. The lateral bands are mobilized. The head of the proximal phalanx is removed preserving the collateral ligaments on either side and the canal of the proximal phalanx is broached. Osteophytes are trimmed from the middle phalanx, particularly on the palmar lip. If excessive bone is left on the palmar lip of the middle phalanx, there will be impingement when the joint is flexed, limiting motion. The intramedullary canal of the midphalanx is broached. Enough bone must be removed from the proximal phalanx to allow the prosthesis to fit comfortably between the bones. In a boutonnière deformity, more bone than usual may have to be resected because of soft tissue contracture. Once the prosthesis is in place, the central slip is reattached either by sutures at the base of the middle phalanx or to the stump of insertion which had been preserved. The lateral bands are sutured to the central slip dorsal to the mid-axis of the joint. The lateral bands may have to be rebalanced because of the shortening of the bone. The PIP joint should now lie between neutral and 10° of flexion. It should not be hyperextended and should not lie at rest in more than 15° of flexion. The finger is immobilized in extension for 10 d when active motion is started. The joint must be protected for 5–6 weeks as the extensor mechanism heals. Vigorous motion too soon after surgery could obviously disrupt the central slip repair. The present author has enjoyed some success with this technique in selected cases. Results can be superior to arthrodesis when a procedure is performed for the correct indications. However, even in a busy rheumatoid practice, arthroplasty for severe boutonnière deformities in rheumatoid arthritis is only occasionally performed.

Treatment: swan-neck deformity

Mild. In the early stages of swan-neck deformity, the finger assumes a posture of flexion at the distal joint and hyperextension at the PIP joint. On examination, there is full active and passive motion at the PIP joint with no evidence of intrinsic tightness. There is no destruction of the joint surface on X-ray. The deformity may be secondary to rupture or attenuation of the terminal extensor tendon with hyperextension of the PIP joint due to synovitis of the joint and laxity of the palmar plate (see Fig. 8.3).

If the problem is primarily at the PIP joint, the distal joint flexion will partially correct if the PIP joint is brought into flexion because the tendon system is rebalanced. In patients with early swan-neck deformity, if the surgeon feels that the deformity is in part due to disruption of the extensor mechanism over the distal joint, treatment must be directed at stabilizing the distal joint in the extended position and restoring palmar stability of the PIP joint. These two goals can be achieved by arthrodesis of the distal joint in extension and flexor superficialis tenodesis on the palmar aspect of the PIP joint. The distal joint is approached through a dorsal H-shaped incision. A 4–5 mm skin bridge must be left between the nail and the skin incision to ensure blood supply to the distal flap. The cartilage is removed with a rongeur. Two Kirschner wires are passed through the distal phalanx, one longitudinally and one obliquely. The bones are impacted in a position of 0–5° of flexion. The Kirschner wires are then driven across the arthrodesis site and cut off below the skin. Superficialis tenodesis is then performed through a palmar Bruner-type incision. One slip of the flexor digitorum superficialis is isolated, detached proximally and left attached to its distal insertion. The cut proximal end may then be interwoven through the A-2 pulley under the proper tension to gain the tenodesis effect. Millender & Nalebuff (1975) recommend putting the tendon end into bone, as originally described by Swanson (1972). In setting the tension, the surgeon attempts to create a flexion contracture of 10–15°. Both the arthrodesis and tenodesis must be protected for 6 weeks, but active flexion of the PIP should be started early.

Other procedures that have been recommended are dermadesis of the skin palmar to the PIP joint and oblique retinacular ligament reconstruction. Oblique retinacular ligament reconstruction using the ulnar intrinsics or a free tendon graft may be of help to correct the deformity. The present author feels it is difficult to rebalance the finger with this method, especially if more than one finger has to be operated on. The combination of distal joint stabilization and flexor superficialis tenodesis will correct most cases of mild swan-neck deformity.

Moderate. At this stage, in addition to having an abnormal posture, active and passive motion are decreased (see Fig. 8.1). Loss of motion can be made worse by moving the proximal phalanx in a radial and dorsal direction. Intrinsic tightness is now contributing to the deformity. As the severity of the problem increases, flexion of the PIP joint may be completely lost despite good articular surfaces. At this stage, in addition to rebalancing the tendon forces, contractures of soft tissue must be corrected. The operation should consist of an intrinsic release, tenolysis of the extensor mechanism over the proximal phalanx, manipulation of the joint, lateral band mobilization and skin release if necessary. If the loss of flexion occurs only in certain positions (Nalebuff stage II), intrinsic release can be performed and combined with DIP arthrodesis. Intrinsic release is performed through a dorsal incision over the proximal phalanx. The edge of the lateral band on either side of the phalanx is identified and mobilized. The oblique fibres attaching the lateral bands to the central slip are excised. This removes a triangular piece of tissue from the extensor mechanism and decreases the pull on the PIP joint (Fig. 8.10). If the PIP joint has lost motion in all positions of the finger, then tenolysis of the extensor mechanism over the proximal phalanx and PIP joint manipulation may be necessary. This combination should restore PIP passive motion in most patients with good joint surfaces. The joint should be pinned in 40–50° of flexion for 2 weeks. If the skin is tight, the distal portion of the curvilinear incision is left open and

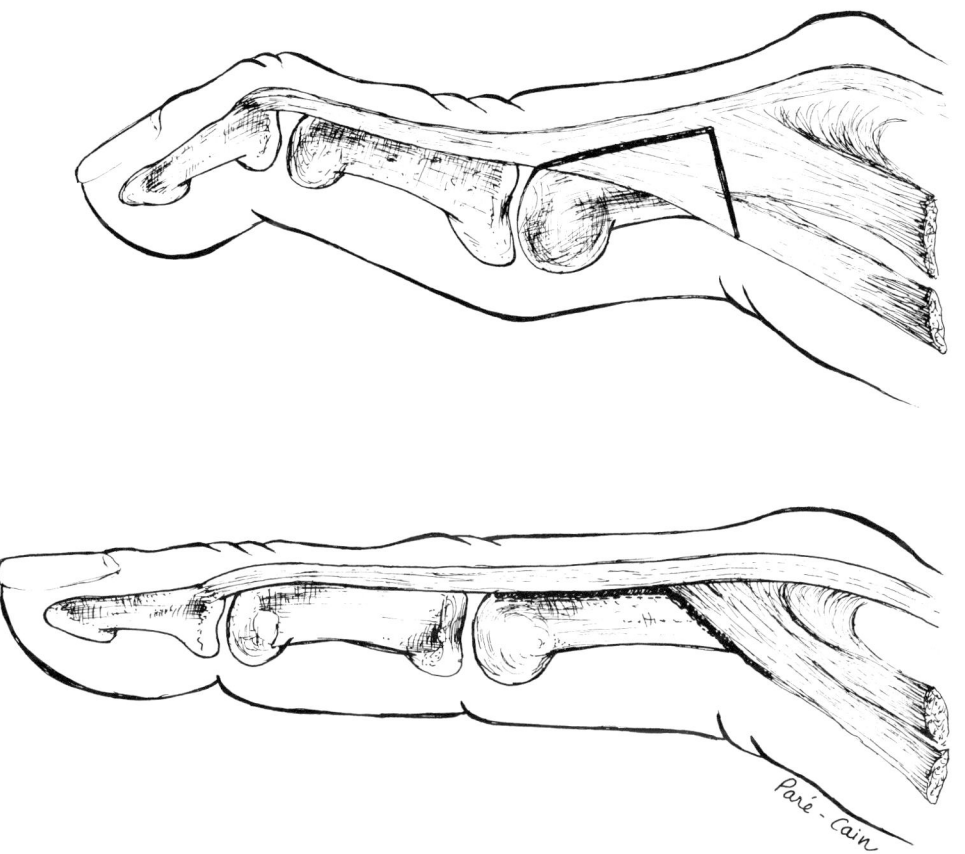

Fig. 8.10 Intrinsic release over the proximal phalanx performed on both radial and ulnar sides.

the wound allowed to granulate (Millender et al 1982) (Fig. 8.11). Occasionally a step cut release of the central slip and surgical release of the collateral ligaments are necessary, but this is rare. When MCP joint arthroplasties are combined with efforts to correct a swan-neck deformity, simple manipulation and pinning of the PIP joint may be of great benefit. The intrinsic release associated with MCP arthroplasty and the necessary shortening of the bony elements aid in the reduction of the extensor forces over the PIP joint. Manipulation and pinning in this situation may be all that is necessary to gain adequate PIP motion.

Severe. All efforts should be made to correct a swan-neck deformity in the mild or moderate stage. Preservation of potential joint motion is always preferred. If the X-ray appearance of the joint is poor, and the joint is stiff, then only arthroplasty or arthrodesis will help (Fig. 8.12). As in severe boutonnière deformities, there are several factors which influence a surgeon's decision. In the index finger, arthrodesis is always preferred because of the stability provided to the finger. If the surgeon can anticipate that MCP joint arthroplasties will be necessary, then PIP joint arthrodesis is generally the procedure of choice. Angulation deformities with poor ligament support and flexor tendon ruptures would make the surgeon lean toward arthrodesis. In general, the worse the condition of the joint itself and the worse the condition of the hand, the more indications there are to perform an arthrodesis. The technique of arthrodesis in swan-neck deformity is similar to the technique used in boutonnière deformities. After making the incision, the extensor mechanism is split longitudinally. Enough bone is resected to

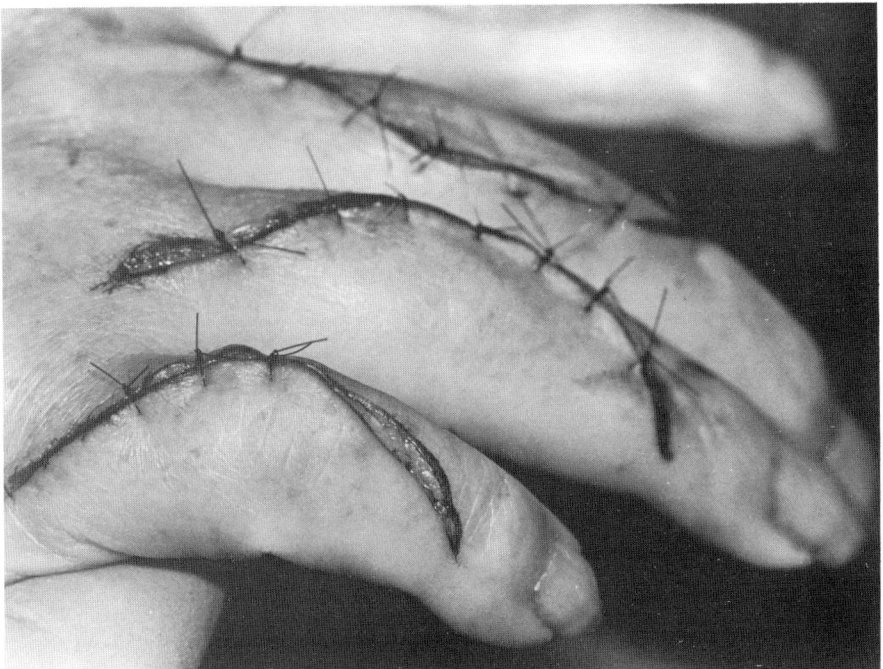

Fig. 8.11 An intrinsic release has been performed. The distal portion of the wound is left open because of skin contracture.

achieve the proper degree of flexion without undue force. Cross Kirschner wires are used for stabilization. Buried pins allow a shorter period of external immobilization which is particularly important if simultaneous MCP arthroplasties are being performed. Healing should be complete in 6–8 weeks. Arthrodesis of the PIP joint in a proper position will rebalance the forces on the distal joint, and most often no further surgery is necessary on the distal joint.

Arthroplasty

Constrained hinge prostheses are not generally used in the rheumatoid PIP joint, either for boutonnière or swan-neck deformities. Flatt (1983c) reported a series of 75 prosthetic replace-

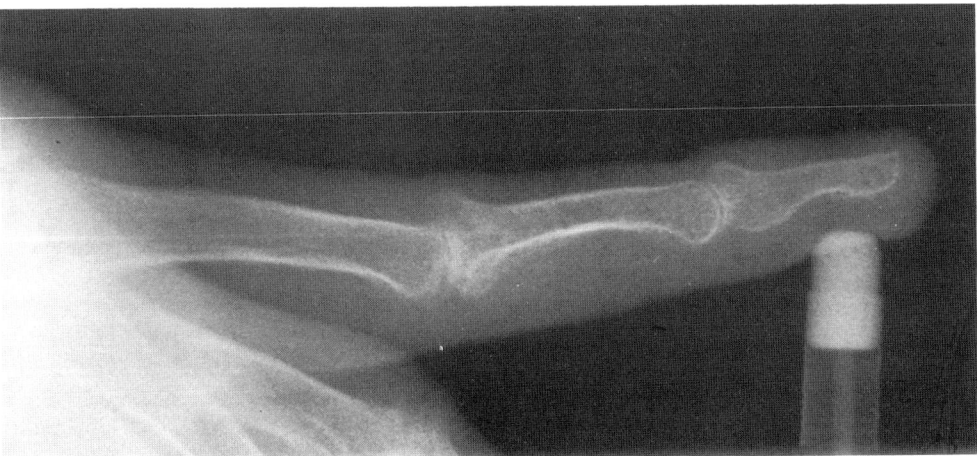

Fig. 8.12 A severe swan-neck deformity with joint destruction. Arthrodesis or arthroplasty are the surgical options.

ments in the PIP joint using a two pronged hinge prosthesis. The majority of these prostheses were inserted for persistent swan-neck deformities. Eleven of the prostheses were later removed. The average motion obtained was approximately 45° in the prostheses which stayed in. Flatt makes the point that there was no recurrence of hyperextension and that he was less pleased with his results using either the Niebauer or Swanson design. Swanson (1973a) reported a series of 61 flexible implants used in swan-neck deformities. The average postoperative arc of motion was 66°. There was a postoperative hyperextension tendency in nine joints averaging 10°.

In performing an arthroplasty for swan-neck deformity, attention should be focused on rebalancing the extensor mechanism and on freeing the flexor tendon to allow active power to be transmitted to the proximal interphalangeal joint. A dorsal curved incision is used and its distal portion may be left open if necessary at the conclusion of the procedure. The extensor mechanism may be split longitudinally or step cut, as described by Swanson. The lateral band should be freed from the central slip if very contracted. The necessary bone shortening required in arthroplasty will take some tension off the soft tissues. Tenodesis or dermodesis may also be used in an attempt to create a flexion posture. Flexor tenolysis may be performed through a separate volar incision if necessary. If the distal joint is in significant flexion, it should be pinned or arthrodesed in a neutral position. This will help to rebalance the finger and, hopefully, provide better flexion of the PIP joint. Advanced disease involving the PIP joint in rheumatoid arthritis remains a major problem for the hand surgeon. New prosthetic replacements are in the process of being developed and hopefully will provide more functional restoration of joint function. At present, the silicone prosthesis designed by Swanson is the most common prosthetic replacement used in the PIP joint. If attention is paid to detail, satisfactory results can be obtained.

JUVENILE RHEUMATOID ARTHRITIS

Juvenile rheumatoid arthritis (JRA) is the most common childhood connective tissue disease. Cassidy (1985) estimated that 250 000 children in the USA have this disease. The aetiology and the pathogenesis are unknown. There are three distinct types of onset of the disease: polyarthritis, oligoarthritis and systemic disease. The polyarthritis type most often affects the small joints of the hand. Histologically, there is villous hypertrophy of the synovium and hyperplasia of the synovial lining. The synovial hyperplasia is similar to that seen in adult rheumatoid arthritis. The early radiographic changes consist of soft tissue swelling, osteoporosis, and periosteal new bone formation (Fig. 8.13). Premature epiphyseal closure may result in stunting of bone growth. In chronic cases, articular erosions are seen followed by narrowing of the joint space. In the late stages, the articular spaces completely disappear obliterated by fibrous or bony ankylosis. Both Calabro (1979) and Cassidy (1985)

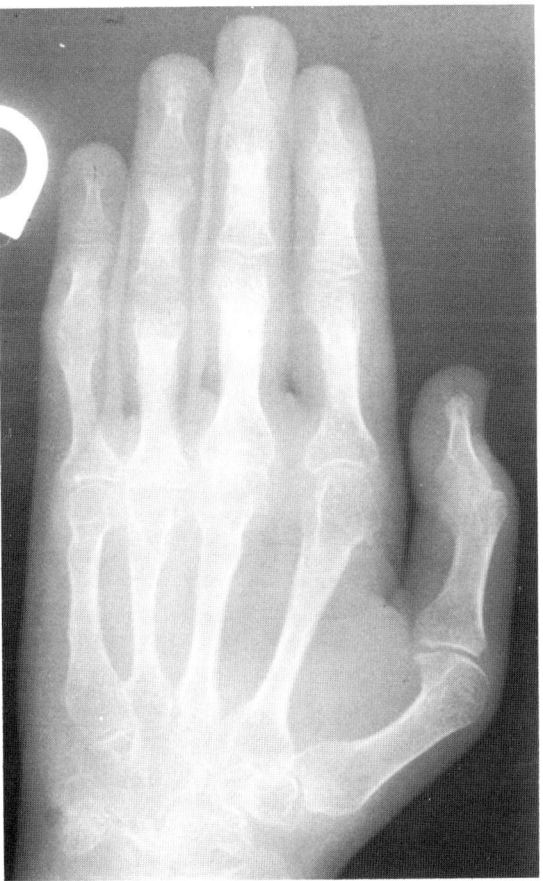

Fig. 8.13 The X-ray of a patient with JRA. Soft tissue swelling, osteoporosis, erosive changes.

estimate that 50% of cases go into a complete remission and 70% of cases regain normal function. Cassidy (1985) states that approximately 10% of children with JRA enter adulthood with severe functional disability. The child most at risk is the one with polyarthritis of late age of onset and early involvement of the small joints of the hands and feet. There is little available information regarding the treatment of the PIP joint deformities in JRA.

Chaplin et al (1969) reviewed 400 patients with JRA. The hand and wrist were involved in 59% of the patients, with 34% having ulnar deviation of the wrist associated with radial deviation of the MCP joints. Flexion deformities of the PIP joints were common, as were boutonnière deformities. Swan-neck deformities were unusual. Granberry & Mangum (1980) performed a clinical review of 100 children with JRA and a radiographic review of 200 cases diagnosed as JRA. In the clinical review, there were 27 PIP joints with decreased flexion, 10 PIP joints with decreased extension, 7 boutonnière deformities and one swan-neck deformity. Intrinsic tightness was not present in this group of children. In the 200 children whose charts and radiographs were examined by Granberry & Mangum (1980), the incidence of PIP joint involvement was 49% with only 6 boutonnière deformities and no swan-neck deformities. This incidence of boutonnière deformities (3%) seems extremely low. Approximately one-half of the patients in these series had PIP joint involvement. Synovitis leading to loss of active range of motion is common and often results in flexion deformities in JRA. Swan-neck deformities are rare in all series. The low incidence of swan-neck deformities may be due to the low incidence of MCP ulnar deviation and the lack of intrinsic tightness.

In general, treatment should be conservative and Granberry & Mangum (1980) feel that surgery is rarely indicated. Eyring et al (1971) reviewed the results of synovectomy in 9 PIP joints. Pain relief was good and joint motion was increased in 6 of the joints. This study does not answer the question of whether or not synovectomy prevents the development of flexion and boutonnière deformities in JRA. In Granberry & Mangum's (1980) series, 10 PIP joint synovectomies were performed in 3 patients. These patients lost motion. They advise against synovectomy of the PIP joint in JRA and recommend physical therapy, splinting and an occasional steroid injection in attempting to maintain motion and prevent deformity. The present author has reconstructed three boutonnière deformities in which the flexion of the PIP joint was greater than 60°. These boutonnière deformities differed from the adult variety in that they were passively much more flexible. Simultaneous synovectomy was performed. The technique used was similar to that described for adults. Over a 2-year period, the joints have maintained a 70° arc of motion with a 10° extensor lag.

In the longstanding fixed flexion deformities seen in JRA, there is very little to offer (Fig. 8.14). Arthroplasties at this stage have not been successful due to the difficulty in regaining extension. Patients feel they are better off maintaining some active flexion at the PIP joint rather than undergo arthrodesis. This is because loss of flexion at the MCP joint also occurs and if the PIP joints are arthrodesed in 45° of flexion, the patient will lose all ability to grasp.

After reviewing the literature, it is impossible to state whether synovectomy of the PIP joints is

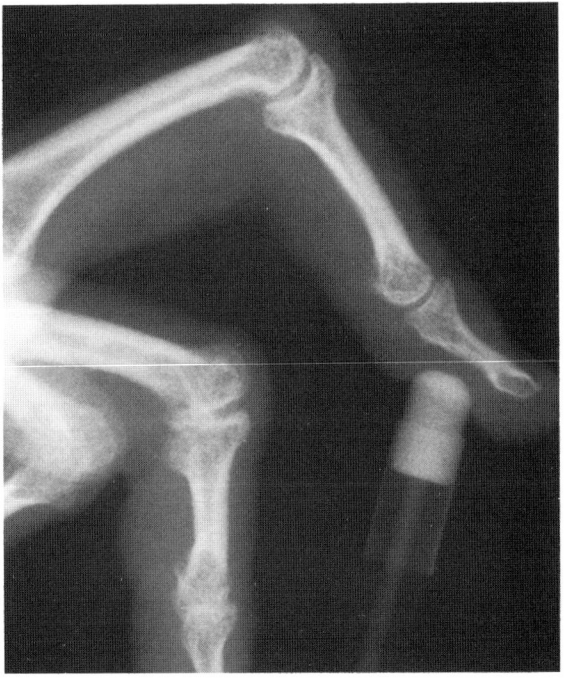

Fig. 8.14 A fixed flexion deformity of the PIP joint in JRA. Attempts at reconstruction of the extensor mechanism are not usually successful.

beneficial in JRA. It is felt that in selected cases, synovectomy and boutonnière reconstruction have been helpful to patients. Reconstruction of chronic fixed flexion deformities secondary to juvenile rheumatoid arthritis is not feasible with the current arthroplastic techniques, and arthrodesis is rarely indicated.

PSORIATIC ARTHRITIS

The association of psoriasis and arthritis was first noted in the early 19th century. With the demonstration of rheumatoid factor in 1947, inflammatory arthritis was divided into two major groups: the seropositive and the seronegative arthritides. It was soon apparent that most patients with psoriatic arthritis were seronegative. Large clinical studies and the confirmation of a familial occurrence established the fact that psoriatic arthritis is a distinct clinical entity. Roberts et al (1976) have defined psoriatic arthritis as an inflammatory disease of joints in a patient with psoriasis usually with a negative serological test for rheumatoid factor.

The inflammatory synovitis is macroscopically similar to rheumatoid arthritis, but there does appear to be less proliferation of the synovium when compared to rheumatoid arthritis. Microscopically, the synovitis is indistinguishable from rheumatoid arthritis. Bennett (1979) reported an excessive fibrosis in the articular soft tissues, and this may account for the stiffness seen in the joints of these patients. Healing of inflamed joints also results in intra-articular fibrosis, leading to stiffness and ankylosis as emphasized by Belsky et al (1982). Clinically, there is a wide spectrum of presentations ranging from mild monoarticular involvement to a rapidly destructive arthritis mutilans. The most common pattern, accounting for 70% of all cases, is an oligoarticular arthritis characteristically asymmetrical in distribution usually affecting scattered DIP, PIP and metatarsophalangeal joints (Wright 1985). In a study of 168 patients (Roberts et al 1976), 26% had distal joint involvement, 50% had PIP joint involvement and 50% had metatarsophalangeal involvement. A commonly held view that psoriatic arthritis has a predilection for the distal joints should probably be revised.

The overall course of the disease is generally less severe and less debilitating than rheumatoid arthritis. Certain characteristic changes are present in the X-rays of patients with psoriatic arthritis. The common findings are:

1. Acro-osteolysis—erosion of the tufts of the distal phalanx
2. Pencil and cup deformity of the small joints in the hand
3. Bony ankylosis—particularly involving the DIP joints
4. A relative lack of osteoporosis (Fig. 8.15)

Flexion contracture is the most common deformity seen in the PIP joints in patients with psoriatic arthritis. The contractures are very stiff and usually are not able to be passively corrected (Fig. 8.16). Instability of the PIP joint, often seen in rheumatoid arthritis, is not a clinical problem in true psoriatic arthritis. Belsky et al (1982) reviewed 25 patients with psoriatic arthritis who required hand surgery. PIP joints were involved in 22 of the 25 patients. No mention is made of either instability or swan-neck deformities. The surgical problem was a destructive arthritis associated with a flexion contracture in 17 patients and a destructive arthritis associated with an extension contracture in 5 patients. The absence of instability is probably attributable to the lack of proliferative synovitis which can destroy ligamentous supporting structures in rheumatoid arthritis.

Medical treatment initially consists of nonsteroidal anti-inflammatory drugs. Local corticosteroid injections using triamcinolone may be helpful in symptomatic treatment of joint complaints. Bennett (1979) states that the use of intraarticular radioactive colloids is not successful in preventing joint destruction. For the fixed flexion contracture which is functionally bothersome or painful, the only solution at present is arthrodesis. The present author has combined arthrodesis of the PIP joint with MCP arthroplasties in psoriatic arthritis with results similar to those seen in rheumatoid arthritis. The success rate of fusion should be high because there is very good bone stock and because the soft tissues provide both support and compression for the arthrodesis. If the joint is fixed in extension, PIP arthroplasty could be considered. The expected motion will be poor.

136 THE INTERPHALANGEAL JOINTS

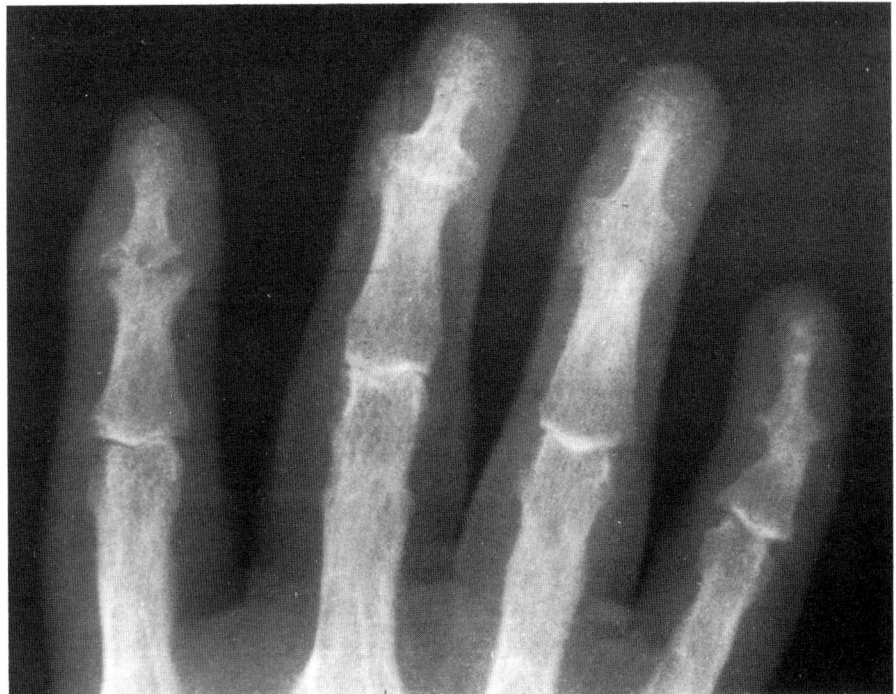

Fig. 8.15 Acro-osteolysis, bony ankylosis (DIP), and joint destruction in psoriatic arthritis.

Eleven arthroplasties were performed in the series of Belsky et al (1982) with an average range of motion of 20°.

Distal joint disease may result in a bony ankylosis or destructive arthritis. If bony ankylosis occurs in a satisfactory position, no further treatment is necessary. If the distal joint has not fused and is painful, then surgical fusion may be necessary. Internal fixation is necessary and bone graft is used if necessary.

In most patients with involvement at the PIP joint severe enough to warrant surgery, arthrodesis

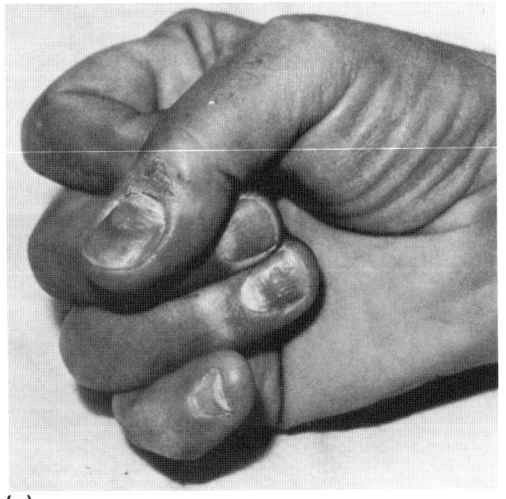
(a)

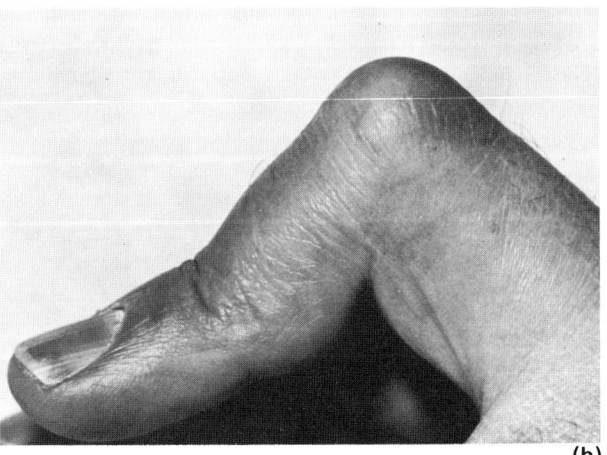
(b)

Fig. 8.16 The hand in psoriatic arthritis. (**a**) Nail changes and (**b**) a fixed flexion deformity of the PIP joint.

is the procedure of choice. A better understanding of the periarticular fibrosis is necessary before arthroplasty may become a good alternative at the PIP joint.

SYSTEMIC LUPUS ERYTHEMATOSUS

The aetiology of systemic lupus erythematosus (SLE) is unknown. Certain laboratory features are recognizable and are associated with autoantibodies to cellular constituents. The reasons for the development of autoantibodies in SLE are unknown, but chronic virus infection, genetic predisposition, environmental factors, and hormonal factors have all been implicated (Rothfield 1979, 1985). Tissue damage is caused by the deposition of antigen–antibody complexes. This is especially true in blood vessels and is the cause of the high incidence of Raynaud's phenomenon. The antigen–antibody complexes are deposited in the vascular endothelium of joints eventually causing biochemical and morphological changes. In Rothfield's (1979) series of 433 patients with SLE, the mean age at the time of diagnosis was 30. Ninety per cent of the patients were female. The most common manifestation of SLE is joint involvement (90%). Joint pain and swelling often precede multisystem disease.

There is no pannus formation in the joints of patients with SLE and the joint cartilage appears to be quite normal, both macroscopically and radiographically (Fig. 8.17). Diffuse synovial lining cell proliferation may be seen, but the hypertrophic synovitis of rheumatoid arthritis is not present. The joint deformities seen in SLE are thought to be secondary to disease within the periarticular tendon structures, ligaments and intrinsic muscles of the hand. The joints most commonly involved are the PIP, knee, wrist, and MCP joints. In Rothfield's (1979) series, there was PIP joint involvement in 82% of patients. Most patients with severe involvement have a typical pattern of deformity (Fig. 8.18). The distal ulna is often subluxed dorsally and there is usually some loss of wrist motion. The extensor tendons are subluxed into the ulnar gutters and the MCP joints are in flexion with or without ulnar deviation. Swan-neck deformities at the PIP joints are common, but boutonnière deformities may occur. Initially, both the MCP flexion deformities and swan-neck de-

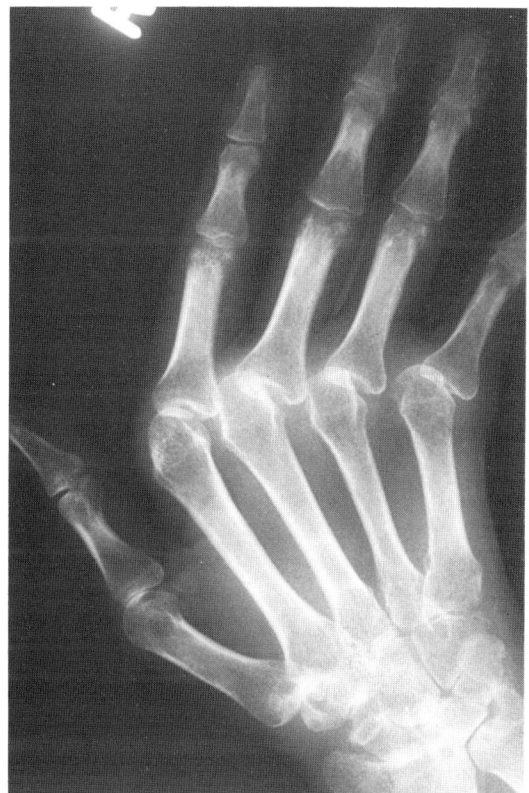

Fig. 8.17 Ulnar deviation and palmar subluxation in SLE. Erosive changes are minimal except in the wrist.

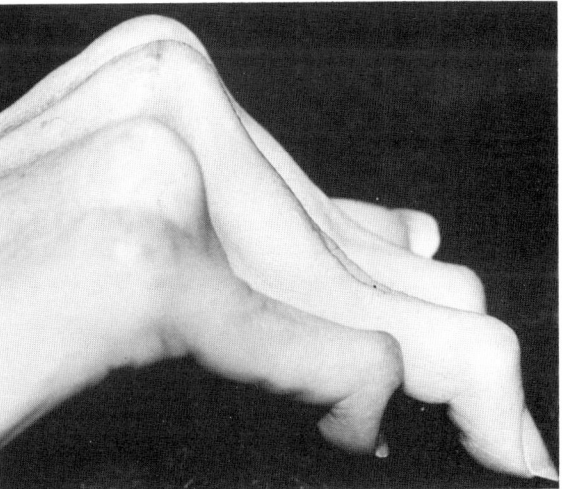

Fig. 8.18 Flexion deformity at the MCP joint and severe swan-neck deformities in a 33-year-old female with SLE.

formities may be passively correctable, but with time these deformities become fixed, especially at the MCP joint. In longstanding disease, the PIP joints have a tendency to lose ligamentous stability and may sublux either dorsally or to either side. Lateral subluxations are not uncommon.

The X-ray appearance of the hand in SLE is also quite typical (see Fig. 8.17). The carpus will often translocate ulnarly and degenerative changes are commonly seen along with evidence of intercarpal instability. Severe radial or ulnar deviation of the carpus and metacarpals is unusual. X-rays of the MCP joints may show subluxation of the joints, but rarely show any erosive or degenerative changes as are seen in the wrist. Likewise, the PIP joint may be in a subluxed position of hyperextension, but does not usually show erosive changes. The PIP joint deformities in SLE appear to be due to two factors: intrinsic tendon imbalance and tightness which is secondary to dislocation of the extensor mechanism and MCP joint flexion deformity; and primary involvement and laxity of the supporting ligaments of the PIP joint. It is rare to see severe involvement of the PIP in SLE without some deformity being present at the MCP joints. In fact, in the early stages of the deformity, one can correct the PIP hyperextension by passively reducing and extending the flexed MCP joints. This fact must be kept in mind if surgical attempts are being made to reverse the deformity of the PIP joint.

The surgical approach to correct the hand in SLE has been outlined by Dray et al (1981). The most important factor in gaining a satisfactory result was correction of the flexion deformity at the MCP joint. Attempts at soft tissue reconstruction at the MCP joint were generally not successful. Twenty-one out of 30 attempts at extensor tendon relocation resulted in recurrent flexion deformity. More success was achieved by performing MCP silicone arthroplasties. Thirteen of 17 patients gained 50° of motion and had correction of deformity.

This correction at the MCP joint will help to rebalance the forces of the PIP joint. If palmar stability is absent at the PIP joint, then a superficialis tenodesis can be performed. If there is lateral instability, then a collateral ligament reconstruction can be done in conjunction with MCP arthroplasty. The soft tissue restraining procedures are performed at the PIP joint as long as the joint surfaces are intact. If there has been post-traumatic destruction of the PIP joint surface, then arthrodesis in the proper position is indicated. In SLE, correction deformity of the MCP joint is mandatory before the surgeon can reasonably construct the PIP joint. If unstable, the PIP joint should be reconstructed early, prior to the post-traumatic degenerative changes which can occur with chronic subluxation.

SCLERODERMA (SYSTEMIC SCLEROSIS)

Scleroderma is a connective tissue disorder characterized by fibrosis and degenerative changes in the skin, synovium, digital arteries, and certain internal organs. Isolated scleroderma can be divided into a rapidly developing, often fatal visceral form and into an indolent and initially more limited form which is labelled the CREST syndrome (for calcinosis, Raynaud's phenomenon, oesophageal hypomotility, sclerodactyly, and telangiectasia (LeRoy 1985)). Peak onset is between 30 and 50 years of age, and the disease is approximately four times as common in women as in men. The aetiology of scleroderma is unknown. Injury to the endothelial cells of the small arteries and capillaries may initiate a reaction which results in increased permeability of vessels, intravascular coagulation, and luminal narrowing. Within the altered vessel, reactive fibrosis begins to occur. As the microscopic fibrosis develops, Raynaud's phenomenon, painless symmetrical oedema, and gradual thickening of the skin of the hand and fingers begins to be seen clinically (Rodnan 1979). These changes are often complicated by arthralgias and stiffness in the finger joints. Hand and finger involvement may be divided into two stages. In the early or oedematous stage, the patient will present with a general swelling of the digits (sausage digits) which is painless. The pitting oedema will interfere with normal motion and there may be complaints of morning stiffness. Most patients will have some degree of Raynaud's phenomenon, even at this early stage.

As the oedema and the initial inflammation subside, they are replaced by a fibrosis resulting in thickening and tightening of the skin. The skin becomes taut, shiny and indurated. Normal skin folds disappear. As the skin fibrosis progresses, joint motion decreases (Fig. 8.19). Typically, the MCP joint develops an extension contracture and the PIP joint, a flexion contracture. The thumb becomes adducted. The rate at which these changes occur is variable. In severe cases, the combination of MCP and PIP contractures result in a claw hand.

The joints themselves are not a major site of involvement of the disease. True inflammatory synovitis is rare (Rodnan 1979). Radiographically, there are no erosive changes in the MCP or PIP joints (Fig. 8.20). The aetiology of joint difficulties in the hand is linked to the presence of ever tightening skin and tendon structures resulting in secondary contracture. The tight skin overlying the bony prominences is particularly vulnerable to injury. The skin on the dorsal surface of the PIP joint will ulcerate if injured, and may not heal because of the pressure from the bone below. These ulcers are due to the pressure on the skin from the underlying bone and are not due to the Raynaud's phenomenon which causes the distal finger tip ulcerations. If the underlying PIP joint becomes exposed, a secondary pyarthrosis and osteomyelitis may develop resulting in destruction of the joint. The severely involved hand becomes almost functionless with fixed extension contractures at the MCP joint, fixed flexion contractures at the PIP joint, and chronic ulcers over the dorsum of the PIP joint. Contributing to loss of function are the painful distal ulcerations secondary to Raynaud's phenomenon and the commonly seen subcutaneous calcification occurring on the volar aspects of the terminal phalanges (see Fig. 8.20).

Medical treatment for this disease is limited. No drugs or combination of drugs have been proved to be of value in adequately controlled trials. No drug is generally accepted as being useful in preventing the deformity. In a large series of patients at the University of Pittsburgh, splinting has been unsuccessful in preventing or correcting joint contractures. Local steroid injections are not indicated. The only treatment for the severely deformed PIP joint is arthrodesis of the joint. This may be combined with resection arthroplasty of the MCP joint if all motion has been lost at the MCP.

The present author's initial exposure to scleroderma patients was prompted by the development of PIP pyarthrosis and secondary osteomyelitis in several scleroderma patients who had non-healing ulcers on the dorsum of the PIP joint. Debridement and primary arthrodesis were successful in these patients and offered relief of local pain and improved function. Arthrodesis of the PIP joint is now recommended prior to the development of chronic infection in patients with flexion contrac-

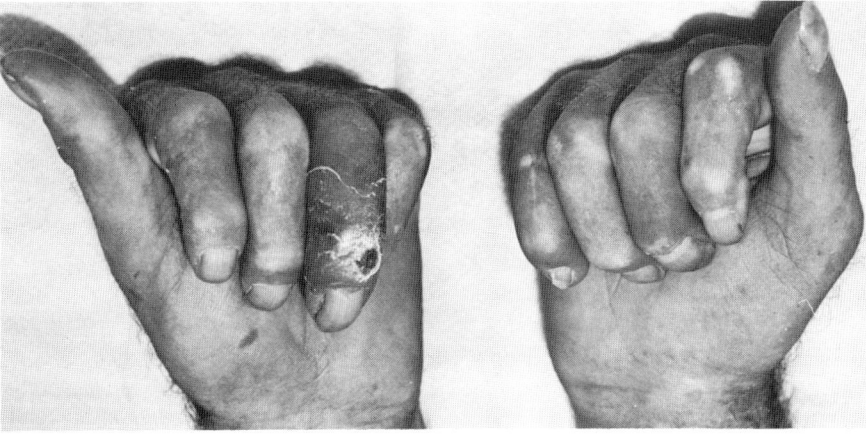

Fig. 8.19 Skin changes in a patient with scleroderma. Note the blanching of the skin over the PIP joint and the ulcer formation.

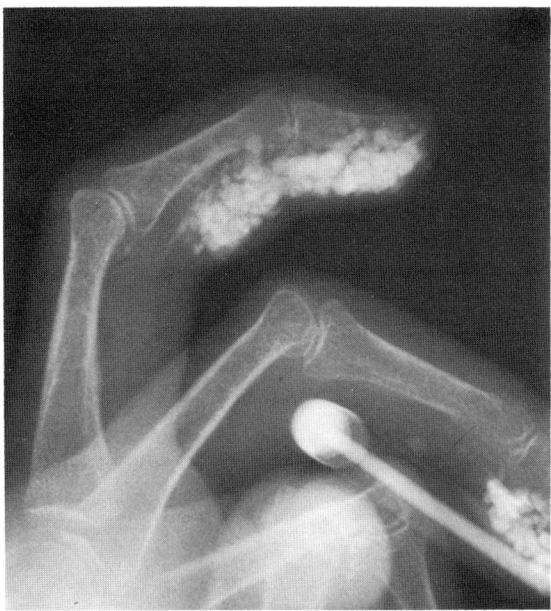

Fig. 8.20 X-ray of a patient with scleroderma. No erosive changes are present but subcutaneous calcification is severe.

tures of the PIP joint greater than 90° who complain of pain and decreased function or who have chronic non-healing ulcers over the dorsum of the joint. Technically, the very thin skin is peeled off the joint, and cartilage is removed. The proximal phalanx must be shortened to allow the skin to be closed and to place the arthrodesis in 55–60° of flexion, as recommended by Lipscomb et al (1969). The joint cannot be brought from a 90° flexion contracture to 55° without some shortening of the bone because of the severe palmar skin and tendon contracture. Internal fixation is achieved with two Kirschner wires which are left in for 6 weeks. The present author has performed this type of arthrodesis in 30 PIP joints of patients with scleroderma. Skin healing has not been a problem, and all joints have fused. Arthroplasty of the PIP joint in scleroderma is not recommended because the periarticular and peritendinous fibrosis would not allow a functional range of motion with the techniques that are presently available.

REFERENCES

Ansell B M, Harrison S H, Little H, Thomas B 1970 Synovectomy of proximal interphalangeal joints. British Journal of Plastic Surgery 23: 380–385

Backhouse K M, Kay A G L, Coomes E N, Kates A 1971 Tendon involvement in the rheumatoid hand. Annals of Rheumatic Disease 30: 236–242

Beckenbaugh R D 1977 New concepts in arthroplasty of the hand and wrist. Archives of Surgery 112: 1094–1098

Belsky M R, Feldon P, Millender L H, Nalebuff E A, Phillips C 1982 Hand involvement in psoriatic arthritis. Journal of Hand Surgery 7: 203–207

Bennett R M 1979 Psoriatic arthritis. In: McCarty D J (ed) Arthritis and allied conditions. Lea & Febiger, Philadelphia ch 43

Calabro J J 1979 Juvenile rheumatoid arthritis. In: McCarty D J (ed) Arthritis and allied conditions. Lea & Febiger, Philadelphia ch 39

Carroll R E, Hill N A 1969 Small joint arthrodesis in hand reconstruction. Journal of Bone and Joint Surgery 36A: 912–920

Cassidy J T 1985 Juvenile rheumatoid arthritis. In: Kelley W N, Harris E D, Ruddy S, Sledge C B (eds) Textbook of rheumatology. W B Saunders, Philadelphia ch 80

Chaplin D, Pulkki T, Saarimaa A, Vainio K 1969 Wrist and finger deformities in juvenile rheumatoid arthritis. Acta Rheumatologica Scandinavica 15: 206–233

Dray G J, Millender L H, Nalebuff E A, Phillips C 1981 The surgical treatment of hand deformities in systemic lupus erythematosus. Journal of Hand Surgery 6: 339–345

Eyring E J, Longert A, Bass J C 1971 Synovectomy in juvenile rheumatoid arthritis. Journal of Bone and Joint Surgery 53A: 638–651

Flatt A E 1983a Soft tissue disease—operative treatment. In: Care of the arthritic hand. 4th edn. C V Mosby, St Louis, ch 6

Flatt A E 1983b Digital joint disease—general considerations. In: Care of the arthritic hand. 4th edn. C V Mosby, St Louis, ch 7

Flatt A E 1983c Joint disease—operative treatment. In: Care of the arthritic hand. 4th edn. C V Mosby, St Louis, ch 8

Granberry W M, Mangum G L 1980 The hand in the child with juvenile rheumatoid arthritis. Journal of Hand Surgery 5: 105–113

Granowitz S, Vainio K 1966 Proximal interphalangeal joint arthrodesis in rheumatoid arthritis. Acta Orthopaedica Scandinavica 37: 301–310

Gschwend N 1985 Synovectomy. In: Kelley W N, Harris E D, Ruddy S, Sledge C B (eds) Textbook of rheumatology. W B Saunders, Philadelphia, ch 113

Helal B 1975 Extra articular causes of proximal interphalangeal joint stiffness in rheumatoid arthritis. Hand 7: 37–40

LeRoy E C 1985 Scleroderma (systemic sclerosis). In: Kelley W N, Harris E D, Ruddy S, Sledge C B (eds) Textbook of rheumatology. W B Saunders, Philadelphia, ch 76

Lipscomb P R 1971 Is early synovectomy of the small joints of the hand worthwhile? In: Cramer L M, Chase R A (eds) Symposium on the Hand C V Mosby, St Louis, ch 3, p 29

Lipscomb P R, Simons G W, Winkleman R K 1969 Surgery for sclerodactylia of the hand: experience with six cases. Journal of Bone and Joint Surgery 51A: 1112

Millender L H, Nalebuff E A 1975 Surgical treatment of the swan-neck deformity in rheumatoid arthritis. Orthopedic Clinics of North America 6: 733–752

Millender L H, Nalebuff E A, Feldon P F 1982 Rheumatoid arthritis. In: Green D P (ed) Operative hand surgery. Churchill Livingstone, New York, ch 37

Moberg E 1960 Arthrodesis of finger joints. Surgical Clinics of North America 40: 465–470

Raunio P 1977 Prophylactic value of synovectomy of the proximal interphalangeal joint in rheumatoid arthritis. Scandinavian Journal of Rheumatology 6 (Suppl. 19): 1–88

Roberts M E T, Wright V, Hill A G S, Mehra A C 1976 Psoriatic arthritis. Annals of Rheumatoid Diseases 35: 206–212

Rodnan G P 1979 Scleroderma, calcinosis, and eosinophilic fasciitis. In: McCarty D J (ed) Arthritis and allied conditions. Lea & Febiger, Philadelphia, ch 6

Rothfield N 1979 Systemic lupus erythematosus: clinical and laboratory aspects. In: McCarty D J (ed) Arthritis and allied conditions. Lea & Febiger, Philadelphia, ch 6

Rothfield N 1985 Clinical features of systemic lupus erythematosus. In: Kelley W N, Harris E D, Ruddy S, Sledge C B (ed) Textbook of rheumatology. W B Saunders, Philadelphia, ch 69

Swanson A B 1973a Proximal interphalangeal and metacarpophalangeal joint flexible implant arthroplasty results. In: Flexible implant arthroplasty in the hand and extremities. C V Mosby, St Louis, ch 11, p 184–207

Swanson A B 1973b Surgical procedures for destroyed interphalangeal joints. In: Flexible implant arthroplasty in the hand and extremities. C V Mosby, St Louis, ch 9, p 160–170

Wilde A H 1974 Synovectomy of the proximal interphalangeal joint of the finger in rheumatoid arthritis. Journal of Bone and Joint Surgery 56A: 71–78

Wissinger H A 1971 Digital flexor lag in rheumatoid arthritis. Journal of Plastic and Reconstructive Surgery 47: 465–468

Wright V 1985 Psoriatic arthritis. In: Kelley W N, Harris E D, Ruddy S, Sledge C B (eds) Textbook of rheumatology. W B Saunders, Philadelphia, ch 66

Dean S. Louis

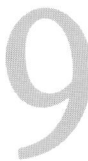

Degenerative arthritis and allied conditions involving the interphalangeal joints

OSTEOARTHRITIS—DEGENERATIVE ARTHRITIS

Biochemistry

The cartilage that covers the ends of the bones forming the adjacent sides of a joint appears to serve two purposes. The congruent mating of the surfaces allows for the smooth gliding of one surface upon the other and, in addition, allows for the distribution of load across the joint.

The chemical composition of normal articular cartilage is quite complex (Brandt 1981). The cellular composition and the macromolecular constituents of the extracellular ground substance are largely responsible for the biomechanical functioning of the joints. The major macromolecules that comprise articular cartilage are collagen and proteoglycans. Collagen accounts for about 50% and proteoglycans for about 10% of the dry weight of articular cartilage. The proteoglycans consist of protein bound to either keratin sulphate or chondroitin sulphate (glycosaminoglycans). The composition of articular cartilage varies from the surface of the joint to the subchondral level so that the relative proportions of these macromolecules may be different from level to level. This variation may be genetically determined or depend upon allied stress. It does not appear to correlate with age or sex. The hydrophilic nature of these macromolecules accounts for the observation that water represents some 70–80% of the total weight of articular cartilage.

Collagen, like the proteoglycans, is not evenly distributed throughout the depth of the cartilage. The proteoglycans, with this high water content, appear to supply resistance to compression, while the collagen appears to provide tensile strength. These constituents of articular cartilage are all synthesized by the chondrocyte which is believed to receive its nutrition from the synovial fluid. Studies in dogs suggest that joint motion is necessary for the satisfactory nutrition of joint cartilage. Prolonged joint immobilization may lead to cartilage degradation and even joint ankylosis (Palmoski et al 1979).

The major biochemical alteration that is measurable in osteoarthritic joints has been the loss of proteoglycans, while the collagen content remains the same (Mankin & Lipiello 1970).

In the canine model, after section of the anterior cruciate ligament, a series of interesting changes occur (McDevitt & Muir 1976). The first of these is an observable increase in the water content of the cartilage. Following this change, there is an alteration in the proteoglycan composition of the subsequently formed macromolecules. There is then a change such that a higher proportion of chondroitin sulphate and a lower proportion of keratin sulphate than normal are noted. These events occur prior to any noticeable morphological change. Subsequent events in this model included cartilage fibrillation, and a decrease in water content.

These latter changes may lead to a loss of compressive stiffness and elasticity of the cartilage, setting in motion the sequence of events that leads to symptomatic osteoarthritis. The aetiology of the subsequent development of marginal osteophytes is still a matter for conjecture (Bland & Stulberg 1981).

Aetiology

The use of the term osteoarthritis (OA) in this chapter is an arbitrary choice by the author, used with the full understanding that some workers prefer the term degenerative joint disease (DJD). Inasmuch as the exact aetiology or aetiologies of osteoarthritis are unknown at this time, any term used to designate the process will carry with it an implied uncertainty.

Clearly all of those structures that comprise a joint—bone, cartilage, synovium, ligaments and musculotendinous units—have a role in the development and progression of OA. Which structures are primarily involved, which ones are early silent witnesses and then later become involved actively is not clearly known at present.

Some researchers believe that wear and tear, as cited in the canine model, is the cause of the observed morphological changes (McDevitt & Muir 1976). Others believe that the process is one of degeneration as the result of a natural ageing process. In addition, hereditary, metabolic, nutritional and biomechanical factors may have an aetiological role in the development of OA. The structural integrity of a joint is clearly necessary for its normal function. Major trauma to the interphalangeal joints is the one recognized and undisputed cause of osteoarthritic change that follows such intra-articular alterations.

There are no serological tests that are confirmatory of the diagnosis of osteoarthritis.

Clinical presentation

The clinical presentation of OA in the interphalangeal joints is that of swelling, which may represent the presence of synovitis as well as osteophyte formation, or a combination of the two. This may be painful or at times remarkably painless in the presence of very significant clinical and radiographic joint deformity. The swelling observed at the distal interphalangeal joints is referred to as Heberden's nodes (Fig. 9.1) and as Bouchard's nodes (Fig. 9.2) when involving the proximal interphalangeal joints. The changes associated with post-traumatic degenerative arthritis of the interphalangeal joints differ from those of degenerative joint disease in that there is a history of acute or chronic trauma, and the changes tend to be isolated to the specific joints so injured, as opposed to the generalized forms of degenerative joint disease which involve similar joints, i.e. proximal or distal, or both, in a relatively symmetrical pattern bilaterally (Staple 1984).

Management

The management of DJD and post-traumatic arthritis is dependent upon many variables. Such

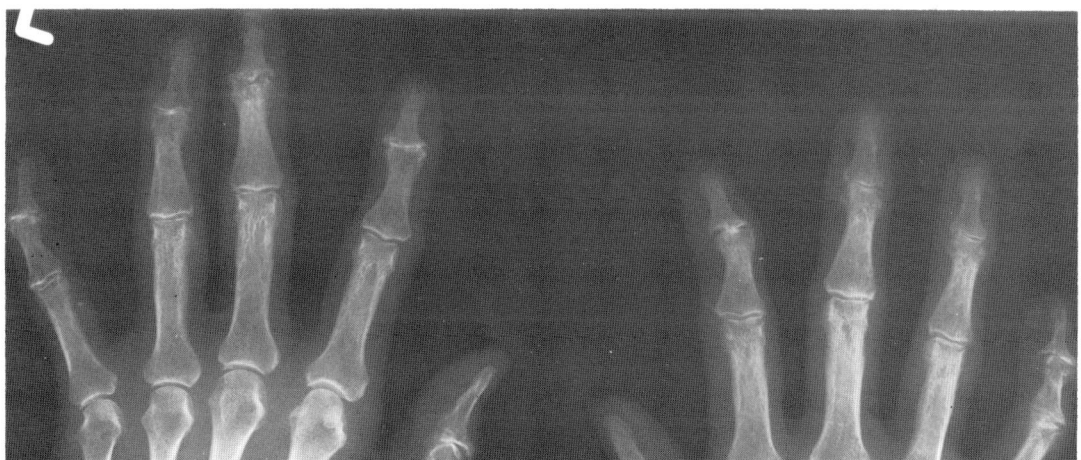

Fig. 9.1 Osteoarthritis—Heberden's nodes. Multiple levels of degenerative change with joint space narrowing, osteophyte formation, and sclerosis can be seen in these radiographs. They are most prominent at the distal interphalangeal joints. The changes can also be seen at the carpometacarpal joints of the thumbs and at the proximal interphalangeal joint of the right little finger. The distal interphalangeal swelling seen most prominently here on both index fingers is indicative of the clinical observation referred to as Heberden's nodes.

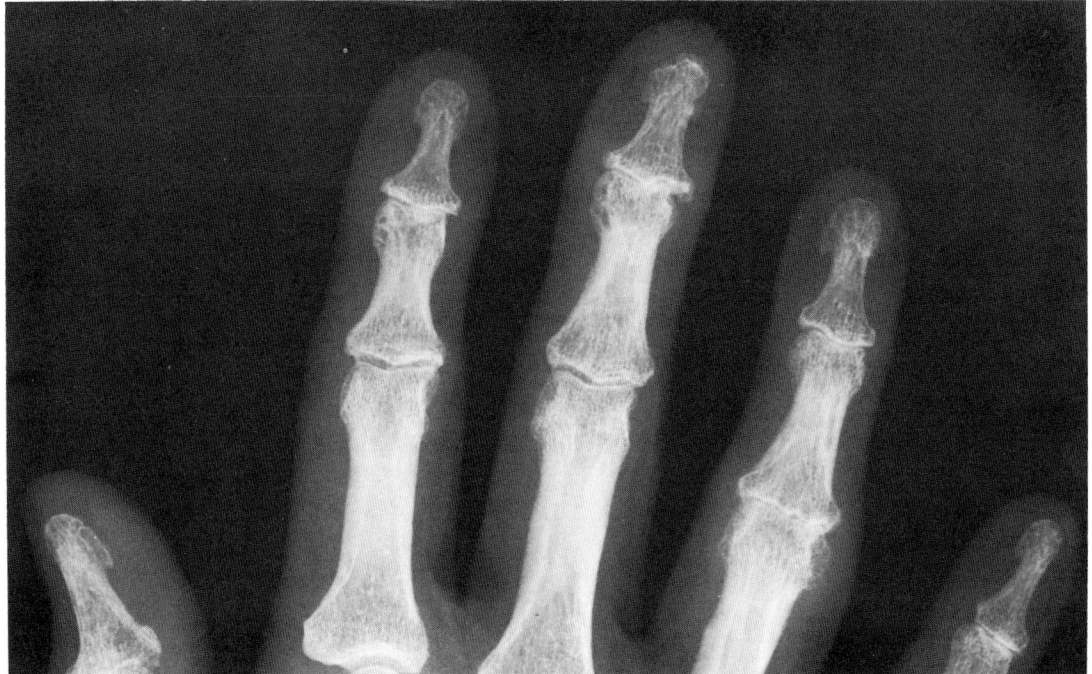

Fig. 9.2 Osteoarthritis—Bouchard's nodes. This radiograph is similar to the one seen in Figure 9.1 and shows degenerative changes present throughout the distal interphalangeal joints. There is also, however, narrowing of the ulnar three proximal interphalangeal joints, most prominently involving the ring finger with the soft tissue enlargement referred to as Bouchard's nodes.

factors are age, the joint or joints involved, the severity of symptoms, and the association of other illnesses, and all may have an influence upon the therapeutic modalities selected in the individual situation. Acetylsalicylic acid, selective splinting, and activity modification are the cornerstones of the early management of these afflictions. When symptoms persist following the use of these methods, any one of the expanding group of non-steroidal anti-inflammatory agents may be used. When non-operative methods have failed, either because of the persistence of symptoms or the presence of significant functional deformity, then operative methods may be indicated. For distal interphalangeal joint involvement, arthrodesis is the method of choice. The techniques involved are discussed in Chapter 13.

From a functional point of view, the loss of distal interphalangeal motion that occurs following arthrodesis is not a severe disability for most individuals. The pain ablation and stability that occur following these procedures may functionally improve the hand which is severely affected with degenerative joint disease. Resection or soft tissue interposition arthroplasty (Carroll & Taber 1954), silicone interposition arthroplasty (Swanson 1973), and arthrodesis (Carroll & Hill 1969) are all applicable methods for management of the affected proximal interphalangeal joint. Soft tissue interposition arthroplasties tend to preserve motion, but lack effective joint stabilization. Silicone interposition arthroplasty, on the other hand, preserves stability as well as motion, and may also effectively alleviate symptoms. Implant breakage, bony atrophy, with collapse of the phalanges about the implant, and silicone synovitis (Smith et al 1985) are all potential problems associated with the use of these devices. In carefully selected patients, however, these implants may last for many years and effectively preserve useful function for a long period of time. In the present author's opinion, there is no current indication for the use of implants that are stabilized by means of polymethyl methacrylate in the management of proximal interphalangeal joint problems. Almost all of the implants of this type have been removed from the market. With the use of silicone interposition arthroplasty technique, should removal be necessary, salvage may be obtained by means of an arthrodesis performed with the use of a bone graft. The necessity for removal of a large amount of bone with the implantation of the cemented prostheses makes retrievability, i.e. arthrodesis, following the removal of one of these implants with its cement, a most formidable surgical task.

Arthrodesis at the proximal interphalangeal joint will effectively eliminate pain and provide stability. However, the loss of motion at this level when arthrodesis is performed is a far greater functional disability than when distal interphalangeal joint arthrodesis is performed. If a single, proximal interphalangeal joint is fused, it will impair the function of the entire hand with grasping activities. When all of the proximal interphalangeal joints are fused, this problem may be compounded. Arthrodesis of the interphalangeal joint of the thumb can effectively improve pinch and grasp when pain and/or instability have been the predominant symptoms. The benefits of such a procedure when the more proximal joints of the thumb are involved with the process is of questionable merit. Arthroplasty of the carpometacarpal joint or at the metacarpophalangeal joint, preserving motion at one or the other level, would be preferable. Fusing the metacarpophalangeal joint of the thumb in the presence of a trapezium implant arthroplasty creates a long lever arm that favours dislocation of such an implant.

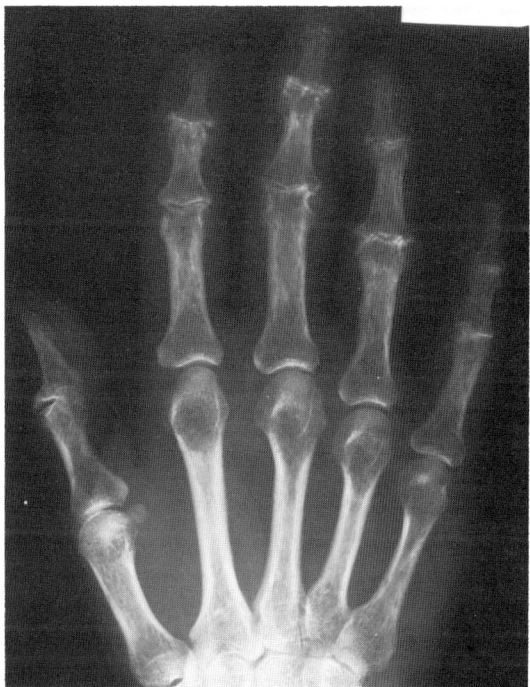

Fig. 9.3 Erosive osteoarthritis. The changes exhibited on this X-ray where there is involvement of both distal and proximal interphalangeal joints and erosive changes seen marginally most prominently on the ulnar side of the proximal interphalangeal joints of the index, middle and ring fingers, is indicative of erosive osteoarthritis. The presence of the erosions, along with the clinical features of painful symmetrical involvement involving only the hand in young or middle-aged women, are the distinguishing characteristics of erosive osteoarthritis from osteoarthritis. However, there is not universal agreement among radiologists and rheumatologists as to the actual existence of this as a separate distinct entity from osteoarthritis.

EROSIVE OSTEOARTHRITIS

Erosive osteoarthritis is primarily a disease that affects the distal and proximal interphalangeal joint of middle-aged women (Swezey & Alexander 1971). It tends to be more rapidly progressive than OA. The acute inflammatory episodes are accompanied by severe pain and may ultimately lead to bony ankylosis. The erosive changes and the lack of sclerosis and osteophyte formation clearly distinguish this radiographically from the more common OA (Fig. 9.3). A recent study by Keats et al (1981) indicates that there may be an association of erosive changes in other large joints, such as the humeral head and the hip, in association with the hand involvement of erosive osteoarthritis. Roh et al (1973) have suggested that classical OA as seen in the hands may also be associated with osteoarthritic changes in the hip to a far greater degree than such hip involvement occurs in the population at large. It would appear that there is a broad spectrum of the presentation of these changes in the hands (Gold et al 1982), that there may be associated involvement of other joints, and that the same is true of both OA and erosive OA. The realm of treatment options that is available for the surgical management of erosive osteoarthritis is similar to that which is applicable in OA. A greater degree of subluxation and loss of bone stock, however, makes arthroplasty procedures less desir-

146 THE INTERPHALANGEAL JOINTS

able and arthrodesis a more suitable option. As with OA, there are no diagnostic laboratory tests.

INFECTIONS

A variety of infections may involve the interphalangeal joints in the hand (Linscheid & Dobyns 1975). Such infections, however, are far less common than those which involve the overlying soft tissues. Pyogenic infections involving organisms such as *Staphylococcus aureus* and *Streptococcus* are most commonly the result of either open wounds to the joint involved (Fig. 9.4), or due to direct inoculation as a result of penetrating injuries. They may also occur as the result of extension from neglected soft tissue infections, such as a paronychia or felon (Fig. 9.5). Infections involving Gram-negative organisms are almost always the result of direct contamination. Infections in drug addicts may be particularly troublesome in that they are often polymicrobial in nature and develop in non-compliant individuals in digits with previously impaired circulatory status (Fig. 9.6). Tuberculosis and atypical mycobacteria, such as *Mycobacterium marinum*, occasionally will involve the interphalangeal joints (Williams & Riordan 1973). Fungal infections such as coccidioidomycosis (Thorpe & Spjut 1985), sporotrichosis (Manhart et al 1970), and rarely blastomycosis may be seen involving the hand and even more unusually involving the joints.

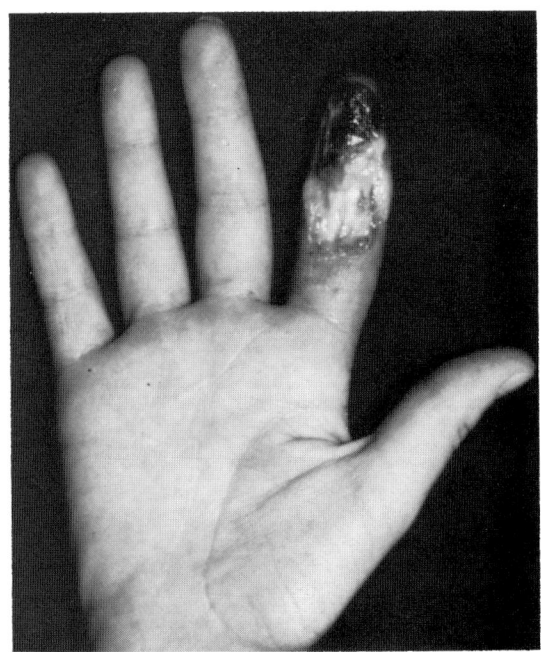

Fig. 9.5 Pyarthrosis. This is another example of an untreated, penetrating injury which occurred when this child was bitten by a pig. The wound was ignored and progressive separation occurred, leading to not only destruction of the joint, but ultimate loss of the finger.

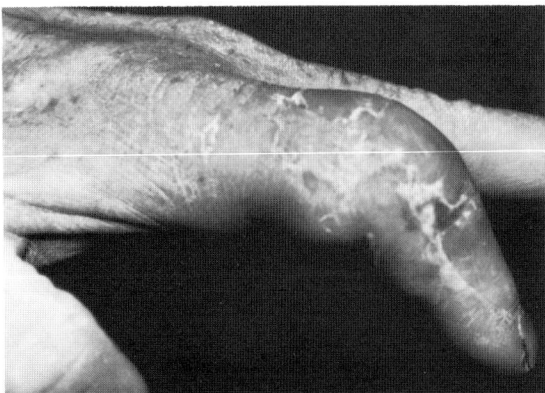

Fig. 9.4 Pyarthrosis. Untreated, penetrating injuries to the interphalangeal joints may lead to severe pyarthrosis and/or osteomyelitis, as seen in this clinical example of an injury that occurred in a barnyard and was polymicrobial in nature. The ultimate result here was marked limitation of motion with loss of cartilage space.

When such infections occur, they most frequently involve tenosynovial tissue, and secondarily extend to involve bone. The diagnosis in all of these circumstances can be made on the basis of the history, physical findings and appropriate radiographs, additionally supplemented by appropriate cultures of joint fluid or synovial tissue.

Most pyogenic infections are evident by an appreciation of the historical data, and the rapidly progressive nature of the tissue destruction. A joint so involved should be thoroughly debrided and left open.

Access is best obtained by a dorsal approach to the joint. In the case of the distal interphalangeal joint a transverse incision at the joint line will expose the extensor tendon. Retraction of the tendon alternately towards the midline of the digit will allow the bulging synovium to be opened on both sides dorsally, permitting drainage. If further exposure is needed, the incision may be extended proximally on one side of the transverse incision and distally on the other. The extensor tendon may then be further retracted for additional access. If

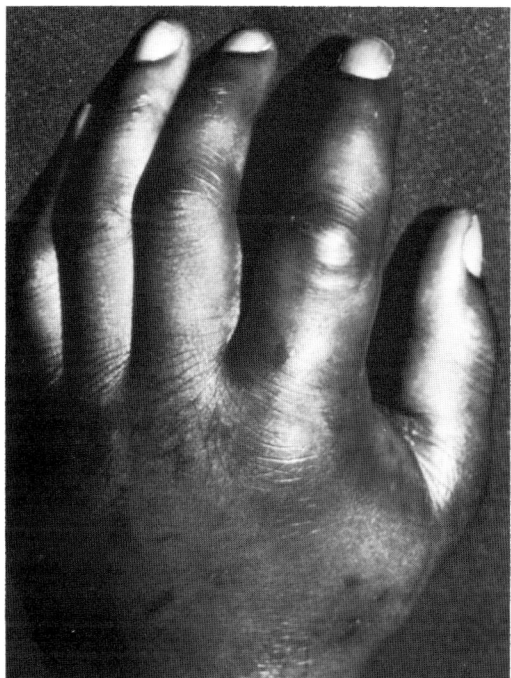

Fig. 9.6 Infection—drug addict. Multiple scars on the dorsum of the left hand of this drug addict are a clue to his addiction. Twenty-two hours previously he had injected a narcotic substance into the dorsum of his index finger directly over the proximal interphalangeal joint. The previous destruction of venous and lymphatic channels led to the ultimate loss of this finger. Early and aggressive therapy with hospitalization and intravenous antibiotics is usually indicated under these circumstances.

deemed necessary the extensor tendon may be divided for a more thorough debridement. Usually, however, a complete irrigation after a Gram stain and culture have been obtained is sufficient. A drain or drains are appropriate for the first 24 h. After this period, the drains are removed and local wound care is instituted. As the infection subsides, the wound will heal satisfactorily by means of secondary intention.

Most street-acquired infections of the hand are resistant to penicillin (Bell 1976). It is therefore proper to begin treatment with intravenous cephalosporins. After definite cultures and sensitivities have been obtained, a change of antibiotics may be indicated. In the case where the initial Gram stain reveals Gram-negative bacteria, one of the aminoglycosides would be appropriate.

Exposure to the proximal interphalangeal joint is made through a gently curved incision that extends from the middle of the proximal phalanx dorsally to the middle of the middle phalanx. Access to the joint is obtained by making parallel incisions on either side of the lateral band of sufficient length to enter the joint. Gram stain, cultures, irrigation, debridement and packing open, as with the distal joint, should follow.

When taking cultures of an unknown infection, especially one that is indolent and chronic, it is important to obtain cultures for mycobacteria, both acid-fast and atypical, and to also culture the material for fungi.

In the case of human bites, *Eikenella corrodens* (Bilos et al 1978) has been a frequent cause of a particularly fulminating infection which may cause extensive cartilage destruction and may even progress to osteomyelitis. This Gram-negative bacteria has fastidious cultural requirements, in particular its growth may be enhanced by increased carbon dioxide concentration in the range of 5–15%.

Pasturella multocida (Lucas & Bartlett 1981) is found in the oral flora of 70% of domestic cats and dogs. It may also lead to a fulminating infection (Fig. 9.7). It is also a Gram-negative bacillus. It may be confused with *Haemophilus influenzae* or *Neisseria* species. When a wound from an animal bite is cultured, the laboratory should be alerted to look for *Pasturella* species. Both *Pasturella* and *Eikenella* are sensitive to penicillin.

When a pyarthrosis has been drained and there has been sufficient resolution of the accompanying soft tissue inflammation, early motion should be begun. The timing of this protected early motion is best considered on an individual basis. It should be remembered, however, that the periarticular structures, including ligaments, tendons, subcutaneous tissue and skin are involved in the inflammatory process. Prolonged immobilization will lead to joint stiffness, even when the articular damage has been minimal. Surgical drainage, appropriate antibiotic treatment and early range of motion are the order of the day for these potentially disabling afflictions. The institution of motion does not need to be preceded by complete wound healing.

As with infections elsewhere, the diagnosis should be based upon a culture of the aspirate from

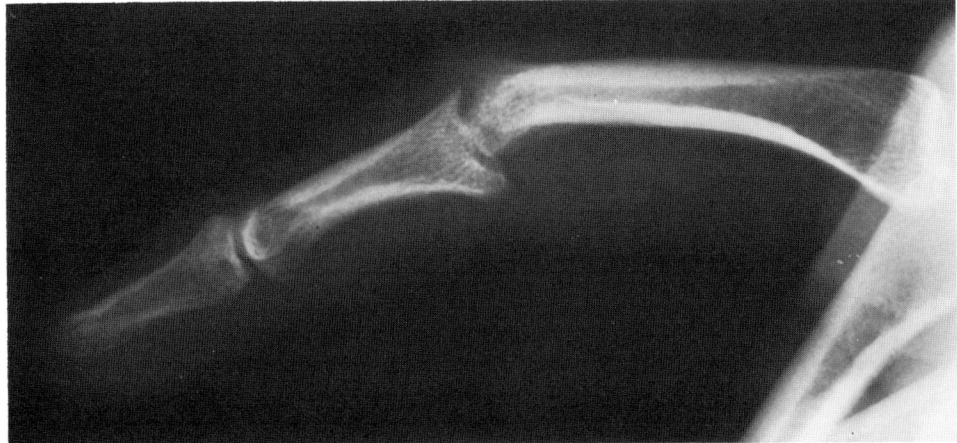

Fig. 9.7 *Pasteurella multocida* pyarthrosis. This 35-year-old right-handed woman was bitten over the area of her proximal interphalangeal joint by a neighbour's cat. This wound was given only local treatment and when swelling ensued, only aspirations of the joint occurred rather than a formal drainage. The patient went on to develop the joint destruction seen here, and ultimately underwent arthrodesis.

the joint and/or tissue obtained at the time of arthrotomy and debridement.

Bell (1976) compared 400 cases of pyogenic hand infection treated in 1947 with a group of similar cases treated in 1974. There were two cases of septic arthritis in 1947 and only one in 1974, indicating the rarity of joint infections when contrasted to the total number of infections in the hand.

GOUT

Definition

Gout is a term which refers to a group of diseases characterized by an elevated serum uric acid concentration; acute attacks of arthritis in which crystals of monosodium urate monohydrate are found in leucocytes in the synovial fluid; and soft tissue deposits of urate crystals about the joints which may lead to severe deformities. There may also be severe renal involvement, impairing all parts of the renal parenchyma and also renal lithiasis (Kelley 1981).

Clinical presentation

Gout is described as progressing through four stages: (1) asymptomatic hyperuricaemia; (2) acute gouty arthritis; (3) intercritical gout; and (4) chronic tophaceous gout.

The problems with tophaceous gout as seen in earlier times fortunately are no longer with us. Occasionally, however, patients will present who have either been non-compliant with their pharmacological regimen, or who have not sought medical attention (Fig. 9.8). Such patients will be seen with involvement of multiple areas in the hand and wrist including the interphalangeal joints (Watt & Middlemiss 1975, Ray & Bassett 1985)

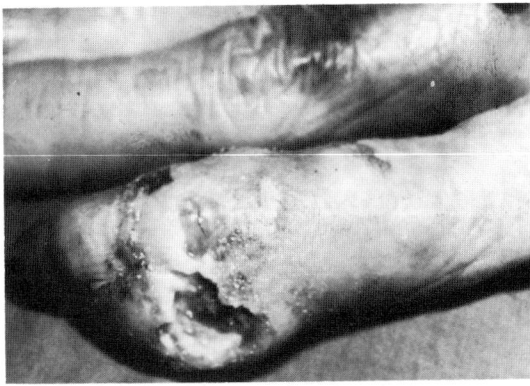

Fig. 9.8 Gout. This 90-year-old woman was brought in by her family because of this erosive lesion involving the distal interphalangeal joint of her index finger. The tophus had eroded through the skin and then become secondarily infected. The distal phalanx and the distal interphalangeal joint were completely destroyed as a result of the deposition of the sodium monourate deposits.

(Fig. 9.9). Involvement of these areas, however, is far less common than involvement of the lower extremities, where the most frequent occurrence is in the metatarsophalangeal joint of the great toe, and then the more proximal joints of the foot and ankle. When a patient presents with untreated tophaceous gout, surgical removal of the deposits may be helpful. The major indications for such

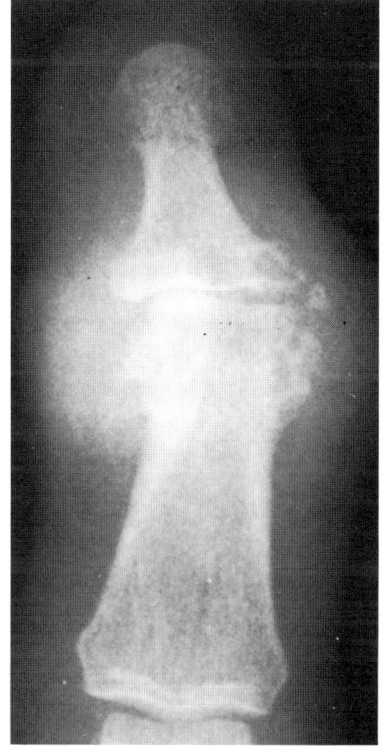

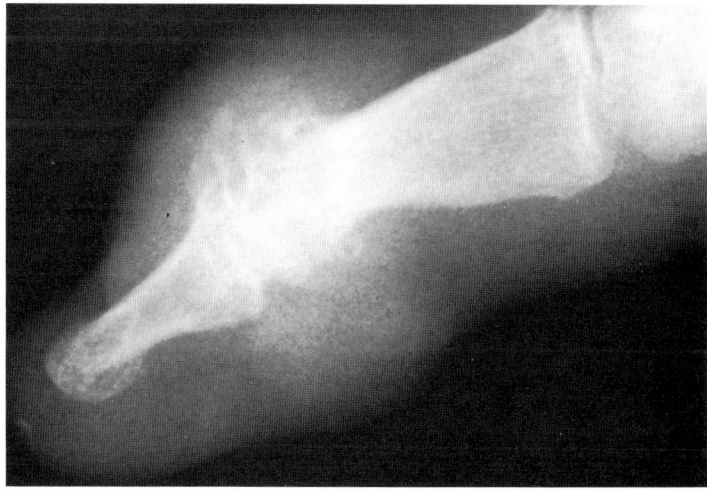

Fig. 9.9 Gout (**a**) This is the distal interphalangeal joint of a 65-year-old man with chronic renal disease and secondary gout. He had multiple tophaceous deposits over his body. The soft tissue aggregations of urate crystals debris are shown in the periarticular region which is partially osseous and marked joint space narrowing, characteristic in far advanced stages as seen here. (**b**) This is a lateral view of the same digit, demonstrating the extensive involvement.

surgery are the failure of resolution of tophaceous deposits under responsible medical management combined with a significant functional limitation of motion. The current use of xanthine oxidase inhibitors and uricosuric agents has made such surgery uncommon except for certain particular situations, as mentioned above and as follows.

In particular, patients with renal disease or allergies to allopurinol may not mobilize tophaceous deposits and thus they may benefit from the surgical excision of the tophaceous deposits. When tophaceous gout is far advanced (Fig. 9.10), there may be intra-articular destruction of the joint requiring arthrodesis. In less advanced cases, the tophaceous deposits may limit joint motion solely by their bulk. Surgical excision of such deposits is not as easy as it might seem initially. There may be extensive involvement of the collateral ligaments and the extensor mechanism as well as the subcutaneous tissue and the skin. The infiltrative nature of these chalk-like deposits makes them extremely difficult to extirpate and requires diligent persistence. Gelberman et al (1980) found it necessary to operate on only two of seven patients with proximal interphalangeal joint involvement which were refractory to medical treatment.

CRYSTALLINE DEPOSITION DISEASE

The intra-articular and extra-articular deposition of sodium urate crystals in gout is the most frequently seen crystalline deposition disease. Calcium pyrophosphate crystals can also cause articular disease presenting as acute and/or chronic arthropathies. In addition, more recent descriptions have included hydroxyapatite crystalline deposition which may cause intra- and extra-articular deposition as well (Howell 1981) (Fig. 9.11). Deposition of these crystalline deposits in and about joints is an infrequent clinical problem, but one which has received increasing attention (Greene & Louis 1980). Involvement of the interphalangeal joints is infrequent although it has been reported. Symptomatic as well as asymptomatic forms of these diseases exist and may be seen in association with numerous other diseases, in particular pseudogout may be seen in conjunction with gout, and other metabolic diseases, such as haemochromatosis and hyperparathyroidism.

The definitive diagnosis in the crystalline deposition disorders, i.e. calcium pyrophosphate deposition disease and hydroxyapatite deposition disease, is based upon recovery of the crystals from the joint synovial fluid or from a synovial biopsy. The radiographic findings in both conditions are similar with peri-articular calcification, joint space diminution, and periarticular erosive changes (Bonavita et al 1980). Multiple other joints may also be involved, including the knees, intercarpal joints, and the distal radioulnar joint.

Treatment in the acute cases is primarily pharmacological with therapeutic doses of phenylbutazone being particularly effective for those individuals who can tolerate the medication. In the event that the patient is unable to tolerate phenylbutazone, then the non-steroidal anti-inflammatory medications are helpful. Joint aspiration has also been reported to give symptomatic relief in acute episodes. Surgery is infrequently indicated.

Haemochromatosis

Idiopathic haemochromatosis is a disorder of iron metabolism which results in deposition of iron throughout many organs in the body. It ultimately leads to deposition of iron deposits within the liver with resulting cirrhosis. Liver biopsy is the definitive diagnostic procedure. Radiographic features of haemochromatosis are chondrocalcinosis (Twersky 1975) and a unique degenerative arthritis (Hirsch et al 1976). Radiographically, changes in the hands most frequently involve the metacarpo-

---

Fig. 9.10 Gout. (**a**) Multiple areas of tophaceous accumulation can be seen in the clinical photograph of this 72-year-old man's hands. Swelling about the wrists and over the metacarpophalangeal joints is suggestive of the inflammatory synovitis and tenosynovitis that is so characteristic of rheumatoid arthritis. (**b**) The radiograph of the same hand demonstrates, however, a rather atypical involvement for rheumatoid arthritis. The metacarpophalangeal joints are relatively spared with the exception of the cystic formation evident on the right small finger. The proximal interphalangeal joints had joint narrowing and erosive changes about the joints with soft tissue accumulation of sodium urate deposits seen most prominently on the radial side of the left index finger here and on the ulnar side of the right index finger. This distribution is characteristic of gouty arthropathy, as are the changes seen on the radiographs.

DEGENERATIVE ARTHRITIS AND ALLIED CONDITIONS 151

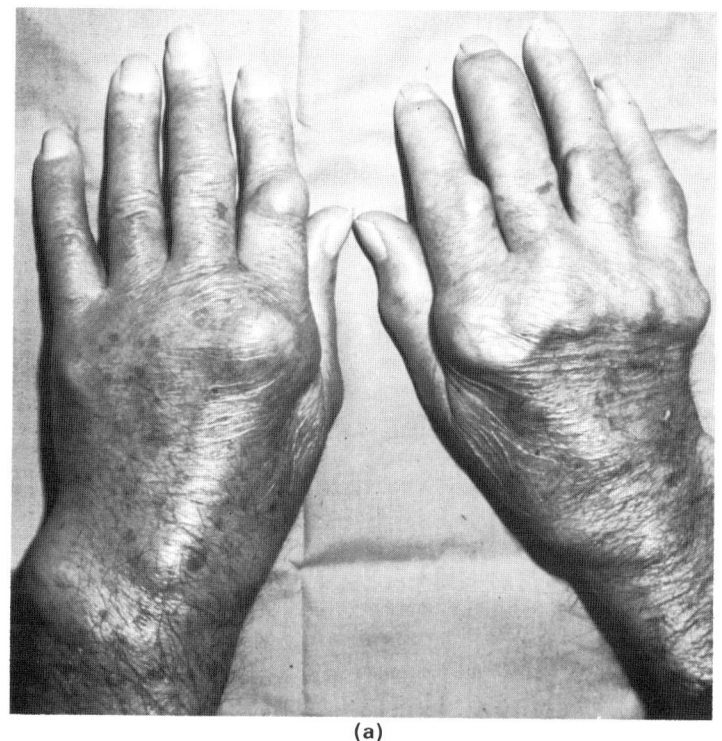

(a)

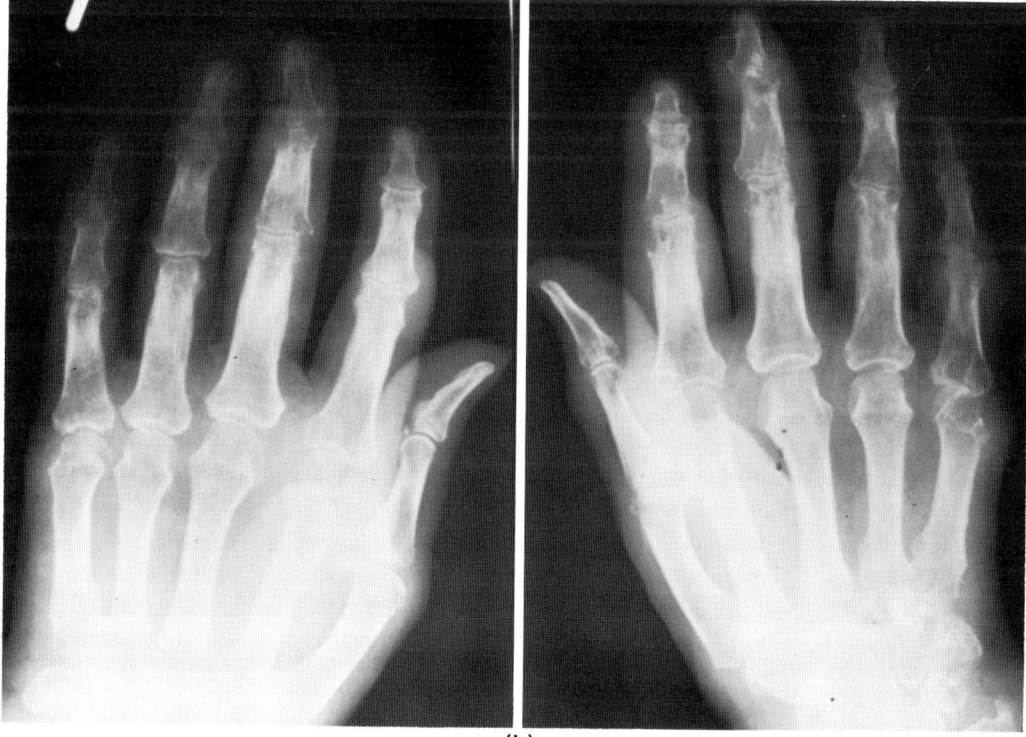

(b)

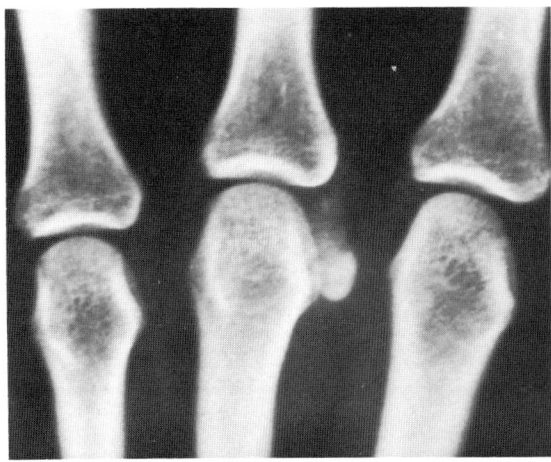

Fig. 9.11 Hydroxyapatite deposition disease. This 35-year-old woman developed acute swelling about her left middle finger metacarpophalangeal joint. The overlying cutaneous changes simulated an acute infectious process. Aspiration was carried out and 4 ml of a chalky white fluid were removed. This material was subsequently identified as hydroxyapatite crystals.

phalangeal joints, but there may be involvement of the interphalangeal joints as well (Fig. 9.12). Calcification of the articular cartilage may be seen and there may be peripheral erosions and a rather diffuse osteopenia. The management of this arthropathy is symptomatic and like the previously mentioned conditions above, surgery is infrequently indicated.

RENAL ARTHROPATHY

Hamilton & Knickerbocker (1982) have recently reviewed the radiographs of 72 patients undergoing haemodialysis for chronic renal failure. Fifteen, or 20% of their patients, showed periarticular erosions in their hands. All of these patients were asymptomatic with regard to the erosions. Twenty additional patients showed evidence of subperiosteal resorption consistent with secondary hyperparathyroidism. With increasing numbers of patients undergoing treatment for chronic renal disease, these observations may be pertinent in the future if the conditions do become symptomatic.

POST-TRAUMATIC ARTHRITIS

Traumatic injuries to the proximal interphalangeal joints are relatively common. They may occur

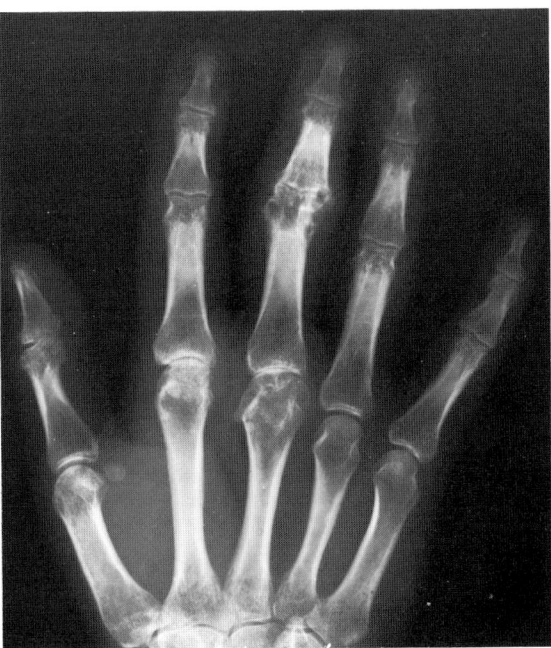

Fig. 9.12 Haemochromatosis. The arthropathy of haemochromatosis has a distribution which is atypical for any of the major, more common arthropathies. The distribution is quite asymmetrical and involves multiple joint levels. Involvement of distal as well as proximal interphalangeal joints is shown with joint narrowing. In addition there is joint narrowing involving the metacarpophalangeal joints, here most prominently seen in the index and long fingers. Calcium pyrophosphate crystal deposition is not always seen radiographically in this disease process, but can be recovered from the synovium by biopsy or sometimes by aspiration.

during a variety of activities including occupational, industrial, and recreational activities. Chapters 4, 5, and 6 detail the panorama of these injuries, in their acute form. There is surprisingly little follow-up of these injuries of a sufficient long-term nature to prognosticate as to which ones will ultimately lead to post-traumatic degenerative changes. In an attempt to evaluate this aspect of the problem, Benke & Stableforth (1979) reviewed 96 joint injuries with an average follow-up of 11 months. Their results were evaluated on the basis of range of motion, stability, symptoms, and function. They divided their patients into three groups: those in group I had a hyperextension-dorsal dislocation but no associated fracture; in group II there was an associated small volar lip fracture at the base of the middle phalanx (Fig. 9.13); those patients in group III had fracture dislocations. Fifty-five per cent of their patients

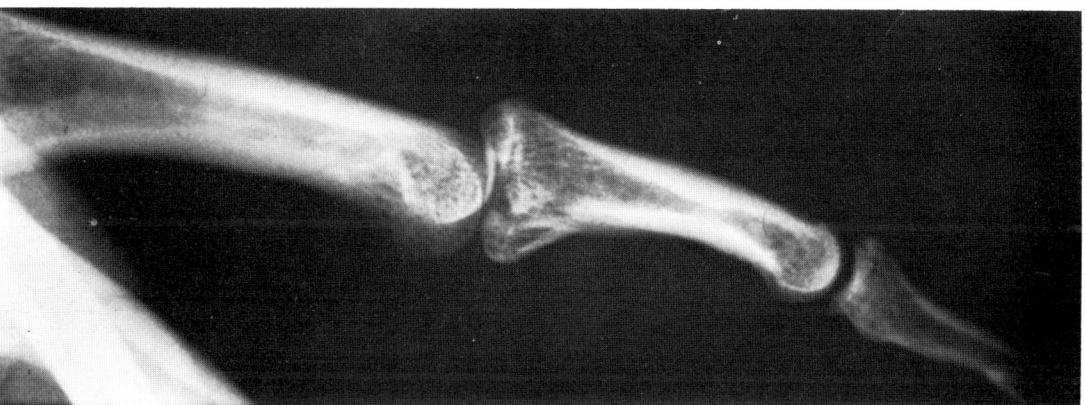

Fig. 9.13 Trauma. This individual sustained a jamming injury to the proximal interphalangeal joint and did not seek treatment until many months later. The incongruous relationship of the joint surfaces is evident. Left unreconstructed, progressive degenerative changes as seen in Figure 9.14 would inevitably ensue.

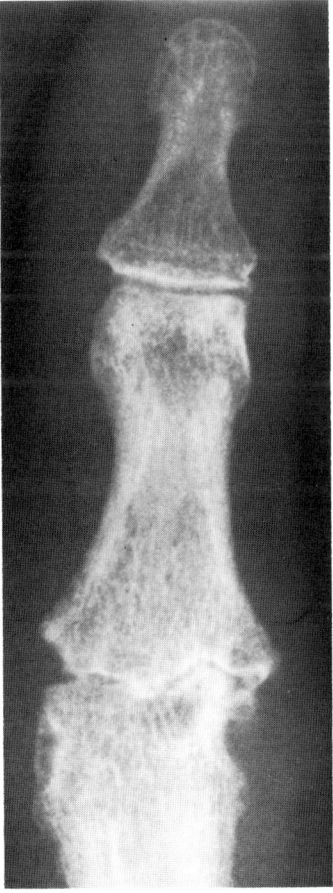

were in the second decade and 85% of their patients were in the second and third decades combined. Their follow-up evaluation assessed symptoms, range of motion, instability and overall hand function. The radiographs were likewise reviewed. Their work suggests that the more severe the initial injury, i.e. their group III, the greater is the likelihood of having a less than satisfactory result by the criteria which they used to assess their patients.

Additional studies of this sort are needed with longer term follow-up and particularly more amplification upon the development of post-traumatic degenerative changes following these injuries. It would seem logical to assume that the dislocating proximal interphalangeal joint is not a desirable fact to have in one's past medical history. Even less desirable would be the affirmation of a previous fracture dislocation. Chronic, repetitive injuries, as well as severe acute injuries may lead to post-traumatic degenerative change (Fig. 9.14).

Post-traumatic degenerative changes in the distal interphalangeal joint would seem to be inevitable sequelae to injuries at this level as well.

Fig. 9.14 Post-traumatic degenerative change. This 55-year-old former baseball player presented with complaints of swelling and limitation of motion of the proximal interphalangeal joint of his index finger. He gave a history of multiple acute episodes related to his athletic endeavours in the past. He had surprisingly little discomfort and was treated with aspirin alone.

It is interesting, therefore, that although many papers have been written about management of the acute mallet finger, and the management of the chronic mallet finger, the present author has been unable to find any series recording post-traumatic degenerative changes occurring at the distal interphalangeal joint as a result of these injuries.

MUCOUS CYST

Mucous cysts were described as early as 1883 (Larsen & Posch 1969). Recent reports (Eaton et al 1973) have suggested that there is a high association of degenerative change in the distal interphalangeal joints so involved. This may be determined radiographically as well as surgically at the time of removal. Eaton and co-workers have suggested that the common cyst (Fig. 9.15) can be effectively removed surgically with a low rate of recurrence if there is marginal osteophyte excision in association with meticulous tracing of this cyst down to its communication with the joint. After removal of the cyst, the resulting wound may be closed by resection of redundant skin, full thickness skin grafting, or by letting the wound heal by secondary intention.

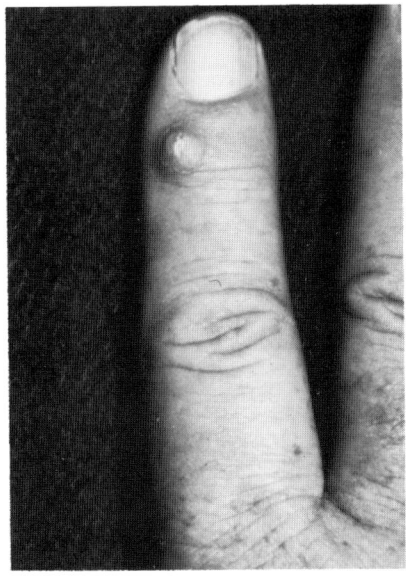

Fig. 9.15 Mucous cysts. This is the dominant index finger of a 65-year-old housewife. This is a characteristic appearance and location of the mucous cyst. Radiographs demonstrated degenerative joint disease at this level with marginal osteophyte formation underlying the area of the cyst.

REFERENCES

Bell M 1976 The changing pattern of pyogenic infections of the hand. Hand 8:298–302

Benke G J, Stableforth P G 1979 Injuries of the proximal interphalangeal joint of the fingers. Hand 11:263–268

Bilos Z J, Kuchanchuk H, Metzger W 1978 *Eikenella corrodens* in human bites. Clinical Orthopaedics and Related Research 134:320–323

Bland J H, Stulberg S D 1981 Osteoarthritis: pathology and clinical patterns. In: Kelley W N, Harris E D, Ruddy S, Sledge C B (eds) Textbook of Rheumatology, W B Saunders Co, Philadelphia, ch 89, pp 1471–1490

Bonavita J A, Dalinka M K, Schumacher H R 1980 Hydroxyapatite deposition disease. Radiology 134:621–625

Brandt K D 1981 The pathogenesis of osteoarthritis. In: Kelley W N, Harris E D, Ruddy S, Sledge C B (eds) Textbook of Rheumatology, W B Saunders Co, Philadelphia, ch 88, pp 1457–1470

Carroll R E, Taber T H 1954 Digital arthroplasty of the proximal interphalangeal joint. Journal of Bone and Joint Surgery 36A:912–920

Carroll R E, Hill N A 1969 Small joint arthrodesis in hand reconstruction. Journal of Bone and Joint Surgery 51A:1219–1221

Eaton R G, Dobranski A I, Littler J W 1973 Marginal osteophyte excision in treatment of mucous cysts. Journal of Bone and Joint Surgery 55A:570–574

Gelberman R H, Doty D H, Hamer M L 1980 Tophaceous gout involving the proximal interphalangeal joint. Clinical Orthopaedics and Related Research 147:225–227

Gold R H, Bassett L W, Theros E G 1982 Radiologic comparison of erosive polyarthritides with prominent interphalangeal involvement. Skeletal Radiology 8:89–97

Greene T L, Louis D S 1980 Calcifying tendinitis in the hand. A report of two cases. Annals of Emergency Medicine 9:438–440

Hamilton S, Knickerbocker J 1982 Periarticular erosions in the hands and wrists in hemodialysis patients. Clinical Radiology 33:19–24

Hirsch J H, Killien F C, Troupin R H 1976 The arthropathy of hemochromatosis. Radiology 118:591–596

Howell D S 1981 Diseases due to the deposition of calcium pyrophosphate and hydroxyapatite. In: Kelley W N, Harris E D, Ruddy S, Sledge C B (eds) Textbook of Rheumatology, W B Saunders Co, Philadelphia, ch 87, pp 1438–1454

Keats T E, Johnstone W H, O'Brien W M (1981) Large joint destruction in erosive osteoarthritis. Skeletal Radiology 6:267–269

Kelley W N 1981 Gout and related disorders of purine metabolism. In: Kelley W N, Harris E D, Ruddy S, Sledge C B (eds) Textbook of Rheumatology, W B Saunders Co, Philadelphia, ch 86, pp 1397–1437

Larsen R D, Posch J 1969 Mucous cysts of the finger. Plastic and Reconstructive Surgery 43: 241–246

Linscheid R L, Dobyns J H 1975 Common and uncommon infections of the hand. Orthopaedic Clinics of North America 6: 1063–1104

Lucas G E, Bartlett D H 1981 Pasturella multocida infection in the hand. Plastic and Reconstructive Surgery 67: 49–53

McDevitt C A, Muir H 1976 Biochemical changes in the cartilage of the knee in experimental and natural osteoarthritis in the dog. Journal of Bone and Joint Surgery 58B: 94–101

Manhart J W, Wilson J A, Korbitz B C 1970 Articular and cutaneous sporotrichosis. Journal of the American Medical Association 214: 365–367

Mankin H J, Lipiello L 1970 Biochemical and metabolic abnormalities in articular cartilage from osteoarthritic human hips. Journal of Bone and Joint Surgery 52A: 424–434

Palmoski M, Perricone E, Brandt K D 1979 Development and reversal of a proteoglycan aggregation defect in normal canine knee cartilage after immobilization. Arthritis and Rheumatism 22: 508–517

Ray M J, Bassett R L 1985 The radiologic manifestations of gout. Orthopedics 8: 95–98

Roh Y S, DeQueker J, Mulier J C 1973 Osteoarthrosis at the hand skeleton in primary osteoarthrosis of the hip and in normal controls. Clinical Orthopaedics and Related Research 90: 90–94

Smith R S, Atkinson R E, Jupiter J B 1985 Silicone synovitis of the wrist. Journal of Hand Surgery 10A: 47–60

Staple T W 1984 Joint disorders. In: Poznanski A K (ed) The Hand in Radiologic Diagnosis, 2nd edn. W B Saunders Co, Philadelphia, ch 20, pp 791–838

Swanson A 1973 Surgical procedures for destroyed interphalangeal joints. In: Flexible Implant Resection Arthroplasty in the Hand and Extremities, C V Mosby Co, St Louis, pp 160–170

Swezey R L, Alexander S J 1971 Erosive osteoarthritis and the main en lorgnette deformity. Archives of Internal Medicine 128: 269–272

Thorpe C D, Spjut H J 1985 Coccidioidial osteomyelitis in a child's finger. Journal of Bone and Joint Surgery 67A: 330–332

Twersky J 1975 Joint changes in idiopathic hemochromatosis. American Journal of Roentgenology 124: 139–144

Watt I, Middlemiss H 1975 The radiology of gout. Clinical Radiology 26: 27–36

Williams C S, Riordan D C 1973 Mycobacterium marinum (atypical acid-fast) bacillus infections of the hand. Journal of Bone and Joint Surgery 55A: 1043–1050

J. S. Thompson

10 Interphalangeal joint arthroplasties

'Snug-fitting joints are stiffened easily'
BUNNELL 1944

INTRODUCTION

Chapters dealing with arthroplasty of the interphalangeal joints almost invariably become historical progressions, chronologically recounting attempts of engineers and surgeons to replace the joint. Although this information is important, it should not be the primary focus when this subject is considered.

Arthroplasty means (in its purest sense) an operation to restore as far as possible the integrity and functional power of a joint. In this age of 'high technology' it is important to resist the natural temptation of equating arthroplasty with joint replacement.

In this chapter, the history of interphalangeal arthroplasty is briefly reviewed, the present author's preferred surgical and rehabilitative technique presented, and other interesting developments influencing interphalangeal arthroplasty are discussed. A short but important section will be devoted to a highly successful soft tissue procedure applicable to specific post-traumatic proximal interphalangeal (PIP) joint problems (Eaton's 'volar plate arthroplasty').

Bunnell (1944) mentioned arthroplasty of the 'middle finger joints' in a single short paragraph in the first edition of his classic text. He stated 'Arthroplasty on a middle finger joint [proximal interphalangeal joint] should be done only when all the other tissues in the vicinity are normal'. In fact, he recommended arthrodesis or amputation in most cases *because* of damage to 'other tissues'. He recognized that the altered condition of periarticular soft issues was *the* major limiting factor in successful interphalangeal arthroplasty. His sage advice deserves consideration, but if taken to the extreme, arthroplasty of the interphalangeal joints would only be feasible in normal fingers. However, the cumulative surgical experience of the past 30–40 years supports a place for interphalangeal arthroplasty in the armamentarium of the hand surgeon, for relief of pain, correction of deformity and restoration of some motion. If preoperative damage to the soft tissue is considered, a surgical procedure that results in a pain-free, stable joint that has reasonable range of motion and satisfactory appearance should be judged extremely successful. The goal of perfectly 'replacing' interphalangeal joints (resulting in normal range of motion) is admirable and worthy of pursuit but the procedure will remain an imperfect one (regardless of technique) due to the soft tissue changes and the inability of any implant to substitute exactly for a normal joint.

To state that arthroplasty of the interphalangeal joint is a challenge from the design, biomechanical, biological, surgical, and rehabilitation standpoint is an extreme understatement. The desire to reproduce a painless range of motion in a diseased interphalangeal joint has fascinated and frustrated many outstanding individuals for many years. Keeping this information in mind, a historical review of the development of interphalangeal joint arthroplasty is appropriate. The PIP joint, being the critical joint of the digit (see Ch. 2) will be the primary focus of the discussion.

HISTORICAL DEVELOPMENT

Prior to the classic paper of Carroll (Carroll & Taber 1954) the entire world's literature concerning arthroplastic attempts at the interphalangeal joints consisted of about 35 cases. Most of these papers were reports of one or two cases using different types of biological interposition material (fat, fascia, etc.). Reports had been made of the use of both Vitallium and lucite for replacing the condylar heads of the proximal phalanx in arthroplastic attempts (Burman 1940, Burman & Abrahamson 1943). In their milestone paper, Carroll & Taber (1954) reported a series of 30 patients treated with resection arthroplasty of the PIP joint. They used three criteria to select patients for the operation: (1) severe deformity of the finger, 'awkward position' [a stiff PIP joint in the position of function was not considered an indication]; (2) no tendon injury about the joint; and (3) 'patient motivation must be high'. Arthrodesis was performed if there was any doubt about the patient's motivation. Old extensive infection or many years of immobility were absolute contraindications for the procedure. Carroll utilized no interposition material other than scar.

The procedure consisted of resection of the distal one-third (or slightly less) of the proximal phalanx followed by Kirschner wire distraction for 6 weeks. Although the majority of the patients in this series were 'improved', there was a significant incidence of problems: (1) shortening of the digit; (2) instability of the resection arthroplasty; (3) angulation at the site of the resection arthroplasty; and (4) less than satisfactory range of motion. These problems with resection type arthroplasties led directly to the next step in the relatively recent evolution of interphalangeal arthroplasty.

Flatt (1961) conducted trials of several metallic prosthetic replacements in the interphalangeal joints. The design used by Flatt was a modification of the metallic Brannon & Klein (1959) prosthesis (Figs. 10.1, 10.2). These prostheses offered the advantage of inherent stability and adequate range of motion (Flatt 1968). However, the biomechanical properties of rigid metallic prostheses resulted in unacceptable difficulties with migration and erosions of the stems through medullary canals and cortices of the typically soft bone of patients with rheumatoid disease. This early work with metallic prostheses represented an important attempt to restore stability and motion in the unstable diseased interphalangeal joint (Flatt & Ellison 1972) but also represented a failure in the choice of biomaterials.

The silicone age of replacement arthroplasty (Fig. 10.2) of the small joints of the hand was introduced in the 1960s by Swanson (1966, 1968, 1973a, b) and Neibauer (Neibauer 1971, Neibauer et al 1968, 1969, 1971). Other surgeons confirmed the successful use of these silastic implants soon after their introduction (Urbaniak et al 1970). Since that time there have been several articulated, semiconstrained designs of replacement prostheses for the interphalangeal joint (primarily the PIP joint) that have had brief periods of enthusiasm (Beckenbaugh & Linscheid 1982). However, follow-up studies on all articulated cemented-in prostheses have revealed problems with implant fracture, loosening from bone erosion at the bone–

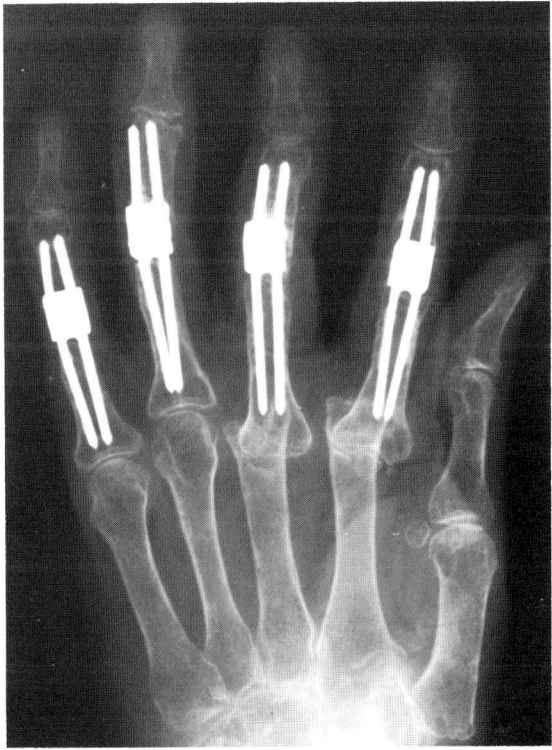

Fig. 10.1 Flatt's PIP prostheses in place. This roentgenogram is of the first patient to receive the Flatt PIP replacement arthroplasties. (Photo courtesy of Adrian E. Flatt, MD.)

158 THE INTERPHALANGEAL JOINTS

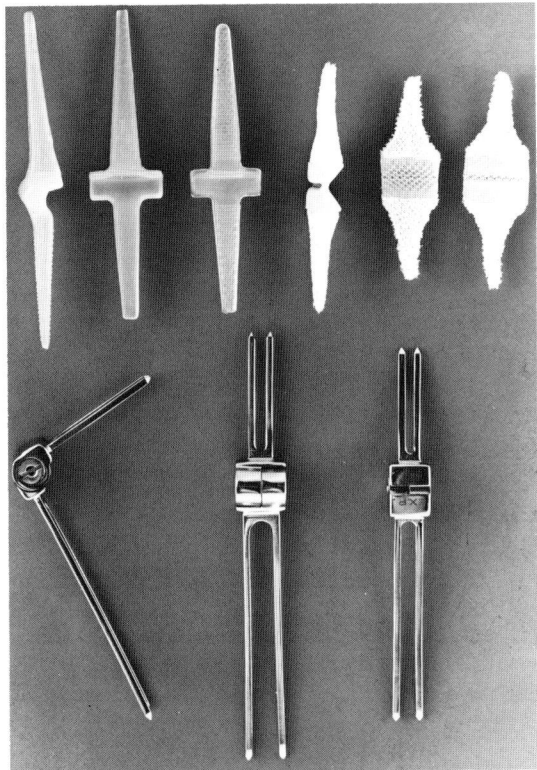

Fig. 10.2 Top row left: Swanson silicone prosthesis (side, dorsal and volar views). Top row right: Neibauer dacron–silicone prosthesis (side, dorsal and volar views). Lower: Flatt prosthesis, same views. (Photo courtesy of Adrian E. Flatt, MD.)

cement interface or loosening at the prosthesis–cement interface.

The standard to which all replacement arthroplasty of the interphalangeal joints must be compared is the silicone spacer arthroplasty developed by Swanson. For almost 20 years this material and technique have endured with an acceptable complication rate and quite satisfactory results in terms of pain relief and adequate range of motion (Blair et al 1984, Swanson et al 1985). However, the silicone replacement arthroplasty is not perfect and further investigation of possible alternatives is continuing at several research and development centres.

Successful arthroplasty of the PIP joint utilizing a silicone 'spacer' implant requires close attention to surgical and rehabilitation detail. Swanson has repeatedly emphasized this fact in the literature (Swanson 1973a, b, 1979, 1980, Swanson et al 1985). It is strongly recommended that all surgeons preparing to perform their first silastic replacement arthroplasty of the interphalangeal joints should review Swanson's teachings. Specific points regarding technique and some modifications proposed by the present author will be discussed later in this chapter.

INDICATIONS

In hand surgery, patient selection and careful, gradual determination of the indications for any surgical procedure are of paramount importance. The surgeons frequently with the most outstanding results are those with the most effective and successful patient selection for any particular procedure. Any surgery on or about the interphalangeal joints (especially the PIP joint) will have a profound influence on the total mechanics of the digit (see Ch. 2). Therefore it cannot be overstressed that interphalangeal arthroplasty is a major procedure on the digit and should be undertaken (ideally) only by an experienced hand surgeon and an intelligent, informed patient who have reached the decision to proceed with this particular operation on a mutual basis. However, this is almost never completely the case because of patient and surgeon bias. It should be remembered that this is, in the vast majority of cases, an elective procedure. Therefore time is available for the education of the patient and thoughtful consideration by the surgeon. The importance of these principles of patient and procedure selection cannot be overstressed.

The obvious major factors entering the indications formula are pain, joint destruction, loss of motion, and deformity. The appearance of the digit (especially the left ring finger) may also be extremely important. Many subjective factors must be considered in the formula such as: patient expectations (frequently unrealistic), motivation, ability to accept perioperative morbidity and the rehabilitation process and effectiveness of the patient–surgeon relationship. The standard areas of age, sex, hand dominance, occupational and recreational requirements should be known and considered. However, even after this process is completed, a predictable excellent result is not possible because of the inability to predict a patient's reaction to the controlled trauma of surgical treatment. Therefore we must attempt to adapt a surgical treatment to the individual needs of each patient using the foregoing process plus careful physical examination and proceed on the statistical basis that the majority of patients will be improved (98% pain free) (Swanson et al 1985).

CONTRAINDICATIONS

The procedure should not be carried out in digits with open epiphyses of the phalanges or in the presence of active infection. It cannot be performed in a digit without functional or potential PIP flexor or extensor tendons. Most factors mitigating against this procedure such as heavy labour-type occupations may be only relative contraindications. Digits with compromised neurovascular status (replants and revascularizations) would be expected to achieve less range of motion but the ability of the spacers to achieve joint pain relief remains satisfactory.

Swanson's most recent review (Swanson et al 1985) has resulted in the stated opinion that: 'We no longer recommend the use of the flexible implant in swan-neck deformities'. This opinion was based upon a high incidence of recurrent hyperextension deformities in fingers of rheumatoid patients surgically treated with PIP replacement and swan-neck reconstruction. A patient with rheumatoid disease and swan-neck deformities of the fingers now represents a contraindication (according to Swanson) in the use of the flexible hinge silicone replacement arthroplasty. In the experience of the present author, most swan-neck deformities in patients with rheumatoid disease do extremely well with soft tissue procedures, since in most cases adequate articular surface is present on the volar 75% of the condyles of the proximal phalanx and the base of the middle phalanx.

Some surgeons feel that PIP replacement of the index finger for post-traumatic arthrosis or osteoarthritis is relatively contraindicated because of the strong likelihood of ulnar angulation deformity developing at the prosthetic joint secondary to the repeated stress of pinch with a strong thumb. However, this can be prevented with careful attention to preservation of the radial collateral ligament (discussed in detail in technique section). Figure 10.3 illustrates such a case.

PREOPERATIVE EVALUATION

Replacement arthroplasty of the PIP joint should be performed only after specific and thorough evaluations have been completed. The neurovascular status should be documented. Denervated or partially innervated digits should be expected to achieve less range of motion since motivation to use the digit will be decreased as a result of diminished sensibility. The intrinsic muscles should be checked for tightness and intrinsic releases performed at the time of PIP replacement if necessary. Active and passive range of motion should be recorded. Angular deformities should be documented. The competence of the collateral ligaments should be checked; this is especially important in the index finger. The extensor and flexor systems should be evaluated for possible adhesions proximal to the PIP joint which might contribute to a decreased range of motion. Routine roentgenograms should be reviewed, specific architectural deformities may necessitate variations in surgical technique (Fig. 10.6).

TECHNIQUE

Surgical exposure for silastic PIP joint replacement may be lateral, volar or dorsal. The approach of choice may vary due to specific circumstances but in general, the dorsal approach with a gentle curvilinear incision is preferred (Fig. 10.4**a**). A little emphasized but important point is the preservation of the central dorsal longitudinal vein. This can be preserved in the dorsal flap and preservation of this structure significantly reduces postoperative oedema. Dissection is carried sharply down to the extensor mechanism and the overlying soft tissue is cleared from the extensor mechanism in a single layer. The extensor mechanism is divided longitudinally and the joint exposed (Fig. 10.4**b**). The collateral ligaments are identified. In the present author's opinion, it is important to preserve the proximal origin of the collateral ligaments. This usually is possible in post-traumatic and osteoarthritic deformities but may be difficult or impossible in severe deformity secondary to rheumatoid disease. The combination of a strong thumb and rheumatoid synovitis or surgical

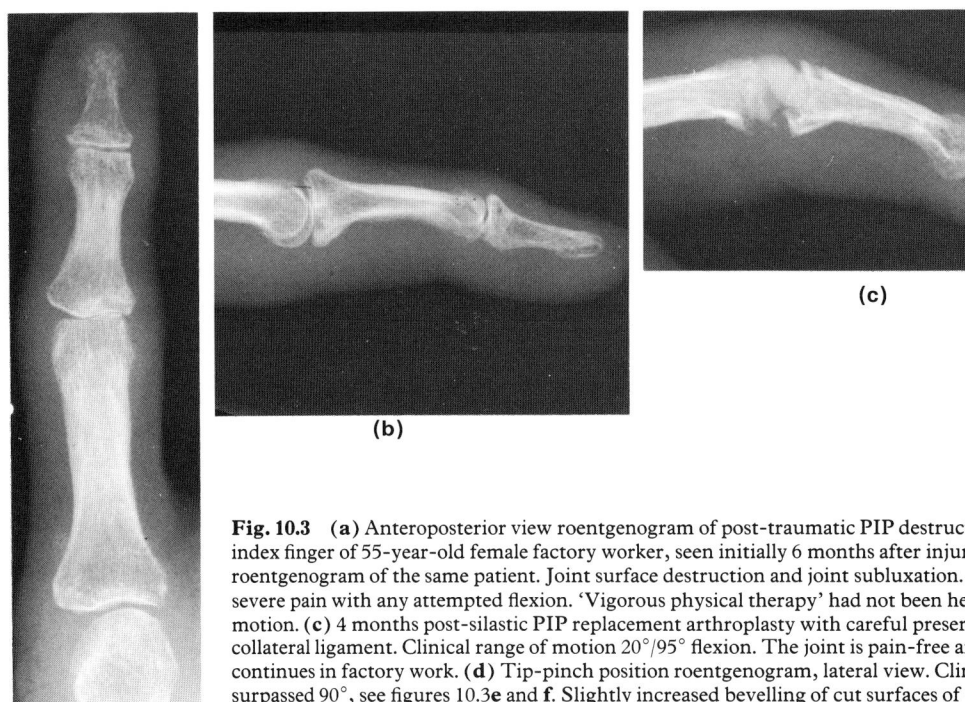

Fig. 10.3 (**a**) Anteroposterior view roentgenogram of post-traumatic PIP destruction in dominant index finger of 55-year-old female factory worker, seen initially 6 months after injury. (**b**) Lateral view roentgenogram of the same patient. Joint surface destruction and joint subluxation. The patient had severe pain with any attempted flexion. 'Vigorous physical therapy' had not been helpful in improving motion. (**c**) 4 months post-silastic PIP replacement arthroplasty with careful preservation of radial collateral ligament. Clinical range of motion 20°/95° flexion. The joint is pain-free and the patient continues in factory work. (**d**) Tip-pinch position roentgenogram, lateral view. Clinically flexion surpassed 90°, see figures 10.3**e** and **f**. Slightly increased bevelling of cut surfaces of proximal and middle phalanges might have increased maximum flexion (see technique section). (**e**) Flexion PIP surpasses 90°. (**f**) Extension lag of 20°. Patient and surgeon satisfaction excellent. Patient is now 2 years after surgery with no problems. Durability of the implant in this worker remains the only potential question.

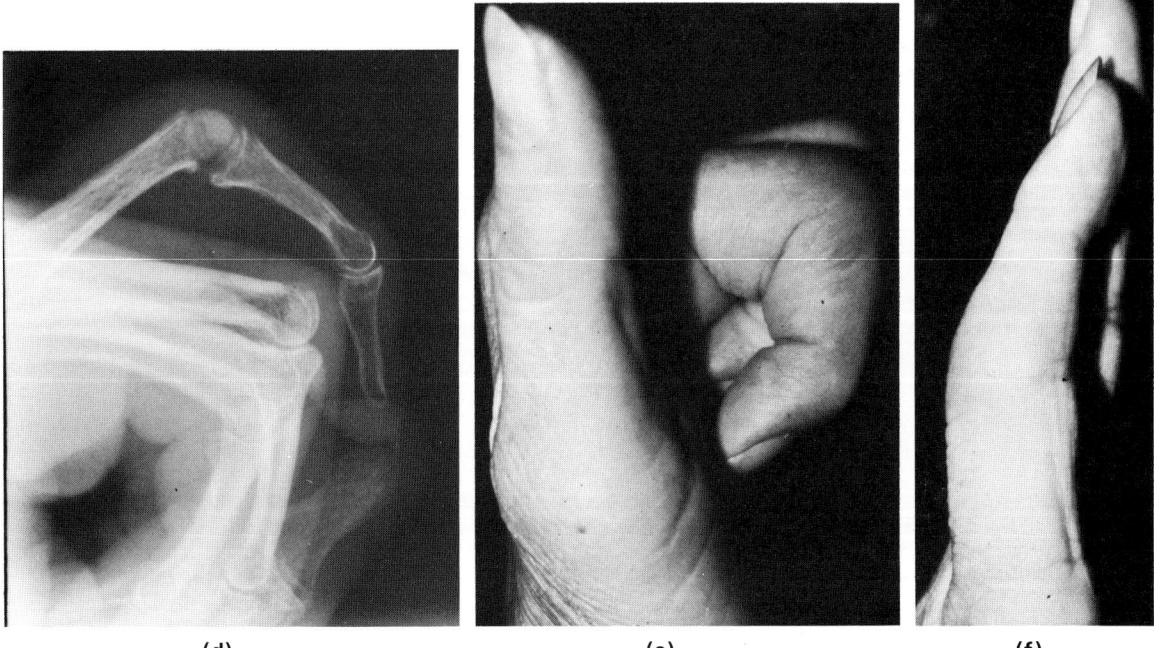

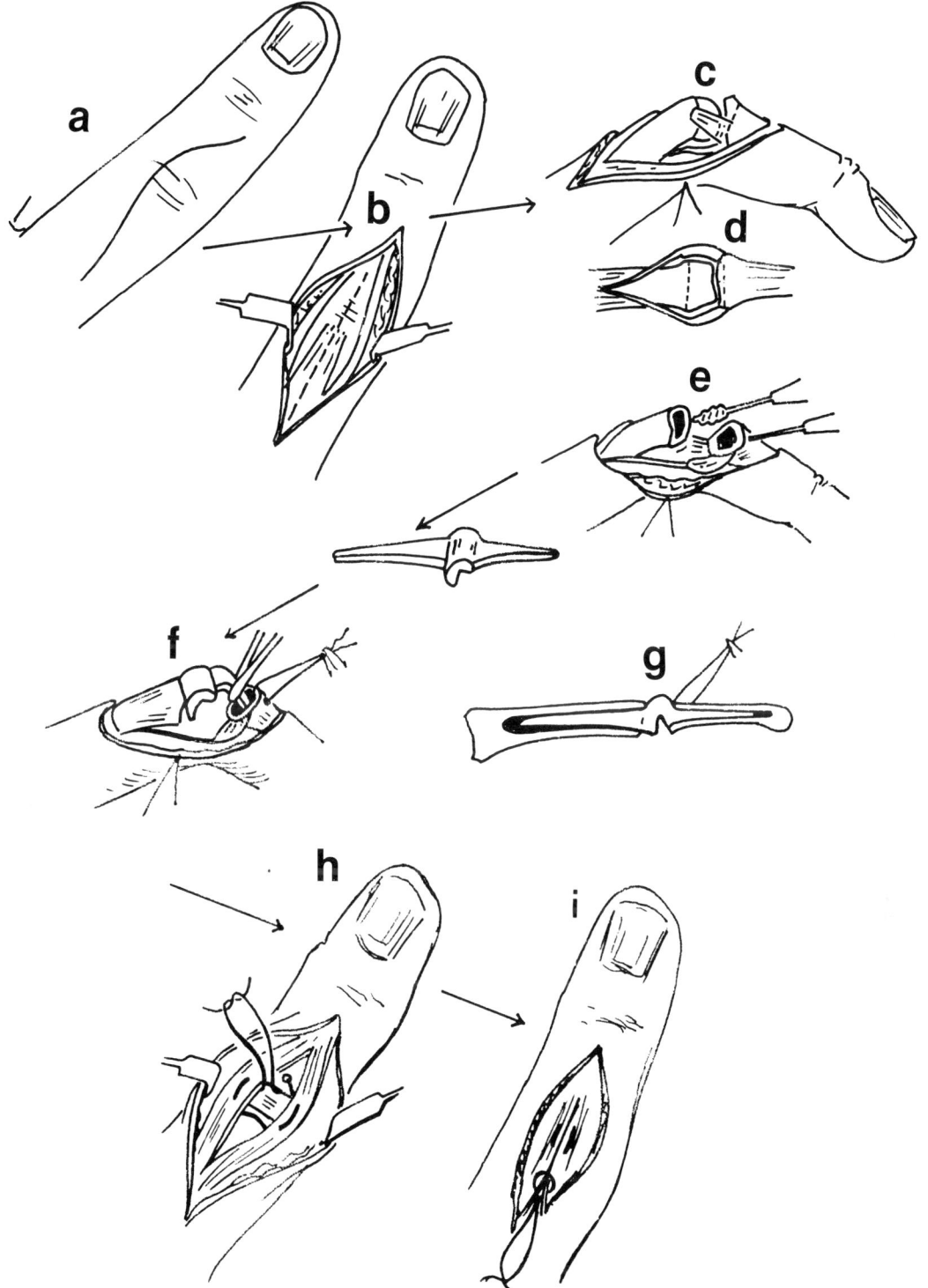

Fig. 10.4 (a) Dorsal incision and exposure of extensor mechanism. (b) Longitudinal division of extensor mechanism. (c) Bony resection, lateral view. (d) Bony resection, anteroposterior view (note preservation of proximal attachment of collateral ligaments with either actual collateral origins or periosteal sleeve tissue). (e) Medullary reaming and dorsal hole placement at dorsal base of middle phalanx. (f) Insertion of the prosthesis, note the bevelled cut surface of the proximal phalanx. (g) Proper fit of the silastic spacer in the medullary canals with at least 1 mm of clearance proximally and distally with the finger in extension. Again note bevelled cuts of proximal and middle phalanx. (h) Reinsertion of the extensor mechanism at the base of middle phalanx. (i) Repair of the central cleft in the extensor mechanism.

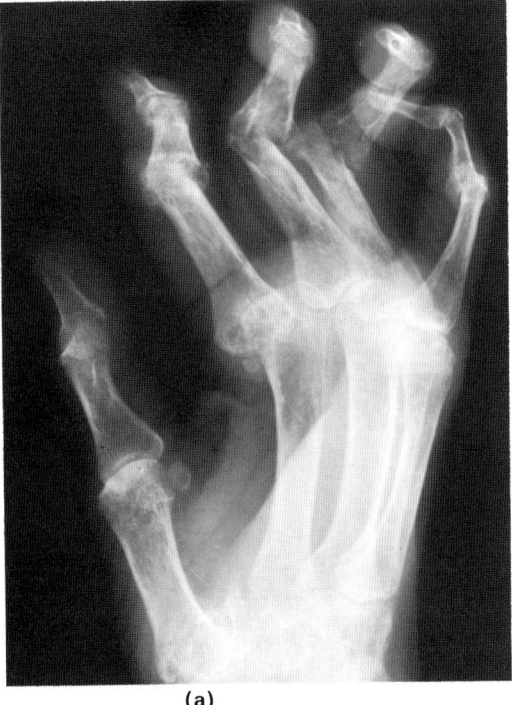 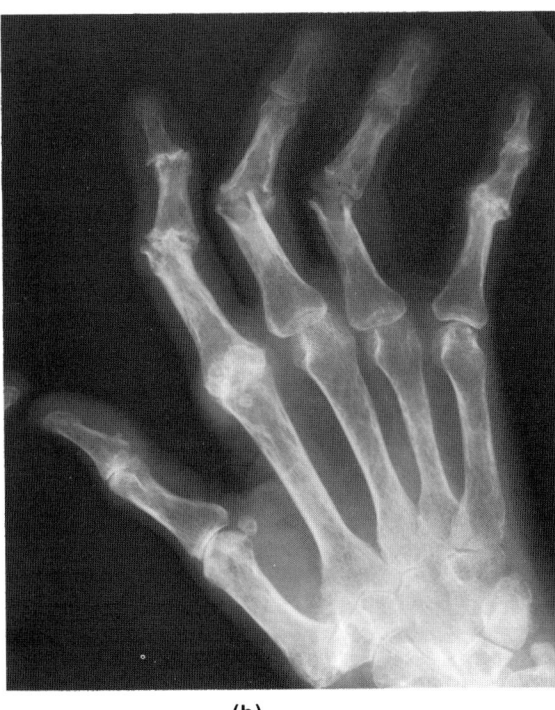

Fig. 10.5 Rheumatoid disease with severe interphalangeal destruction and deformity. PIP joints of middle and ring finger replaced 3 years earlier. The collateral ligaments (radial and ulnar) were released. The combination of a strong thumb plus rheumatoid synovitis of the index PIP and collateral ligament releases of the PIP joints of the middle and ring fingers at the time of silastic replacement arthroplasty has resulted in severe ulnar angulation and hyperextension deformities. The prostheses are fractured.

release of the PIP radial collateral ligaments can be devastating (Fig. 10.5). In most cases with sharp and delicate technique, the fibres of the origin of the collateral ligaments can be preserved. If these fibres must be completely released, an attempt should be made to maintain continuity with a sleeve of periosteal tissue (see Fig. 10.4**d**). The reward for the extra time involved in attention to this detail will be very gratifying to both the patient and surgeon when the operated PIP joint has the inherent stability to withstand power key pinch without ulnar deviation.

When the condyles have been carefully removed in a perpendicular cut to the longitudinal axis of the proximal phalanx, careful attention must be given to the shaping of the bone ends. A shallow bevelled cut of the ends of the proximal and middle phalanx will facilitate the possibility of maximum flexion (see Figs. 10.4**c–g**, 10.7**c**, 10.8). At this point in the procedure the retrocondylar space should be inspected and any osteophytes or prolif- erative synovial tissue removed. Failure to pay attention to this seemingly obvious detail may result in lack of flexion in the 'replaced joint' (Fig. 10.6). Soft tissue release at the volar aspect of the joint may also be necessary, especially in a finger with preoperative flexion contracture. The careful attention to bone end preparation and soft tissue release volarly should prevent placement of the implant in a situation that might cause buckling or pinching of the device (Fig. 10.7). These forces on the implant resulting from placement after inadequate soft tissue release or inadequate bony resection, predispose the implant to stress fracture.

Preparation of the intramedullary canals should be done with the special blunt-ended 'Swanson' burrs (see Fig. 10.4**e**). Even though the tips of the burrs are blunt, it is possible to penetrate the cortex of the phalanges with the burrs (especially in the narrow distal area of the middle phalanx in rheumatoid patients) and this should be carefully avoided. Sizing of the implant requires some

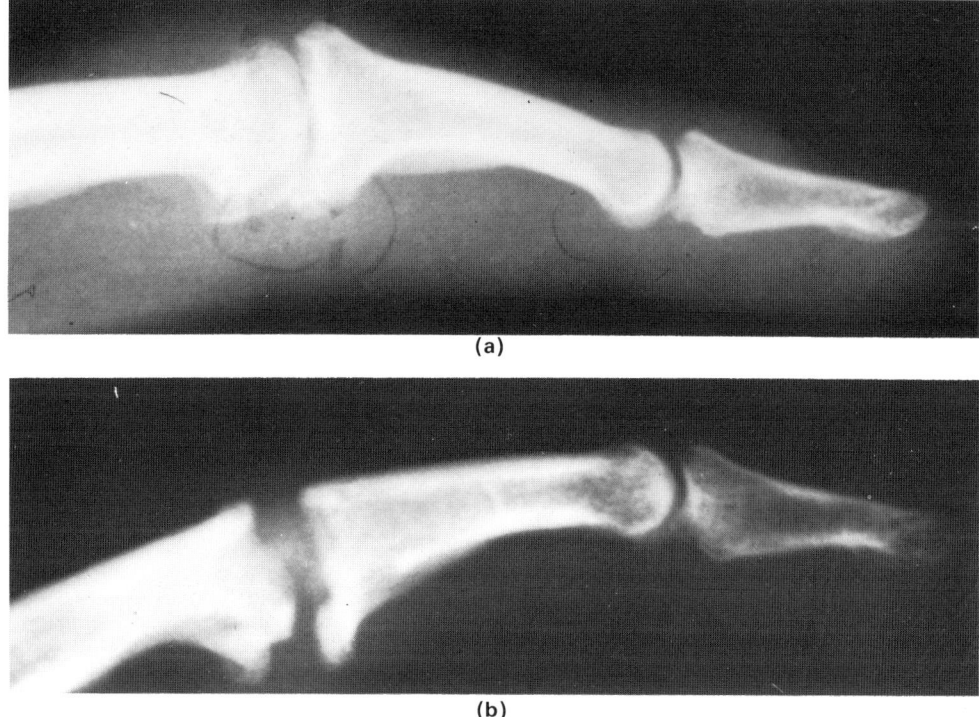

Fig. 10.6 (a) Post-traumatic arthrosis with healing fracture volarly on the middle phalanx and impaction of the proximal phalangeal condyles. This combination produced extensive bone at the volar aspect of the joint. (b) Post-silastic replacement arthroplasty (maximum flexion view). Clear demonstration of the importance of volar clearance for flexion after this procedure.

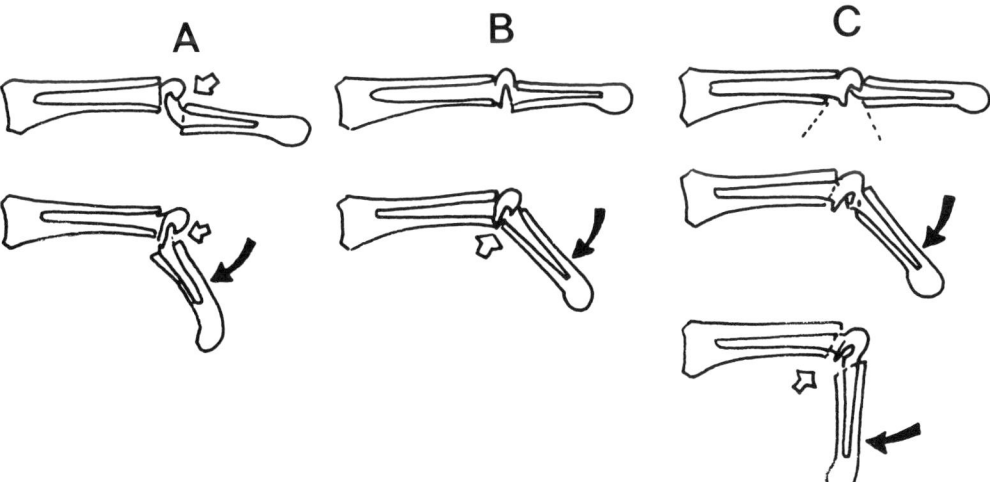

Fig. 10.7 (**A**) Incomplete soft tissue release resulting in subluxed position of the joint and buckling of the implant. This technical error will result in decreased potential motion and increased probability of implant fracture. (Redrawn from Swanson.) (**B**) Proper joint position but inadequate bone removal resulting in a 'pinched' implant. This technical error will reduce flexion by causing impingement of the volar cortices with attempted flexion. This impingement may also be painful. (Redrawn from Swanson). (**C**) Proper position, proper bone removal and bevelled cuts of bone ends. This allows proper sliding of the middle phalanx around the end of the proximal phalanx and prevents volar abutment. (Modified from Swanson.)

judgement, since the proper implant should fit snugly at the joint and be wide enough to abut both bone ends at its mid-section. Frequently it will be found that the implant that seems to be the most appropriate for proper joint fit in terms of size of the hinge area has stems that are too long. Therefore it is common practice to trim stems for proper length within the intramedullary canals. The stems should be 1 mm shorter than the reamed canal (Fig. 10.8). This space within the canal allows pistoning of the implant and the sliding/gliding action of the hinge will therefore allow the middle phalanx to circumscribe the proximal phalanx. The implant does not function as a true hinge and if it is implanted so that pistoning is not possible (the implant itself truly flexing and extending), it is too tight (see Fig. 10.7).

Prior to the final insertion of the implant, small holes should be made and sutures passed for reattachment of the extensor mechanism and collateral ligaments (if necessary) (Fig. 10.9). The dorsal periosteum and collateral ligament edges should be closed with fine suture to provide a smooth surface for the extensor tendon (Fig. 10.9c). At this point, prior to reattachment of the extensor tendon, an important technical detail should be carried out. In patients with long-standing extension contracture, adhesions beneath the extensor mechanism may develop. Using a small blunt freer-elevator the space beneath the extensor proximally should be explored and these adhesions lysed if they are present. After this has been done, the central slip is reattached under proper tension with 3–0 non-absorbable suture (see Fig. 10.4h). Inverted sutures are then used to repair the extensor tendon (see Fig. 10.4i).

A few variances in the reconstructive technique that are necessary in the presence of preoperative boutonnière deformity should be mentioned. The central slip will need advancement, the lateral bands may require step-cut lengthening and the distal interphalangeal (DIP) joint may require a transarticular Kirschner wire in the neutral position.

Finally, if there is any question as to the adequacy of flexor tendon excursion, the tendons should be exposed through a small transverse incision in the palm (just proximal to the A–1 pulley) and using a blunt probe, the tendons should be individually tested for excursion, adhesions frequently will be felt to lyse during this manoeuvre.

The wounds are closed over small rubber drains (rubber vessel loops preferred) which are removed after 48 h. The hand is carefully dressed in a conforming dressing supported by a volar splint from finger tip to mid-forearm. The PIP joint is placed in extension and the metacarpophalangeal joints are flexed. The wrist should be in a position of comfortable extension. It is noteworthy that this procedure can be carried out as an outpatient operation and over the past several years, the majority of these cases have been done in that manner. This places further emphasis on careful technique and attention to detail in order to minimize postoperative complications.

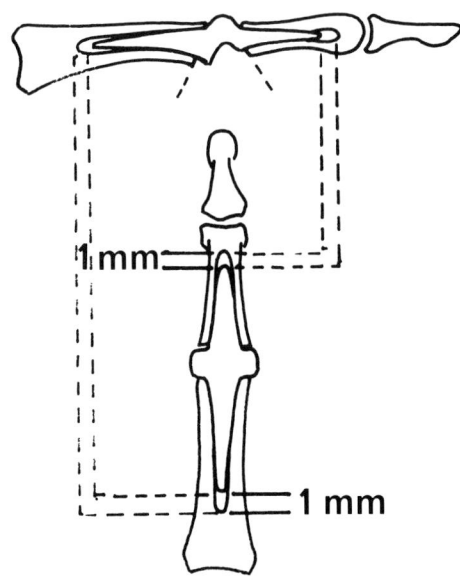

Fig. 10.8 Correct intramedullar canal preparation and shortening of implant stems if necessary should result in 1 mm space at the tips of both stems in extension. Pistoning of the implant must occur for optimal range of motion. Note bevelled cuts of proximal and middle phalangeal ends. (Modified from Swanson.)

POSTOPERATIVE CARE/ REHABILITATION

The general principles of all hand reconstruction should be followed. Elevation and rest of the

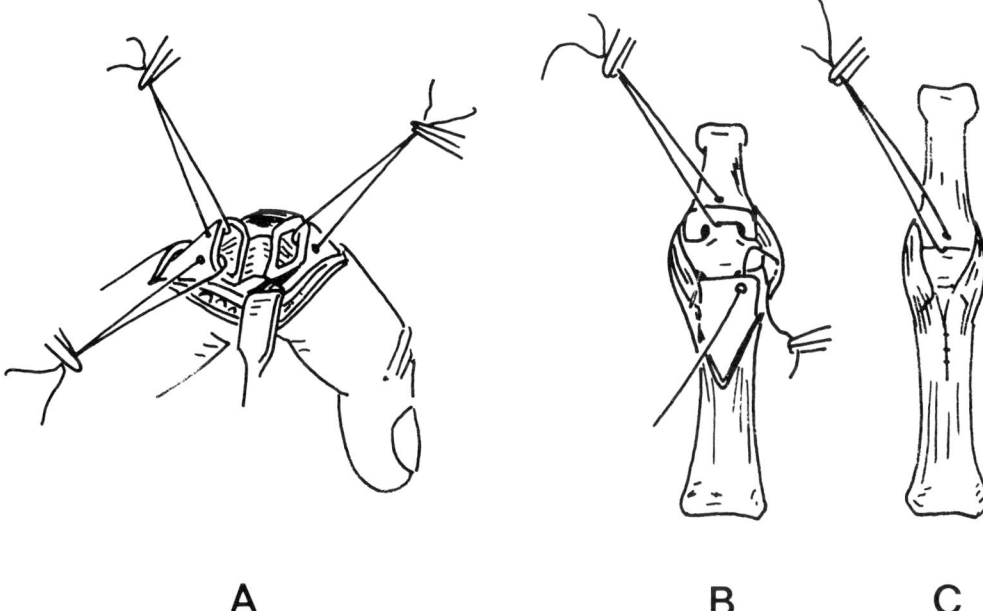

Fig. 10.9 (**A**) Sutures placed to reattach collateral ligament—periosteal sleeve to proximal phalanx and central extensor to middle phalanx. (**B**) The suture for reapproximation of the collateral ligament—periosteal sleeve may be used to change the tension of the ligaments if necessary. (**C**) Reattachment of periosteum and collateral ligaments completed. In most cases of post-traumatic arthrosis and osteoarthritis, it is possible to preserve some of the proximal fibres of the collateral ligaments. Sutures may not be necessary in these cases depending on the radial/ulnar stability with the implant in place.

operated extremity are important. Inordinate pain during the immediate postoperative period should be a warning sign initiating wound inspection (haematoma beneath the dorsal flap may cause wound problems, flap necrosis and delayed rehabilitation due to increased pain and fibrosis).

These guidelines vary somewhat from those proposed by Swanson et al (1978) and have been effective in the present author's experience. The splint maintaining the PIP joint in extension is kept in place for 2 weeks. At that point gentle active flexion exercises (within limits of discomfort) are begun. This process is carefully monitored and supervised by the surgeon and a trained hand therapist. Removable static splints are fabricated for rest and sleeping. The exercises should be two or three times a day for short periods of time with few repetitions followed by return to the resting extension splint. This should continue until 4 weeks after the operation. The ever present danger in the early postoperative period is overzealous flexion exercises (usually by a patient in a hurry) resulting in loss of extension. Careful observation on *any* extension deficit should be a part of each examination and the pace and course of rehabilitation must be guided by the balancing of any extension lag against the increase in flexion. The weakest part of the periarticular tissues at this point is the extensor repair and reattachment. Rupture or attenuation of this structure can doom the procedure, thus attention to its protection until 6–8 weeks after the operation is imperative. At this point, the extension splint for the PIP can be reduced to night-only use, if the extension lag is less than 15° and shows no increase when it is removed during the day. If it does increase, the extension splint should be used during the day (when not exercising) for another 2 weeks.

Depending upon the condition of the extensor, light hand use without the splint can be allowed at 6–8 weeks after the operation. The amount of active and passive flexion may gradually increase for several months. An active exercise programme should be followed for at least 1 year. The programme should include flexion/extension exercises of the interphalangeal joints with the metacarpophalangeal joint stabilized in both extension and flexion. Active assistive and gentle passive range of motion exercises are also permitted. However, these are not allowed until at least 6–8 weeks after surgery depending again upon the status of the PIP extensor. Night extension splinting should continue for at least 3–6 months. The optimum results depend upon the combination of careful surgery, balanced rehabilitation and patient understanding and cooperation.

RESULTS

The largest series of patients reported is that of Swanson et al (1985). They noted greater than 40° arc of motion in the majority of patients and a rate of complete pain relief of 98.3%.

In general, a range of motion of 40–60° is about the average expected in reported series. These results should be presented in both active and passive terms. The pre- and postoperative arc of motion should be compared because even though 40–60° may not be a great deal of motion, if it is in a more functional arc and painless, the patient will be greatly improved. Swanson does not specifically mention stability but if attention is directed at the preservation or reconstruction of the collateral ligaments, stability should be satisfactory. Probably the greatest value of this prosthesis is its ability to relieve predictably debilitating joint pain. This is vividly demonstrated in patients such as the one shown in Figure 10.10. The functional importance of pain-free stable joints in the patient disabled by painful osteoarthritis in terms of improved ability in the activities of daily living cannot be overstated.

PROBLEMS

Infection is rare, and usually occurs in rheumatoid patients with poor soft tissue coverage. It is (as

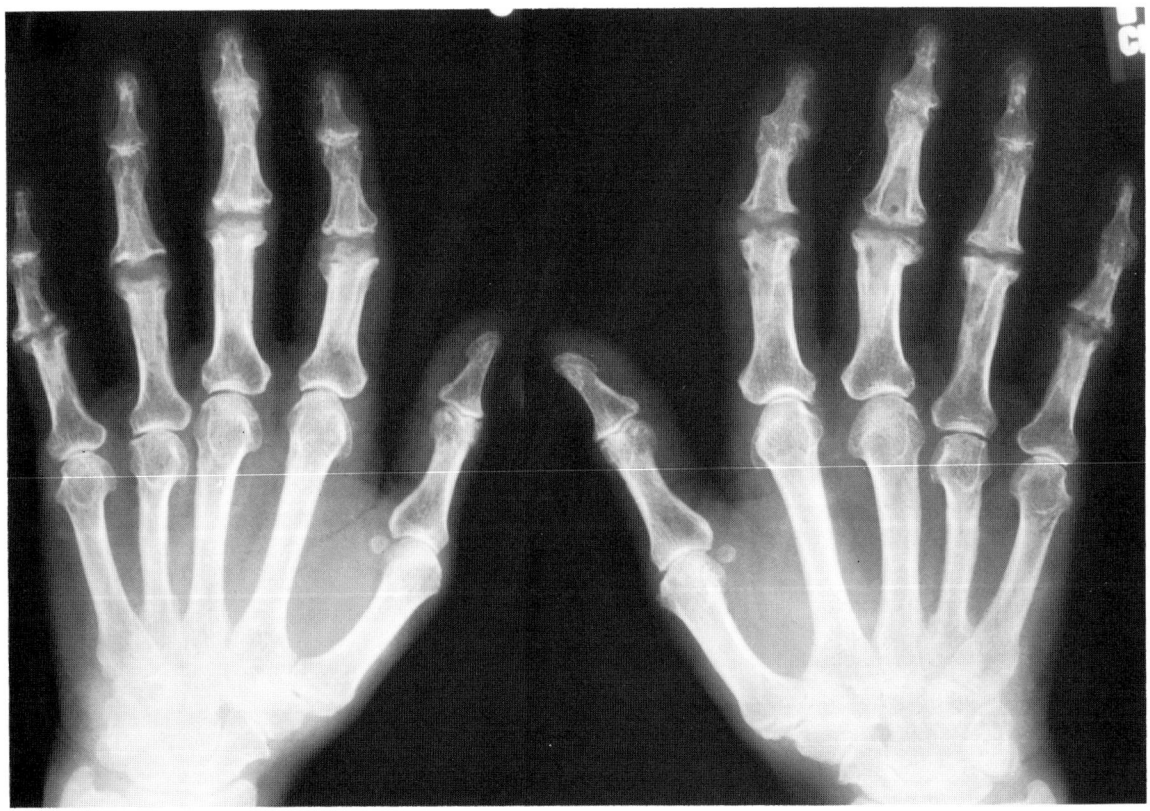

Fig. 10.10 A 55-year-old female waitress disabled with painful osteoarthritis of the PIP joints. In a staged reconstruction, all PIPs were replaced. She is pain-free, has an average arc of motion of 55° and the joints are stable. She continues to work.

INTERPHALANGEAL JOINT ARTHROPLASTIES 167

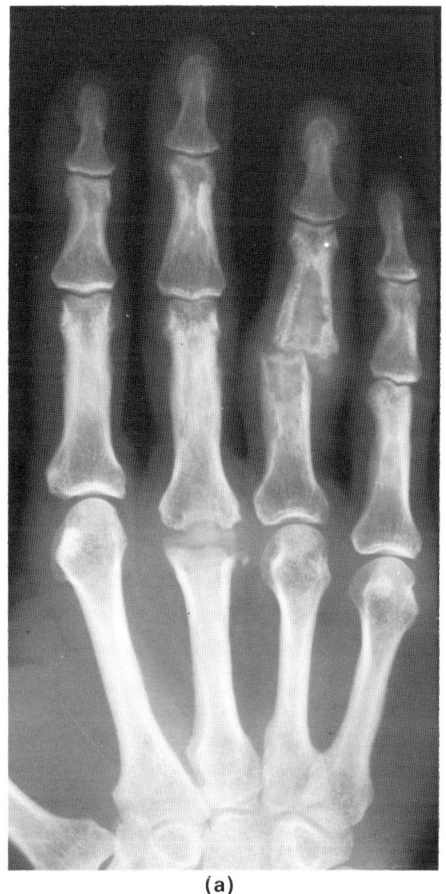

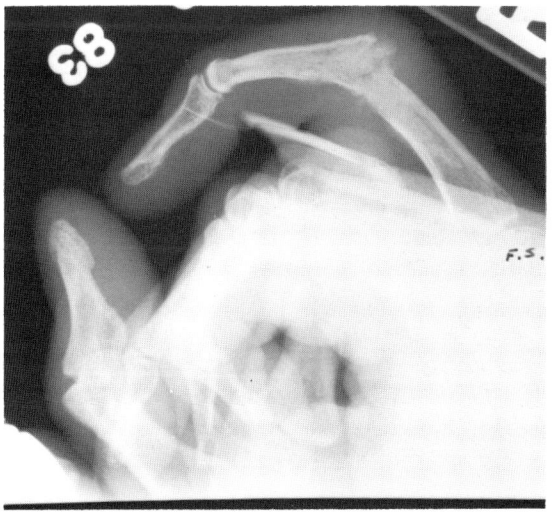

with the implantation of any permanent foreign body) more a potential hazard in immunosuppressed patients. Unless specifically contraindicated, broad-spectrum antibiotics should be used perioperatively in patients undergoing this procedure.

Implant fracture may be expected in a smaller number of patients (Fig. 10.11). Usually these are rheumatoid patients with an excellent postoperative range of motion. Fewer fractures have occurred since the introduction of 'high performance silicone' but they still occur. Swanson reported a 5% fracture rate in his latest review (Swanson et al 1985).

Bony overgrowth (Fig. 10.12) may also occur. An arthrodesis that develops when an arthroplasty was planned can be most frustrating, especially to the surgeon. An incidence of bony overgrowth of 4.2% in a review of 424 PIP silicone arthroplasties was recently reported (Swanson et al 1985). The patients most likely to exhibit this phenomenon are those with either post-traumatic arthrosis or hypertrophic osteoarthritis. If the arthrodesis occurs in a satisfactory position, it is usually painless and should be accepted by the patient and surgeon. Careful surgical technique with vigorous irrigation of the small bone chips and dust (especially the intramedullary debris caused by reaming) may decrease the possibility of this complication.

Silicone synovitis is a complication that is receiving increased attention. Cyst formation and reactive synovitis seem to be a significant complication when the material is placed under compressive load in the presence of shear forces (Gordon & Bullough 1982, Peimer et al 1986). This is most commonly seen in the silicone carpal replacement arthroplasties, particularly the scaphoid, lunate and trapezium. Indeed, this problem may lead to a significant alteration in the frequency with which these particular implants are used. It is known that the synovitis results from a reaction to particulate silicone (Worsing et al 1982). Therefore there should be little problem in the hinged replacements

Fig. 10.11 (a) A 50-year-old male with rheumatoid disease. Isolated joint destruction of middle metacarpophalangeal joint and ring PIP joint. The patient had strong grip and excellent range of movement (0–100°). The implant fractured (ring PIP) at about 6 months after surgery. Thus far the patient has declined revision. Anteroposterior view. (b) Lateral view.

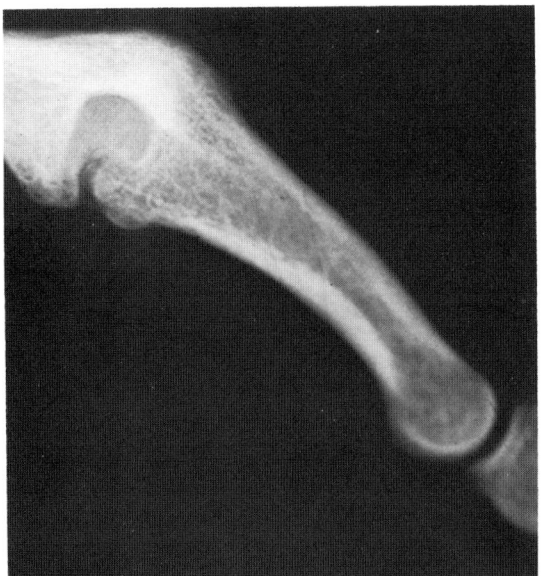

Fig. 10.12 Complete bony arthrodesis occurring around implanted silastic PIP replacement arthroplasty. (Photo courtesy of James F. Murray, MD.)

for joints unless bony impingement on the implant or implant fracture contribute to small particle formation. Very few cases of silicone synovitis at the interphalangeal joints are known or have been reported at the time of writing. However, it deserves mention in preoperative counselling as a possible complication of the permanent implantation of silicone in any location. It should be noted that the host response to silicone particles has been thoroughly studied and found to be uniformly benign in nature (Nalbandian et al 1983).

In our increasingly liability and litigation laden society, careful discussion of these specific complications in addition to the usual potential hazards attendant to any surgical procedure, will only contribute to the long-term satisfaction of both the patient and the surgeon. Overall there was a 10.9% revision rate in the large series reported by Swanson et al (1985) covering a 15-year period (1966–1981). Despite this fact, no procedure compares to the silicone replacement arthroplasty of the PIP joint for reliability in attaining pain-free functional motion.

A silicone replacement is available for the DIP joint. Experience with this implant is limited (Swanson's personal series is about 50 cases over a 20-year period). The procedure may retain some DIP motion and improve the appearance of the finger, but in view of the contribution of the DIP joint to the flexion arc (see Ch. 2), it is debatable whether it represents a clearly superior alternative to DIP arthrodesis in the vast majority of cases.

VOLAR PLATE ARTHROPLASTY

This procedure, first used by Eaton in 1967 (Eaton & Malerich 1980), has proven useful in the PIP joint for the treatment of dorsal fracture dislocations in which the volar articular surface of the middle phalanx has been destroyed but the condyles of the proximal phalanx have been preserved (Fig. 10.13). The technique of volar plate arthroplasty (VPA) is exacting and satisfactory results depend upon adherence to Eaton's technique (Eaton & Malerich 1980) and carefully monitored rehabilitation. This is not a procedure that will succeed without careful attention to detail. One of the greatest challenges confronting hand surgeons is restoration of motion to a stiff PIP joint. The most difficult portion of this technique is ascertaining and maintaining reduction of a PIP joint that possibly has been dislocated for many months.

The details of the technique are clearly stated in Eaton's definitive paper (Eaton & Malerich 1980). The approach is volar (Fig. 10.14**a**) and involves excision of the flexor sheath from the distal edge of the A-2 pulley to the proximal edge of the A-4 pulley. The collateral ligaments are excised, the volar plate is detached, elevated proximally and the joint is hyperextended (Fig. 10.14**b, c**). The base of the middle phalanx is debrided of fracture fragments and a smooth symmetrical transverse trough is created (Fig. 10.14**d**). Pull-out wires are used to advance the volar plate into the deficit (Fig. 10.14**e**). It is extremely important to inspect, and debride if necessary, the space between the extensor mechanism and the proximal phalanx dorsally. This can easily be done from the volar approach with the joint hyperextended. If the extensor is tethered in this area by scar, it may prevent accurate reduction of the remaining articular surface of the middle phalanx onto the proximal phalangeal condyles. Contracture of the

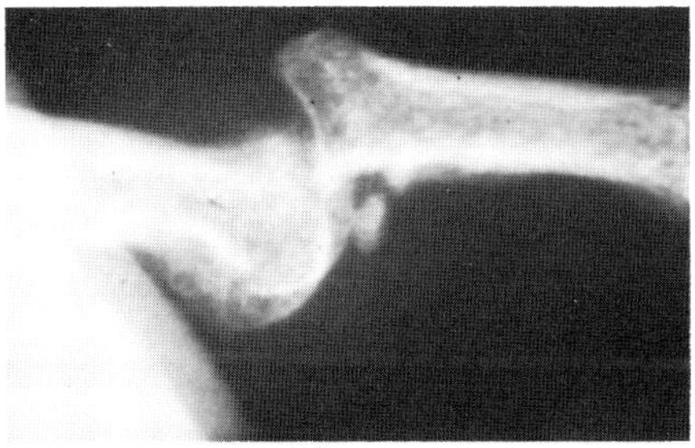

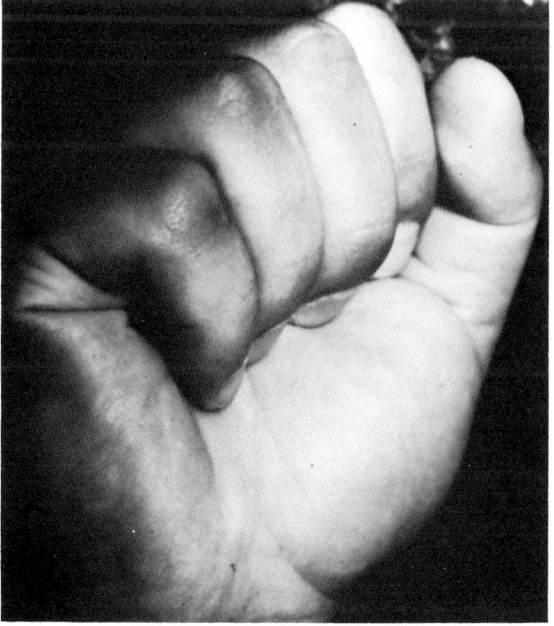

Fig. 10.13 (**a**) Dominant little finger in a 24-year-old male high school coach who sustained the injury 6 months prior to presentation. His own attempted reduction was unsuccessful. Constant pain and absent PIP flexion were present. A true example of 'coach's finger'. (**b**) Five months after volar plate arthroplasty (VPA), the joint is reduced. There is a measurable 40° extension deficit at PIP joint and 20° hyperextension of the DIP. (**c**) Flexion film taken same time as Fig. 10.13(**b**). Flexion is 95° at PIP and 40° at DIP. Motion is painless. Note defect in dorsal condylar area secondary to erosion by the base of the middle phalanx with forced flexion attempts while in the dislocated position (Fig. 10.13**a**). (**d**) Clinical photo-extension and appearance of digit. (**e**) Clinical photo-flexion. Patient and surgeon satisfaction excellent.

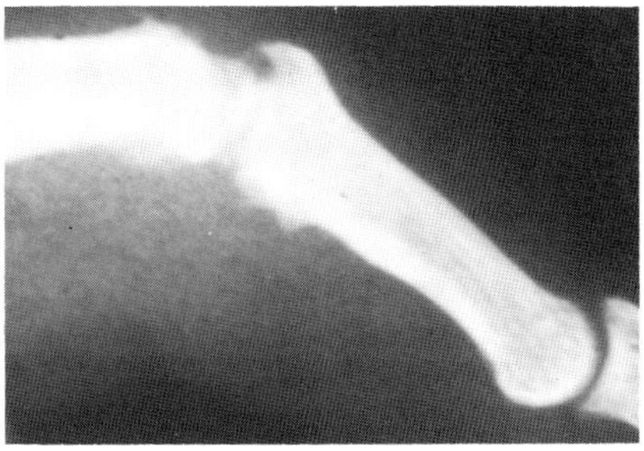

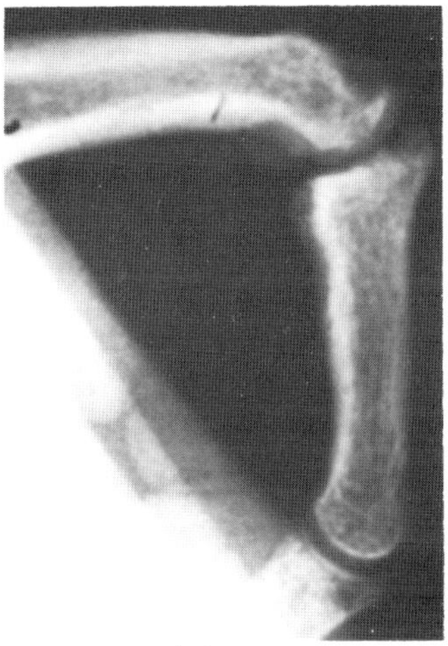

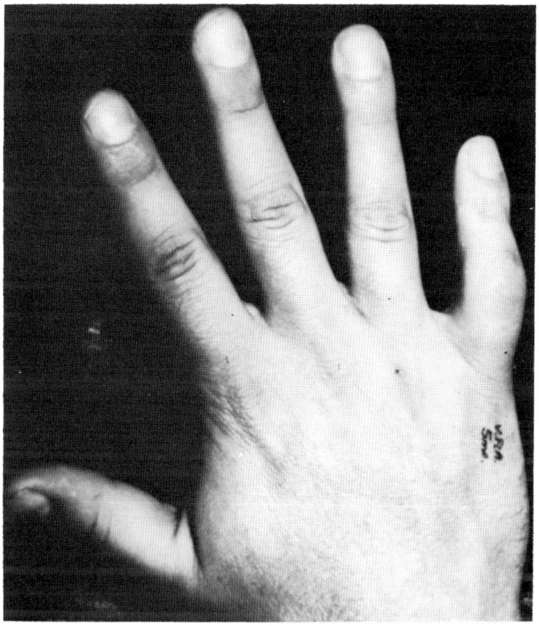

collateral ligaments may also prevent reduction and it is for this reason that either partial or complete excision is recommended. After reduction has been confirmed by a true lateral roentgenogram taken in the operating room, the joint is transfixed with a small calibre transarticular Kirschner wire and the volar plate advanced into the volar defect in the middle phalanx by tightening the pull-out wires which exit at the dorsal base of the middle phalanx (Fig. 10.14**f**). These wires are then tied over a pad or button.

Postoperatively the transarticular wire is left in place for 2–3 weeks. At that time the Kirschner wire is removed and a dorsal PIP block splint applied. The maximum extension allowed in the splint must be determined by the surgeon and may vary from case to case depending on stability or instability of the reduced joint at the time of surgery. The pull-out wire is removed at 4 weeks and the dorsal block splint is modified each week to allow more potential extension. Hand therapy with the therapist twice a week and on a daily basis at home may be necessary for 8–12 weeks before the maximum range of motion is achieved. A dynamic splint for PIP extension might be considered if PIP extension is not satisfactory after 6–8 weeks. Many of these patients do not achieve full PIP extension. However, their functional arc of motion is markedly improved in spite of a varying PIP extension deficit. Flexion is usually excellent and strength is markedly improved. The joints are usually pain-free and this procedure has proven to be very beneficial in reconstruction of the commonly seen dorsal fracture dislocation of the PIP joint. Certainly in this situation, this procedure should be considered before replacement arthroplasty or arthrodesis. The condition of the condyles of the proximal phalanx is a critical factor in predicting the success of the volar plate arthroplasty, probably equally as important as an accurate anatomical reduction of the joint at the time of surgery.

RECENT DEVELOPMENTS

The dream of the reconstructive surgeon is the perfect reconstitution of nature. Although it is difficult to believe that this dream will ever be realized, several newer techniques with specific indications are exciting. The first and most dramatic development is the application of microvascular technique to joint reconstruction. Buncke et al (1967) demonstrated experimentally that whole joints transferred with microvascular anastomoses maintained normal joint architecture and function. These experiments utilized the Rhesus monkey as a model, included finger and toe joints and extended to 2 years' post-microsurgical digital replantation. Autogenous microvascular transfer of joints from the toe (usually second toe) have been reported from several centres (Tsai et al 1982, O'Brien et al 1984, Kuo et al 1984). Indeed Tsai has reported a double transfer of PIP and DIP joint from the second toe to the index finger (Tsai & Singer 1984). The goal of these procedures was perhaps best summarized by O'Brien et al (1984) when they stated: 'Free vascularized digital joint transfers should provide joint stability, painless functional range of motion, tolerance of normal stresses without degeneration, and growth potential in children'. Although the question of the influence of the presence or absence of joint reinnervation in these clinical applications remains, it has not been reported to be a problem. At the present time these procedures remain in the realm of clinical experiments performed by expert microsurgeons in cases inappropriate for established reconstructive methods. Remarkable digital salvage has resulted in several otherwise unsalvageable situations (Tsai & Singer 1984).

These results are encouraging in terms of maintaining growth potential in children, maintaining a joint surface of normal cartilage to tolerate the stress of hand use and maintaining stability through the transferred collateral ligaments. However, the results in terms of active and passive movement in these joints have not been as encouraging (O'Brien et al 1984). This may be related to the decreased range of motion potential of the toe joints or the methods of fixation utilized. Many of these cases had composite tissue loss and composite transfers, especially extensor mechanism and dorsal skin. The motion therefore, in many cases, is probably decreased because of periarticular soft tissue changes (remember Bunnell's admonition). Thus the ideal candidate for

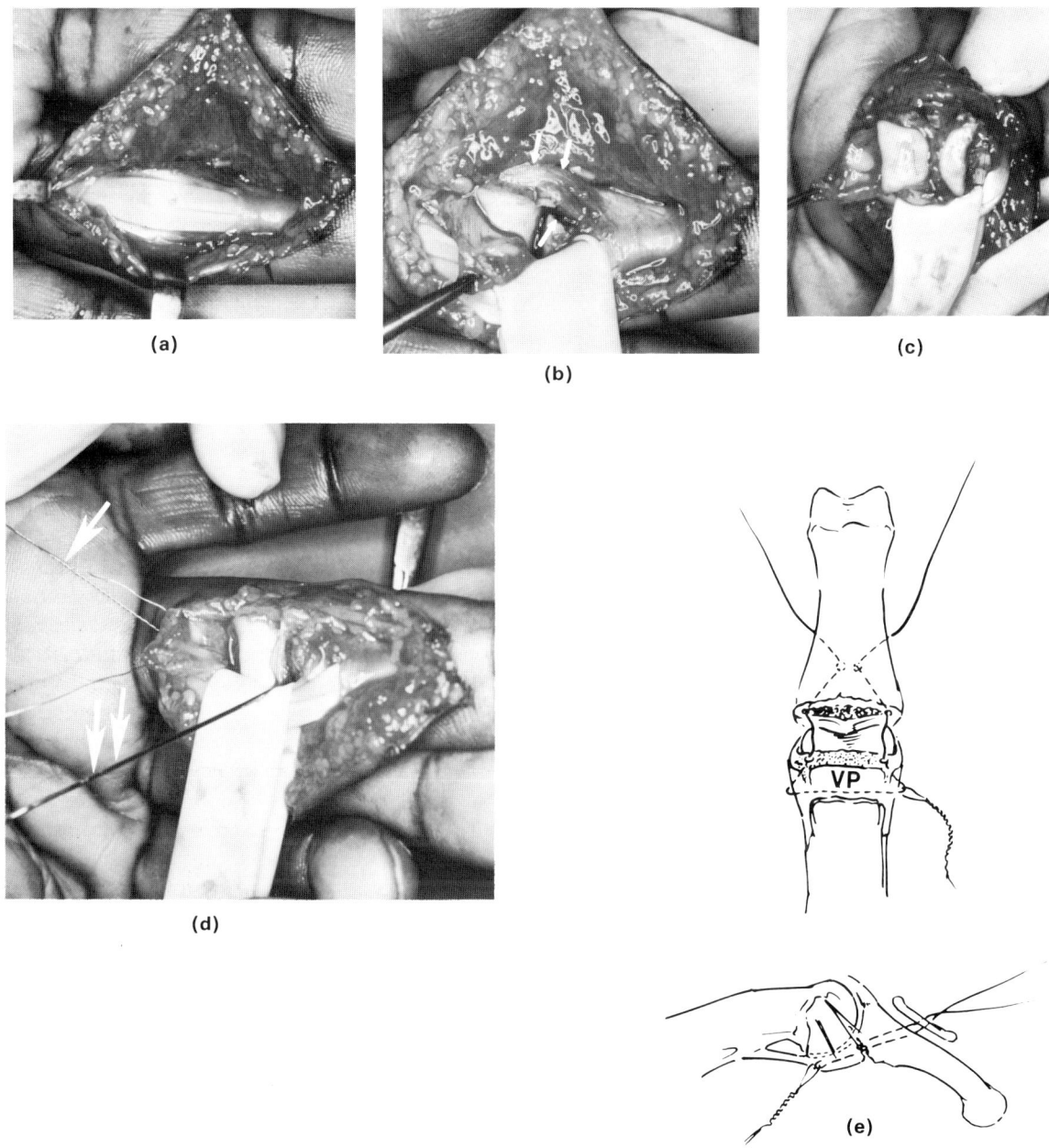

Fig. 10.14 (**a**) Surgical approach for volar plate arthroplasty (VPA). Flexor sheath excised from distal A-2 pulley to A-4 pulley. (**b**) PIP joint exposed. Volar plate elevated in hook, fracture site visualized (arrow). Flexor tendons are retracted in penrose drain. Collateral ligament (double arrows) has not been excised. (**c**) The PIP joint is 'shotgunned' (maximum hyperextension after collateral ligaments excised) and the condyles of the proximal phalanx are viewed directly end-on. The trough for the volar plate advancement has been created. Volar plate is held in forceps. Deeply embedded fragments of the base of the middle phalanx are left in place. (**d**) Pull-out wire in place in the volar plate (arrow). A straight needle (double arrows) is used to pass the pull-out wire through the middle phalanx. See Fig. 14(**e**). (**e**) Diagram of pull-out wire technique for VPA. (Reproduced with permission of R G Eaton, 1968, Journal of Hand Surgery, 5.)

the dream result would be a patient with a destroyed joint and normal periarticular tissue—extremely rare. Microvascular joint transfers are best considered in children who have joint and soft tissue deficits but satisfactory neurovascular function. In these cases this procedure does offer a true advantage by the provision of growth potential and elimination of bone and soft tissue deficits. The procedure will not be the perfect arthroplasty however, because of its inability to provide maximum motion.

In individuals under the age of 40 with no history of infection, tendon involvement or systemic disease with joint involvement, perichondral arthroplasty of the PIP joint might be indicated (Seradge et al 1984). This procedure is mentioned in the interest of completeness and the fact that it may be useful in young active individuals who have sustained intra-articular trauma, especially osteochondral fractures. The satisfactory results in this rather select patient population probably result from the ability of rib perichondrium to regenerate cartilaginous tissue after free non-vascularized transfer. The nature of the regenerative tissue is fibrocartilage rather than articular cartilage as clearly documented by biopsies of perichondrial arthroplasties (Seradge et al 1984). The procedure is most indicated in metacarpophalangeal and PIP joints in which only one side of the joint requires resurfacing, there is no subchondral deformity, there is no prior history of infection or systemic disease causing the joint destruction, and the patient is under 40 years old. These limiting criteria dictate that the indications for this procedure are narrow indeed.

CONCLUSION

The quest for the perfect arthroplasty continues. It is being pursued by many entities, collective and individual, proceeding along a great variety of investigational avenues. Surgeons who perform this procedure frequently (career hand surgeons) know the limitations and challenges of this procedure intimately. Therefore they are deeply involved in development of new techniques, materials, and postoperative management in order to improve the results of arthroplasties (all types) of the interphalangeal joints.

At the present time, hand surgeons know that in most cases the statistical probability is good (positive risk/benefit ratio) that pain can be relieved, some motion can be retained, deformity can be corrected, and adequate stability can be preserved or reconstructed. The best results of this operation continue to improve and with attention to surgical detail probably will continue to do so. The dream of a 'perfect' arthroplasty may never be achieved but it remains a powerful motivation to the surgeon devoted to hand reconstruction. Thus we as hand surgeons continue to enjoy the challenge of the ongoing quest which may be much more exciting than the ultimate goal. We may not achieve perfection but the attempt do do so adds great interest and stimulation to the daily practice of hand surgery.

REFERENCES

Beckenbaugh R D, Linscheid R L 1982 Arthroplasty in the hand and wrist. In: Green D P (ed) Operative hand surgery. Churchill Livingston, New York, Ch 6, pp 146–147

Blair W F, Shurr D G, Buckwalter J A 1984 Metacarpophalangeal joint implant arthroplasty with a silastic spacer. Journal of Bone and Joint Surgery 66A: 365–370

Brannon E W, Klein G 1959 Experiences with a finger-joint prosthesis. Journal of Bone and Joint Surgery 41A: 87–102

Buncke H J, Daniller A J, Shulz W P 1967 The fate of autogenous whole joints transplanted by microvascular anastomoses. Plastic and Reconstructive Surgery 39: 333–342

Bunnell S 1944 Surgery of the hand. J B Lippincott, Philadelphia, p 215

Burman M S 1940 Vitallium cap arthroplasty of metacarpophalangeal and interphalangeal joints of the fingers. Bulletin of the Hospital for Joint Disease 1: 79–89

Burman M S, Abrahamson R H 1943 The use of plastics in reconstructive surgery. Lucite in arthroplasty. Military Surgeon 93: 405–414

Carroll R E, Taber T H 1954 Digital arthroplasty of the proximal interphalangeal joint. Journal of Bone and Joint Surgery 36A: 912–920

Eaton R G, Malerich M M 1980 Volar plate arthroplasty of the proximal interphalangeal joint: a review of ten years' experience. Journal of Hand Surgery 5: 260–268

Flatt A E 1961 Restoration of rheumatoid finger-joint function. Interim report of trial of prosthetic replacement. Journal of Bone and Joint Surgery 43A: 753–774

Flatt A E 1968 The care of the rheumatoid hand, 2nd edn. C V Mosby, Louis, ch 5, pp 84–85

Flatt A E, Ellison M R 1972 Restoration of rheumatoid finger joint function. III. Journal of Bone and Joint Surgery 54A: 1317–1322

Gordon M L, Bullough P G 1982 Synovial and osseous inflammation in failed silicone rubber prosthesis. Journal of Bone and Joint Surgery 64A: 574–580

Kuo E T, Ji Z L, Zhao Y C, Zhang M L 1984 Reconstruction of metacarpophalangeal joint by free vascularized autogenous metatarsophalangeal joint transplant. Journal of Reconstructive Microsurgery 1: 65–74

Nalbandian R M, Swanson A B, Maupin B K 1983 Long-term silicone implant arthroplasty. Journal of the American Medical Association 250: 1195–1198

Neibauer J J 1971 Dacron–silicone prosthesis for the metacarpophalangeal and interphalangeal joints. In: Cramer L M, Chase R A (eds) Symposium on the hand. C V Mosby, St Louis vol III: 96–105

Neibauer J J, Landry R M 1971 Dacron–silicone prosthesis for the metacarpophalangeal and interphalangeal joints. Hand 3: 55–61

Neibauer J J, Shaw J L, Doren W W 1968 The silicone–dacron hinge prosthesis: design, evaluation and application. Journal of Bone and Joint Surgery 50A: 634

Neibauer J J, Shaw J L, Doren W W 1969 Silicone–dacron hinge prosthesis. Design, evaluation and application. Annals of Rheumatic Disease suppl. 28: 56–58

O'Brien B M, Gould J S, Morrison W A, Russell R C, MacLeod A M, Pribaz J J 1984 Free vascularized small joint transfer to the hand. Journal of Hand Surgery 9A: 634–641

Peimer C, Medige J, Wright J 1986 Reactive synovitis following silicone arthroplasty. Journal of Hand Surgery (in press)

Seradge H, Kutz J A, Klenert H E, Lister G D, Wolff T W, Atasoy E 1984 Perichondrial resurfacing arthroplasty in the hand. Journal of Hand Surgery 9A: 880–886

Swanson A B 1966 A flexible implant for replacement of arthritic or destroyed joints in the hand. New York University Interclinical Information Bulletin 6: 16–19

Swanson A B 1968 Silicone rubber implants for replacement of arthritic or destroyed joints in the hand. Surgical Clinics of North America 48: 1113–1127

Swanson A B 1973a Flexible implant resection arthroplasty in the hand and extremities. C V Mosby, St Louis, ch 11, p 184

Swanson A B 1973b Implant resection arthroplasty of the proximal interphalangeal joint. Orthopedic Clinics of North America 4: 1007–1029

Swanson A B 1979 Flexible implant arthroplasty of the proximal interphalangeal joint. Annals of Plastic Surgery 3: 346–354

Swanson A B 1980 Surgical techniques for flexible implant arthroplasty in the MP, PIP, DIP joints of the hand. Grand Rapids, Michigan

Swanson A B, Swanson G de G, Leonard J 1978 Postoperative rehabilitation program in flexible implant arthroplasty of the digits. Rehabilitation of the Hand. C V Mosby, St Louis pp 31–69

Swanson A B, Maupin B K, Gajjar N V, Swanson G de G 1985 Long-term review of flexible implant arthroplasty in the proximal interphalangeal joint of the hand. Journal of Hand Surgery 10A: 796–805

Tsai T M, Jupiter J B, Kutz J E, Kleinert H E 1982 Vascularized autogenous whole joint transfer in the hand—a clinical study. Journal of Hand Surgery 7: 335–342

Tsai T M, Singer R 1984 Elective free vascularized double transfer of toe joint from second toe to proximal interphalangeal joint of index finger: a case report. Journal of Hand Surgery 9A: 816–820

Urbaniak J R, McCollum D E, Goldner J L 1970 Metacarpophalangeal and interphalangeal joint reconstruction: use of silicone rubber–dacron prostheses for replacement of irreparable joints of the hand. Southern Medical Journal 63: 1281–1290

Worsing R A, Engber W D, Land T A 1982 Reactive synovitis from particulate silastic. Journal of Bone and Joint Surgery 64A: 581–585

G. Hooper

11
Techniques of interphalangeal arthrodesis

Arthrodesis of an interphalangeal (IP) joint has the inevitable disadvantage that movement in the joint is lost. However, many patients and surgeons are happy to accept this disadvantage in the knowledge that arthrodesis is a once and for all procedure that will provide stability and relief from pain in a high percentage of cases without the prospect of further revisional surgery being necessary.

INDICATIONS

The indications for arthrodesis of an IP joint overlap with the indications for other procedures such as arthroplasty. As the relative merits of the various available procedures for dealing with specific conditions are discussed elsewhere in this book they will not be considered further here. Suffice it to say that arthrodesis of an IP joint is the procedure of choice when the joint is painful, unstable, flail or deformed and these problems cannot be overcome by other means. Even when other means of joint reconstruction are feasible, arthrodesis may still be considered as an alternative. The conditions in which arthrodesis may be indicated are listed in Table 11.1.

POSITION OF ARTHRODESIS

A useful guide to the desirable degree of angulation of an IP arthrodesis is that given by Straub (1959): the IP joints should be fixed in the position most readily adopted by these joints when the hand is held in the position of rest. This implies that the angle of the arthrodesis is greater in the more ulnar digits to provide a normal cascade of the fingers and to preserve a strong power grip, for which flexion of the little and ring fingers is so important. Lister (1984) has recommended that a proximal IP joint in one of the ulnar three digits should be fused at an angle that allows the finger to be brought into a power grasp but that does not result in malalignment of the pulp of the finger with the others when the hand is fully extended. As the ability of the metacarpophalangeal joints to hyperextend increases from the radial to the ulnar border of the hand it is possible to fuse the proximal IP joints of the ulnar digits in more flexion to preserve power grip and yet still allow the pulp of the finger to come out to the plane of the palm when the hand is extended.

Table 11.1 Indications for arthrodesis of an IP joint

General indications	
Malposition of fingers	
Flail uncontrolled IP joint	
Painful destruction of a joint	
Indications in specific conditions	
Acute trauma	Severe joint destruction
Osteoarthritis (primary or secondary)	Pain and deformity
Rheumatoid arthritis	Pain and deformity
Psoriatic arthropathy	Pain and deformity
Extensor tendon injuries	Symptomatic late mallet deformity
	Rigid boutonnière deformity
Flexor tendon injuries	Unstable terminal phalanx due to cut profundus tendon in finger or thumb
Scleroderma	Deformity
Burns	Deformity
Dupuytren's disease	Deformity
Septic arthritis	Joint destruction

The distal IP joints are usually fused at slightly lesser angles than the proximal IP joints, although a fairly wide range of angles is permissible provided that there is full active motion at more proximal joints.

In the IP joint of the thumb only slight flexion is needed so that the thumb can easily be put through ring-handled tools such as scissors, and the span of the hand is preserved. In practice a considerable variation in the angle of arthrodesis can be tolerated in the thumb.

A final decision about the angle of arthrodesis will of course depend on an analysis of the individual patient's requirements, but Table 11.2 provides a summary of recommended angles of arthrodesis that will be found to be suitable for the majority of patients.

Table 11.2 Recommended angles for arthrodesis

Thumb	MCP	20°	IP	10–20°
Index finger	PIP	20°	DIP	10°
Middle finger	PIP	20°	DIP	10–20°
Ring finger	PIP	40°	DIP	15–30°
Little finger	PIP	50°	DIP	20–40°

MCP: metacarpophalangeal joint
PIP: proximal interphalangeal joint
IP: interphalangeal joint
DIP: distal interphalangeal joint

SURGICAL TECHNIQUES

The object of any technique of digital arthrodesis is to achieve a stable and painless union in a proper position within a reasonable space of time (Moberg & Henrikson 1960). In addition, the technique should be within the capabilities of most surgeons, require the minimum of specialized equipment and allow early mobilization of the hand, without external support if possible. Although many methods of IP arthrodesis are available, few fulfil all these criteria. All the methods are similar in that the remains of the articular cartilage are removed, the joint is placed in the desired position and held in that position until bony union has occurred. They differ in the preparation of the bony surfaces and the technique of stabilizing the phalanges during the period to union (see Table 11.3).

Incisions

Most surgeons prefer to expose the proximal IP joint through a longitudinal or curved dorsal skin incision with longitudinal division of the extensor apparatus over the joint. It is important to resect both collateral ligaments to allow exposure of the joint surfaces, but it is not necessary to interfere with the volar plate. The extensor apparatus should be repaired with fine sutures.

Although the midline approach has proved satisfactory in patients affected by rheumatoid arthritis (Granovitz & Vainio 1966), Flatt (1983) recommends that the extensor apparatus be reflected laterally, rather than divided in the midline, when performing IP arthrodesis is this condition.

Hill (1982) exposes the joint by a mid-axial skin incision; the collateral ligament is resected and the extensor hood is reflected laterally. This allows the distal part of the finger to be deviated laterally, thus delivering the articular surfaces into the incision.

The distal IP joint can be exposed through a chevron incision with its apex pointing distally. The extensor insertion is divided in the line of the skin incision and should be repaired when closing the wound. It practice this gives a rather inadequate exposure of the joint and Lister (1978) prefers an H-shaped incision with the vertical limbs placed midlaterally; it is important to dissect the distal flap deeply close to bone to ensure its viability.

The IP joint of the thumb can be exposed through any of the incisions described for the distal IP joint of a finger. The metacarpophalangeal joint of the thumb is readily exposed by a straight dorsal incision passing between the extensor pollicis longus and brevis tendons.

Surgical exposure is a matter of personal preference, but it should be appropriate to the method chosen to stabilize the arthrodesis. Any method of stabilization can be used when the joint is exposed through a dorsal approach but a lateral skin incision limits the surgeon to the use of Kirschner wires.

Preparation of bone surfaces

For a successful arthrodesis it is essential that good contact between cancellous bone surfaces is obtained.

The joint surfaces may be squared off by cuts made with a power saw at angles that will place the

176 THE INTERPHALANGEAL JOINTS

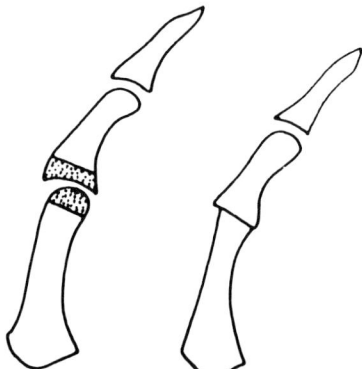

Fig. 11.1 Preparation of bone surfaces by excision of joint surfaces by flat cuts. Provided the surfaces remain in contact the angle of the arthrodesis is determined by the angles of the cuts.

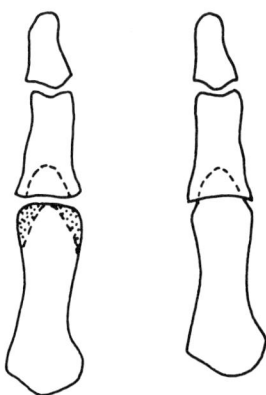

Fig. 11.3 Preparation of bone surfaces by cup and cone method, which allows adjustment of position in three planes.

arthrodesis in the desired position of flexion when the bone surfaces are brought into contact (Fig. 11.1). In practice it can be difficult to make the cuts accurately and, furthermore, the flat bone surfaces will lose contact if the relative position of the phalanges changes even slightly, as it so frequently does when fixation is applied.

The chevron method described by Omer (1968) (Fig. 11.2) is slightly more forgiving than cutting the opposing surfaces flat, but once again it can be difficult to cut the bone ends accurately.

Carroll & Hill (1969) have described a simple cup and cone technique: the head of the proximal phalanx is shaped with rongeurs to produce a convex surface and the articular surface of the distal phalanx is removed with gouges to provide a corresponding concave surface (Fig. 11.3). Making a circle of holes with an awl around the periphery of the articular surface of the distal phalanx facilitates its removal with a gouge, but difficulty may be experienced because of the small size of the bone and its hardness. It is feasible to make a central hole in the base of the phalanx with an awl and then remove the rest of the articular surface with an angled rongeur or the tip of a 0.6 cm ($\frac{1}{4}''$) or 1.3 cm ($\frac{1}{2}''$) bit on a power drill (Watson & Shaffer 1970).

This cup and cone method allows the arthrodesis to be positioned in three planes. Most often it is necessary to adjust the position in the sagittal plane of the finger only. If this is the case the adjacent bone surfaces can be shaped with rongeurs into a simple tongue and groove configuration, which provides stability and good bone contact (Fig. 11.4).

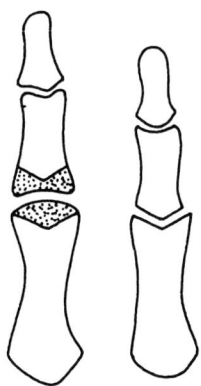

Fig. 11.2 Preparation of bone surfaces by chevron cuts.

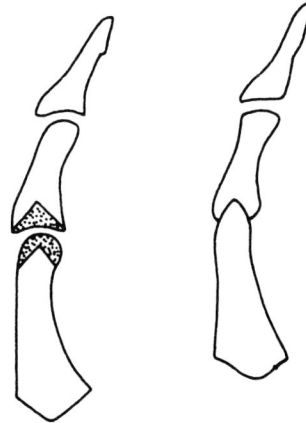

Fig. 11.4 Preparation of bone surfaces by tongue and groove method. Simple and stable.

If there has been bone destruction, for example in rheumatoid arthritis, it may be necessary to shape the remains of the head of the proximal phalanx into a point to fit into the base of the adjacent phalanx (Granovitz & Vainio 1966). Even more severe bone loss, usually the result of arthritis mutilans (Vainio & Pulkki 1959) or severe trauma (Allende & Engelem 1980), may have to be overcome by inserting a corticocancellous bone graft between the phalanges.

The method of preparation of bone surfaces should be appropriate to the method of stabilization that will be used. For example, it is difficult or impossible to use the compression screw or bone graft techniques described below if much of the head of the proximal phalanx has been destroyed by disease or damaged during preparation of the bone surfaces.

Stabilization

The various methods available for stabilizing an IP arthrodesis during the period of union are given in Table 11.3.

Table 11.3 Methods of stabilizing an IP arthrodesis

Internal fixation
  Kirschner wires
  Compression screw
  Plate
  Tension band wiring
  Intraosseous wiring
  Medullary peg

Bone graft

External fixation

Kirschner wires

Carroll & Hill (1969) described the use of one oblique Kirschner wire driven retrograde from the joint surface and then back across the joint after obtaining the correct position in their cup and cone arthrodesis (see Fig. 11.3). After surgery the finger and the adjacent finger were incorporated in a plaster dressing extending from the antecubital fossa and holding the metacarpophalangeal joints flexed. The dressing was maintained for 6 weeks. The authors reported on arthrodesis of 635 joints using this technique: there was a pseudarthrosis rate of 5% and four revisions were necessary for rotational errors.

A single Kirschner wire does not provide good rotational stability (Fyfe & Mason 1979) and the use of two crossed wires is preferred by many (Granovitz & Vainio 1966, Boyes 1970, Watson & Shaffer 1970, Edwards et al 1982). There is a danger that two wires can hold the joint surfaces distracted from each other, but this danger can be avoided if one wire is placed longitudinally and the other obliquely (Fig. 11.5). Both wires are driven-retrograde from the joint; the longitudinal wire is driven back across the joint first and then the oblique wire is driven back while the bones are held firmly together (Boyes 1970). Ideally the wires should cross within bone rather than at the level of the arthrodesis (Watson & Shaffer 1970), and this requires very careful positioning of the wires. Usually there is only one opportunity to place them in the correct position. Repeated attempts invite frustration because the wire may take the same track again, or damage the remaining bone stock close to the joint. In order to obtain the correct position at the first attempt the following points of technique are recommended:

1. A lightweight power drill should be used to drive the wires
2. A double-ended Kirschner wire of 0.9 mm diameter is used
3. A 'preview' wire should be laid across the arthrodesis external to bone to gauge the correct angle

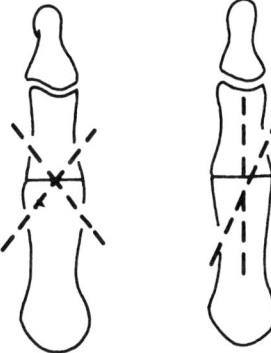

Fig. 11.5 Correct and incorrect positioning of Kirschner wires. The configuration on the left may hold the bone surfaces apart.

4. A needle from a 14-gauge intravenous catheter can be used as a 'drill guide' for an 0.9 mm wire and will prevent the wire skating from the surface of cortical bone (Edwards et al 1982)

Hill (1982) recommends that the ends of the Kirschner wires be left long and bent over outside the skin to prevent migration; he states that infection is less common when this is done. Leaving the wire outside the skin does have the advantage that another operation is not necessary for removal. However, wires outside the skin are liable to catch on objects and clothing and Lister (1978) has pointed out that this might result in a wire being withdrawn accidentally if only one end is outside the skin.

Excellent results have been reported using crossed wires for stabilization. Watson & Shaffer (1970) reported a 100% rate of union in 40 IP joints. External support (unspecified) was used for around 5 weeks and the wires were removed on average 6 weeks after surgery. Granovitz & Vainio (1966) used the technique in 122 IP joints affected by rheumatoid arthritis. External support was not used and there were eight non-unions. They stressed the importance of retaining the head of the phalanx if possible, since if it is resected or already destroyed by disease it is not possible to bring cancellous bone surfaces into contact at the site of arthrodesis and the risk of non-union is increased. If there is significant loss of bone the insertion of a corticocancellous graft may be necessary (Vainio & Pulkki 1959) and it may then be difficult or impossible to stabilize the arthrodesis by the use of crossed wires.

Compression screws

The small ASIF (AO) screws can provide great stability and compression of bone surfaces in IP joint arthrodesis (Narakas 1976, Gschwend 1980, Heim & Pfeiffer 1982).

These screws are of most value in arthrodesis of the proximal IP joint. After removal of the joint surfaces, either by cutting them flush with a power saw at the desired angle of arthrodesis or by the tongue and groove method, a hole is drilled with a 2 mm drill, retrograde from the joint, to emerge on the dorsum of the proximal phalanx (Fig. 11.6). The angle of this hole relative to the long axis of

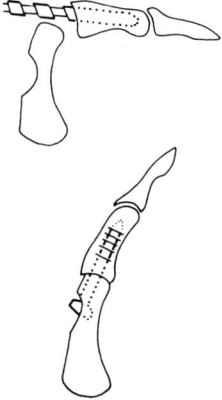

Fig. 11.6 Technique of arthrodesis using compression screw. Tapping of the bones has not been illustrated. For details see text.

the proximal phalanx will determine the angle of the arthrodesis. The intermediate phalanx is then drilled with a 2 mm bit and both drill holes are tapped with the 3.5 mm tap. Before inserting a small cancellous lag screw of suitable length, a trough is prepared on the dorsum of the proximal phalanx to avoid prominence of the head of the screw. In patients with small phalanges it may be necessary to use smaller ASIF screws with their appropriate drills and taps.

Very stable fixation is obtained by this method and external splintage after surgery may be minimal or even dispensed with altogether. There is, however, no margin for error and if the arthrodesis is made at the wrong angle it will not be possible to correct it. It is also easy to damage soft bone with the drill and then the technique must be abandoned. Although compression screw arthrodesis has been used with success in joints affected by rheumatoid arthritis (Gschwend 1980), great care is necessary and it is difficult or impossible to use this method if there has been much destruction of bone by disease.

A similar technique can be used in the distal IP joint, but the small size of the bones makes it difficult and it is not recommended. Instead a small screw can be driven from the finger tip into the intermediate phalanx. Great stability is achieved (Engle et al 1977), but no angulation of the arthrodesis is possible. Furthermore, the head of the screw lies superficially and the screw may have to be removed because of discomfort. To avoid this the screw can be driven proximally to bury the head in the terminal phalanx but this runs the risk of splitting the bone. The great advantage of this technique is that external splintage is not needed; the rate of union is similar to that obtained with crossed Kirschner wires (Engle et al 1977).

Instead of an ASIF small fragment screw, Faithfull & Herbert (1984) have used the Herbert double-ended scaphoid compression screw to stabilize small joints in the hand, with promising results in their pilot series.

Plate

Paneva-Holevich (1977) has used a special 90° blade plate with a spiked blade and two hole plate to stabilize phalangeal fractures or IP joint arthrodeses. Compression is applied on the dynamic compression plate (DCP) principle by tightening the two screws in the oval holes of the plate. Five cases of arthrodesis of the proximal IP joint for severe intra-articular fractures were reported with good results. Clearly this technique requires special equipment and would appear unduly finicky in comparison with some of the other methods available. It might also prove difficult to control the angle of the arthrodesis with such a device.

Tension band wiring

As the flexors of the fingers are stronger than the extensors, a tension band placed on the extensor aspect of the finger will result in compression of the bone surfaces at the arthrodesis when attempts are made to flex the finger.

The tension band technique is mainly applicable to fusion of the proximal IP joint. After removing the joint surfaces, a length of 24-gauge wire is passed through a transverse drill hole in the intermediate phalanx. Two parallel 0.9 mm Kir-

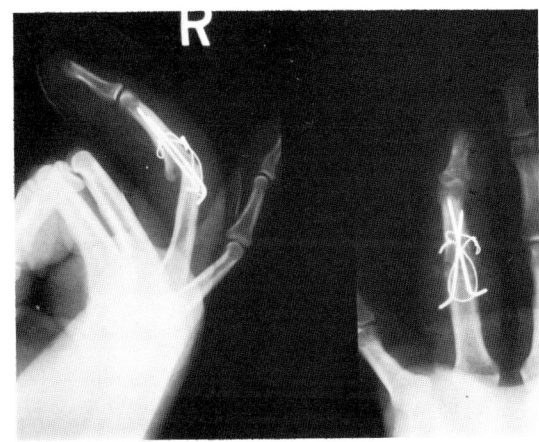

Fig. 11.7 Fixation by tension band wiring.

schner wires are then driven retrograde through the head of the proximal phalanx at the desired angle of arthrodesis and then back up the intermediate phalanx. The wire is tightened as a figure-of-eight loop around the protruding ends of the Kirschner wires, which are bent to a right angle (Fig. 11.7). No external splintage is necessary as the fixation is very strong (Gould et al 1984).

Allende and Engelem (1980) used this technique in 26 joints in patients who had mostly sustained open articular fractures; there were 2 infections, 2 lateral deviation malunions and one delayed union. They did not advise the use of this method when the bones were osteoporotic or when there was severe joint destruction, although it is possible to insert a corticocancellous bone block between the bone ends to gain length if necessary. In contrast, Narakas (1976) has specifically recommended the use of the tension band technique when the bones are osteoporotic.

This is a reliable and simple technique. Its main disadvantage is the inevitable interference with the extensor mechanism by the wires, which must be removed later.

Intraosseous wiring

Robertson (1964) described a method of IP stabilization using two parallel loops of wire inserted through holes drilled proximal and distal to the joint in an anteroposterior direction. The technique was used mainly to obtain arthrodesis of distal interphalangeal joints and there were no failures in 63 IP joints in 52 patients.

Lister (1978) reported the use of a modified technique of intraosseous wiring (Fig. 11.8). After preparation of the bone ends a single loop of no. 0 (BS gauge 26) monofilament stainless steel wire is passed through two parallel holes drilled transversely with a 0.9 mm diameter Kirschner wire 0.5 cm on either side of the joint. A 0.9 mm Kirschner wire is then driven retrograde from the joint. This wire may lie either parallel or oblique to the long axis of the finger, depending on the need to avoid transfixing soft tissues; it is usually oblique at the proximal IP joint and in the longitudinal axis at the distal IP joint. The exposed cancellous bone surfaces are carefully opposed, holding the phalanges at the desired angle relative to each other, and then the Kirschner wire is driven back across the joint to stabilize it. The wire loop is then tightened and, to prevent irritation of soft tissues, its twisted end is buried in a hole in the bone drilled with a Kirschner wire. No external support is needed after operation and mobilization of the hand is commenced at 3 days.

Lister reported on 53 arthrodeses using this method. The mean time to union was around 10 weeks. The Kirschner wire was removed when there was clinical evidence of union, judged by lack of pain on stressing the joint. There was a failure of union in 5 cases and these were attributed to failures in essential elements of the technique, such as congruity of bone surfaces and maintenance of fixation until there was clinical evidence of union.

A similar method of intraosseous wiring has been used by others. Høgh & Jensen (1982) reported their experience gained in the arthrodesis of 43 joints over a 10-year period. They preferred to use two Kirschner wires to ensure rotatory stability, although this is in fact good in the simpler method described by Lister (Fyfe & Mason 1979). Holes for the cerclage wires were drilled with hypodermic needles into which the wire could be inserted to facilitate its withdrawal through bone (Fig. 11.9). External splintage was used, generally for 6 weeks, and all wires were removed in most patients. Union was not obtained in 7 joints, but in only 3 patients was the non-union symptomatic.

The technique of intraosseous wiring is simple, quick and reliable. It allows early mobilization free of external support. No special instruments are needed and several joints can be stabilized in one patient at the same sitting. In addition the strength of fixation is better than that obtained with crossed Kirschner wires and is strong enough to withstand the flexor forces involved in pinching (Fyfe & Mason 1979, Massengill et al 1979, Vanik et al 1984). Unlike fixation with crossed Kirschner wires, there is no risk of distraction of the bone surfaces; indeed, if the cerclage wire is placed dorsal to the axis of the joint a tension band compression effect is obtained.

Medullary peg

Harrison & Nicolle (1974) designed a simple polypropylene peg to stabilize arthrodeses in the

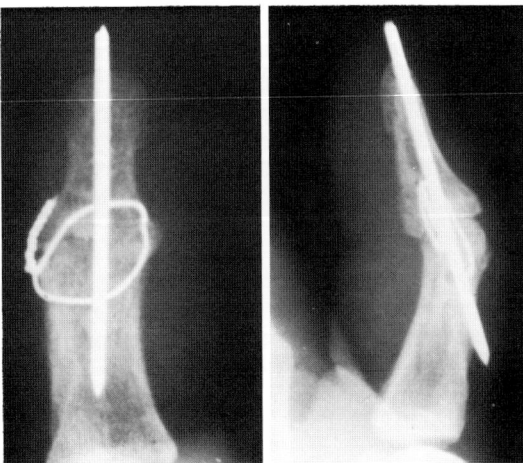

Fig. 11.8 Fixation by intraosseous wiring.

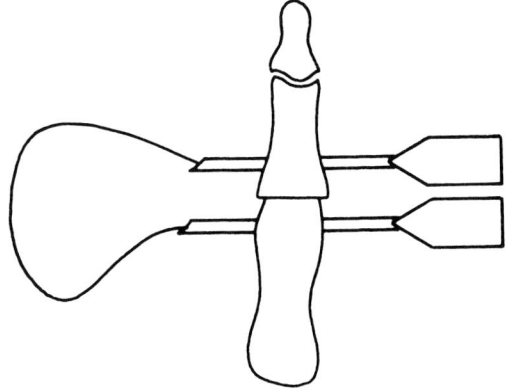

Fig. 11.9 In the technique of intraosseous wiring hypodermic needles can be used to drill the phalanges and facilitate the passage of the wire loop through bone.

TECHNIQUES OF INTERPHALANGEAL ARTHRODESIS 181

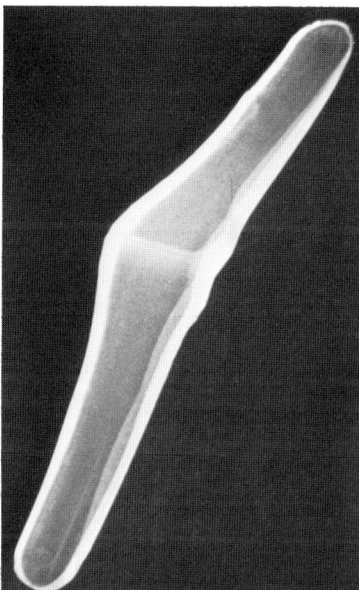

Fig. 11.10 Harrison-Nicolle polypropylene peg.

rheumatoid hand (Fig. 11.10). The peg is tapered at either end and is made in different sizes with various angles to suit the particular joint involved. The technique is very simple: after nibbling away the remains of the joint surface, the medullary cavity of each phalanx is prepared with a hand reamer and the peg is inserted. No external splintage other than a dressing is used.

Although the aim of this technique was to obtain an arthrodesis, early follow-up of the first patients indicated that a pain-free, stable, fibrous union was the more usual result (Harrison 1974). A longer review has however shown that, in time, bony union does occur in the majority, with a satisfactory fibrous union in the remainder (Harrison et al 1977).

This simple, quick technique is certainly of value in the rheumatoid hand and can be used for other indications (Harrison 1974). It is perhaps best regarded as a means of obtaining pain relief and stability in joints, rather than a technique of arthrodesis, and it does have the disadvantage that specialized equipment is needed.

Bone graft

The use of a corticocancellous bone graft to stabilize an IP arthrodesis gives good results in terms of union but is technically very demanding.

Brittain (1952) described an ingenious method in which a graft was inlaid in the medullary cavity and placed under compression when attempts were made to flex the joint. He noted that IP joints were most difficult to fuse successfully and concluded that his technique was indicated for use only in the thumb.

A medullary peg of the type described by Brittain precludes accurate fixation of an IP joint in flexion. This objection has been overcome by the method described by Moberg & Henrikson (1960) (Fig. 11.11). After preparing the joint surfaces, a drill hole is made in the proximal phalanx, entering the dorsum of the phalanx about 1 cm proximal to the joint at the angle required for the arthrodesis. Alternatively, the hole can be drilled retrograde from the joint, as is done in an ASIF compression screw arthrodesis. A further drill hole is made in the medulla of the more distal phalanx. A matchstick corticocancellous graft, 1.5–3 cm in length, is obtained from the dorsum of the ulna just below the olecranon. The round hole in the head of the proximal phalanx is squared off with a small file and the graft is shaped to allow it to be driven through the hole and up into the medullary cavity of the distal phalanx. After operation the finger is enclosed in a well-moulded plaster cast extending up the forearm. The cast is retained for 4–6 weeks. Moberg (1960) reported good results: out of 50 joints there was failure of union in only 2 when the correct technique had been used. The average healing time was less than 6 weeks.

Potenza (1973) described a similar technique, but with further stabilization provided by crossed Kirschner wires passing through the phalanges and peg graft to allow earlier mobilization free from support. The graft was taken from the dorsum of the proximal phalanx, eliminating the need for a separate incision over the ulna but requiring a

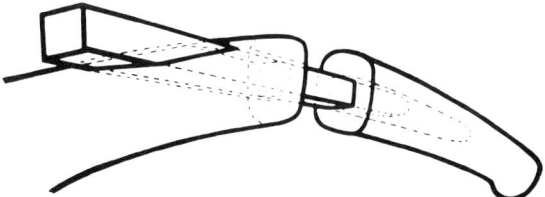

Fig. 11.11 Stabilization of arthrodesis by bone graft. (From Moberg E, Henrikson B 1960 Acta Chirugica Scandinavica 118: 331–338, by kind permission).

longer incision on the finger and producing greater interference with the extensor mechanism. There were no failures in 40 IP joints.

The graft techniques can be combined with intraosseous wiring to provide greater stability and place the joint surfaces and graft in compression. An intraosseous wire loop is passed through the phalanx and graft proximally, but only the phalanx distally, and then tightened (Lister 1978).

The bone peg technique requires patience and skill. Because of the time needed to carry out the procedure it cannot be used in several joints in the same hand at one sitting. It is easy to damage the head or dorsum of the proximal phalanx when making the initial drill hole and then it will be difficult to stabilize the arthrodesis by any method. There is no chance of correcting the angle of arthrodesis if this is wrongly judged initially.

The limitation on the number of joints that can be done at one sitting and the risk of damage to soft bone limit the usefulness of this technique in the hand affected by rheumatoid arthritis. It can be used in this condition, but is applicable only when the bone stock is good and one joint must be fused (Flatt 1983).

External fixation

The benefits of compression in obtaining early union were demonstrated by Charnley (1953). Compression does not accelerate osteogenesis but is effective because it provides stability and maintains close apposition of adjacent bones. Compression is provided by the tension band and intraosseous wiring techniques, blade plates applied on the DCP principle and also by external fixation devices.

There are some disadvantages to using external fixation devices in the fingers. Most obviously the device gets in the way of other fingers and, although a single plane fixation device can provide an acceptable degree of stability for arthrodesis of joints such as the knee where broad cancellous surfaces are apposed, stability is poor in small joints and the bones can angulate forwards or backwards as compression is applied (Fig. 11.12). To overcome the problem of angulation in IP joints Charnley (1953) recommended that the device be applied in the sagittal plane of the finger; this has the

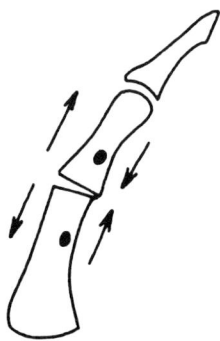

Fig. 11.12 It is difficult to position the transverse Kirschner wires of an external fixation device so that bone contact is not lost when the device is tightened. An axial wire will prevent this problem.

disadvantage that the tendons or the nail bed may be transfixed. Others have preferred to stabilize the joint with an axial Kirschner wire before the external fixation device is compressed (Leonard & Capen 1979, Ferlic et al 1983).

The most widely used external compression device is based on the well-known Charnley knee clamp. After preparing the bone surfaces, clamps are applied to the ends of 1.6 mm Kirschner wires placed transversely above and below the joint (Micks & Hager 1968). Using this type of device (Fig. 11.13) in conjunction with a longitudinal stabilizing Kirschner wire, Leonard & Capen (1979) obtained fusion in 49 of 54 IP joints. The longitudinal wire was removed 6 weeks after

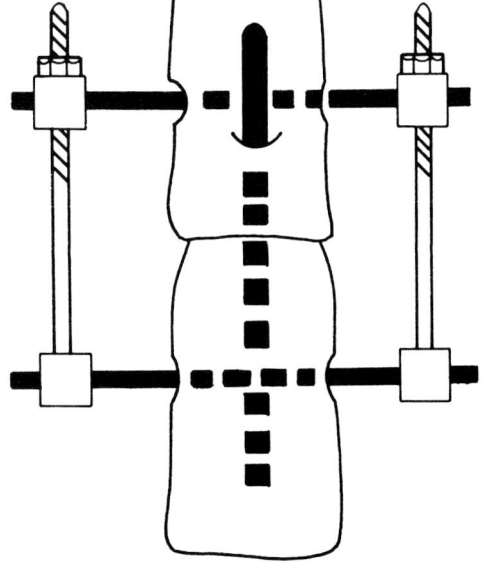

Fig. 11.13 A 'mini-Charnley' external fixation clamp. Note the axial Kirschner wire to maintain stability.

surgery and the external fixation retained for a further 2 weeks.

External fixation devices are satisfactory for use in the thumb, because they do not interfere with the movement of the fingers. Ferlic et al (1983) had good results using the Micks and Hager compression system in 82 arthrodeses of small joints in the thumb. Most of the operations were done on joints affected by rheumatoid arthritis. A sound fusion was obtained in 81 joints, although reoperation for delayed or non-union had been necessary in 3. There were 8 pin track infections which resolved when the wires were removed. The authors stressed that if the parallel wires are placed too close together it will not be possible to put on the compression clamps and that, if a longitudinal Kirschner wire is not used, the transverse wires must be placed midlaterally to prevent backwards or forwards angulation when the clamps are tightened.

Compression may be applied in other ways if the 'mini-Charnley' clamps are not available. Tupper (1972) described an ingenious method using orthodontic traction screws attached to two eye holes made in the external ends of two parallel 0.9 mm Kirschner wires which had been driven into, but not through, the phalanges above and below the excised joint. More than one screw could be applied in different planes. Wexter et al (1977) reported an even simpler method using elastic bands to obtain compression between Kirschner wires driven in a dorsoventral direction above and below the joint, after removal of the surfaces. They believed that transfixion of the tendons aided stability, but advised the use of an axial Kirschner wire if the joint appeared unstable. Compression was maintained for only a short time (2.5–4 weeks) and good fusions were obtained in 42 out of 46 joints. Malunion occurred in 4, skin necrosis in 2 and infections in 5. Four of the infections occurred in burned hands and the authors concluded that post-burn deformity was a relative contraindication to this method. No mention was made of elastic band failure!

COMPLICATIONS OF ARTHRODESIS

A surgical teacher was fond of saying, 'Arthrodesis of an interphalangeal joint is one of the most difficult operations in surgery.' This opinion may seem strange in view of the 90% or more good results that have been reported using available techniques. The fact is that such good results can only be obtained by strict attention to the details of the technique, whichever method is chosen (Fig. 11.14). Failures are not uncommon and the result of failure is a disability that is often greater than that produced by the condition for which surgery was undertaken (Robertson 1964). Mention of some of the complications of arthrodesis has already been made but they will be summarized here.

Non-union

This is said to be more common in attempted fusion of the distal IP joint (Nevaiser & Adams 1978). A stable fibrous union may give acceptable function, but this is not to be relied upon. Non-union can best be avoided by ensuring that congruent cancellous bone surfaces are placed in close apposition and stabilized, preferably by some method that ensures that the bone surfaces are in compression.

Reoperation is necessary for a symptomatic non-union. It may be possible to freshen the bone ends;

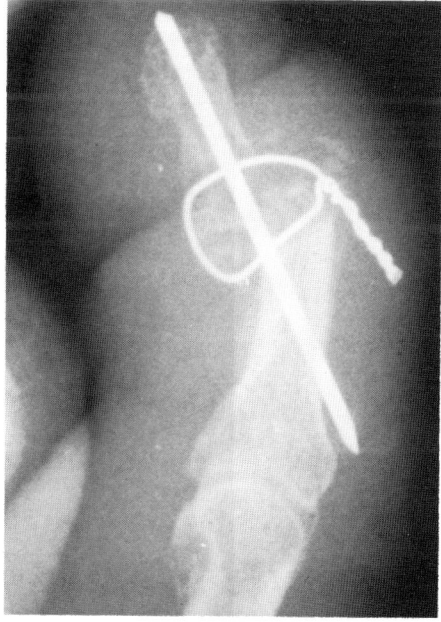

Fig. 11.14 Failure is usually attributable to inadequate attention to details of the chosen technique. In this example the axial Kirschner wire had not been placed accurately in the intermediate phalanx and cut out.

as an alternative a Moberg-type graft can be driven across the sclerotic bone ends and then placed under compression by the use of an intraosseous wire as described above. If non-union is the result of poor bone stock at the arthrodesis site, a corticocancellous bone graft can be inserted and stabilized by the tension band method.

Malunion

It can be extraordinarily difficult to maintain the desired angle of the arthrodesis when applying the fixation device, be it Kirschner wires, screw, bone graft or external fixation clamp. Angulation is not always preventable by cutting the joint surfaces off flat so that the bones lie flush at the desired angle (see Fig. 11.2); indeed, this has the additional complication that small alterations in angulation, which may be clinically acceptable, can cause loss of bone contact and may result in non-union.

Malunion can be prevented by using a method in which the correct angle is maintained by a single axial or oblique Kirschner wire while compression is applied to the joint. If the correct angle has not been obtained it is possible to remove and resite a single wire after adjusting the angle. Malunions should therefore be uncommon if the techniques of intraosseous wiring, tension band wiring, or external fixation supplemented by an axial Kirschner wire are used.

An established, troublesome malunion of an IP joint must be taken down and refashioned.

Infection

Arthrodesis of an IP joint with rigid internal fixation has been recommended as a primary treatment for septic arthritis (Høgh & Jensen 1982). Infection is not a major complication of IP arthrodesis itself, provided the skin is in good condition. It appears to be much more common when the skin has been burned (Wexter et al 1977).

Pin track infections have been reported when external fixation devices have been used, but appear to settle rapidly when the pins are removed. As noted, Hill (1982) has stated that infections related to Kirschner wires are *less* common when the ends of the wires are exposed rather than cut off beneath the skin.

Vascular problems

The circulation in the finger may be compromised if a flexion contracture is corrected by arthrodesis without resecting an adequate amount of bone. This is a particular risk if the condition causing the flexion contracture is one that is associated with poor peripheral circulation, for example scleroderma (Lipscomb et al 1969).

SUMMARY

The variety of methods of IP arthrodesis that are available allows the surgeon to choose an appropriate technique to suit the individual patient's problem. Any of the techniques reviewed here can be relied upon to produce a satisfactory arthrodesis if carried out with care, and if the method chosen is appropriate to the problem. Important principles in all techniques are correct preparation of the joint surfaces to ensure a large area of contact between cancellous bone surfaces, and stabilization of the arthrodesis in the desired position. For the majority of IP arthrodeses the present author's own preference is to prepare the bone ends by the tongue and groove method and to stabilize the phalanges by intraosseous wiring. This method is simple to perform, reliable in obtaining solid union in the desired position and allows early mobilization of the hand free of external splintage. It has the additional advantages that the position of the arthrodesis can be altered fairly easily during the operation, if necessary, and that several joints can be dealt with at the same sitting.

REFERENCES

Allende B T, Engelem J C 1980 Tension band arthrodesis in the finger joints. Journal of Hand Surgery 5:269–271
Boyes J H 1970 Bunnell's surgery of the hand, 5th edn. J B Lippincott, Philadelphia, p 310
Brittain H A 1952 Architectural principles in arthrodesis, 2nd edn. Livingstone, Edinburgh, pp 134–138

Carroll R E, Hill N A 1969 Small joint arthrodesis in hand reconstruction. Journal of Bone and Joint Surgery 51A:1219–1221
Charnley J 1953 Compression arthrodesis. Livingstone, Edinburgh, p 172
Edwards G S, O'Brien E T, Heckman M M 1982 Retrograde

cross-pinning of transverse metacarpal and phalangeal fractures. The Hand 14:141–148
Engle J, Tsier H, Farin I 1977 A comparison between Kirschner wire and compression screw fixation after arthrodesis of the distal interphalangeal joint. Plastic and Reconstructive Surgery 60:611–614
Faithfull D K, Herbert T J 1984 Small joint fusions of the hand using the Herbert bone screw. Journal of Hand Surgery 9B:167–168
Ferlic D C, Turner B D, Clayton M L 1983 Compression arthrodesis of the thumb. Journal of Hand Surgery 8:207–210
Flatt A E 1983 Care of the arthritic hand, 4th edn. C V Mosby, St Louis, pp 193–196
Fyfe I S, Mason S 1979 The mechanical stability of internal fixation of fractured phalanges. The Hand 11:50–54
Gould W L, Belsole R J, Skelton W H 1984 Tension band stabilisation of transverse fractures: an experimental analysis. Plastic and Reconstructive Surgery 73:111–115
Granovitz S, Vainio K 1966 Proximal interphalangeal joint arthrodesis in rheumatoid arthritis. Acta Orthopaedica Scandinavica 37:301–309
Gschwend H 1980 Surgical treatment of rheumatoid arthritis. W B Saunders, Philadelphia, pp 132–136
Harrison S H 1974 The Harrison-Nicolle intramedullary peg. Follow up studies of 100 cases. The Hand 6:304–307
Harrison S H, Nicolle F J 1974 A new intramedullary peg for arthrodesis. British Journal of Plastic Surgery 27:240–241
Harrison S, Smith P, Maxwell D 1977 Stabilisation of the first metacarpophalangeal and terminal interphalangeal joints of the thumb. The Hand 9:242–249
Heim U, Pfeiffer K M 1982 Small fragment set manual. Technical recommended by the ASIF group, 2nd edn. Springer Verlag, Berlin
Hill N A 1982 Small joint arthrodesis. In: Green D P (ed) Operative hand surgery. Churchill Livingstone, New York, p 113–125
Høgh J, Jensen P Ø 1982 Compression-arthrodesis of finger joints using Kirschner wires and cerclage. The Hand 14:149–152
Leonard M H, Capen D A 1979 Compression arthrodesis of finger joints. Clinical Orthopaedics 145:193–198
Lipscomb P R, Simons G W, Winkelmann R K 1969 Surgery for sclerodactylia of the hand: experience with six cases. Journal of Bone and Joint Surgery 51A:1112–1117
Lister G D 1978 Intraosseous wiring of the digital skeleton. Journal of Hand Surgery 3:427–435
Lister G D 1984 The hand: Diagnosis and indications, 2nd edn. Churchill Livingstone, Edinburgh, pp 144–145
Massengill J B, Alexander H, Parson J R, Schecter M J 1979 Mechanical analysis of Kirschner wire fixation in a phalangeal model. Journal of Hand Surgery 4:351–356
Micks J E, Hager D L 1968 A method of accelerating fusion of small joints. Journal of Bone and Joint Surgery 50A:1269
Moberg E 1960 Arthrodesis of finger joints. Surgical Clinics of North America 40:465–470
Moberg E, Henrikson B 1960 Technique for digital arthrodesis. Acta Chirugica Scandinavica 118:331–338
Narakas A 1976 Les arthrodèses interphalangiennes par vissage. Annales de Chirugie 30:913–916
Nevaiser R J 1978 Complications of treatment of injuries of the hand (part 2). In: Epps C H (ed) Complications in orthopaedic surgery. J B Lippincott, Philadelphia, p 393
Omer G E 1968 Evaluation and reconstruction of the forearm and hand after acute traumatic peripheral nerve injuries. Journal of Bone and Joint Surgery 50A:1154–1177
Paneva-Holevich E 1977 Compression osteosynthesis in the hand using a small nail plate. Journal of Bone and Joint Surgery 59A:464–466
Potenza A D 1973 A technique for arthrodesis of finger joints. Journal of Bone and Joint Surgery 55A:1534–1536
Robertson D C 1964 The fusion of interphalangeal joints. Canadian Journal of Surgery 7:433–437
Straub L R 1959 The rheumatoid hand. Clinical Orthopaedics 15:127–139
Tupper J W 1972 A compression arthrodesis device for small joints of the hand. The Hand 4:62–64
Vainio K, Pulkki T 1959 Surgical treatment of arthritis mutilans. Annales Chirurgiae et Gynaecologiae Fenniae 48:361–368
Vanik R K, Weber R C, Matloub H S, Sanger J R, Gingrass R P 1984 The comparative strengths of internal fixation techniques. Journal of Hand Surgery 9A:216–221
Watson H K, Shaffer S R 1970 Concave-convex arthrodesis in joints of the hand. Plastic and Reconstructive Surgery 46:368–371
Wexter M R, Rousso N, Weinberg H 1977 Arthrodesis of finger joints by dynamic external compression using dorsoventral Kirschner wires and rubber bands. Plastic and Reconstructive Surgery 60:882–885

SECTION 4

Congenital and Developmental Conditions

D. Buck-Gramcko

12 Congenital and developmental conditions

The interphalangeal joints of the digits are involved in numerous congenital malformations. In many instances the deformity is a minor part of a congenital malformation syndrome, in others it is the only manifestation of an anomaly. The marginal digital rays are much more involved than the central one; an affection of all five digits is extremely rare.

Deformities of the bones adjacent to the two distal joints of the fingers and the interphalangeal joint of the thumb are seen in many malformation syndromes (Table 12.1) as well as in special congenital deformities. The most common malformations are described in this chapter; rare conditions are mentioned only in a short paragraph.

In cases of *syndactyly* with distal bony fusion a convergence of the involved digits is seen. This is especially remarkable in syndactyly between the ring and little fingers where the shorter finger leads to a severe deviation of the other. In the most frequent syndactyly between the middle and ring fingers such a deviation in the interphalangeal joints can occur by distal bony fusion (Fig. 12.1). Early separation is indicated in these cases to avoid uncorrectable bone deformity. *Hyperphalangy*, a rare condition, shows joint deformities not only in the metacarpophalangeal joint (predominately in the index finger), but also in the interphalangeal joints—caused by oblique articular surfaces on one or both ends of the short middle phalanx and by a joint laxity. Unstable joints are frequently seen in the brachydactyly type of *symbrachydactyly*, while in the true *brachydactyly* the joints are usually stable. In this anomaly there is a great variety of bone deformations: short phalanges in rectangular or trapezoid shape, missing epiphyses, pseudoepiphyses, missing phalanges or the composition of a phalanx out of two short bones which fuse in

Table 12.1 Malformation syndromes in which interphalangeal deformities occur

Achondroplasia
Acrocephalopolysyndactyly (Carpenter's syndrome)
Acrocephalosyndactyly (Apert's syndrome and other forms)
Chondroectodermal dysplasia (Ellis–van Creveld syndrome)
Cleidocranial dysplasia (dysostosis)
de Lange syndrome
Diastrophic dwarfism
Metatropic dwarfism
Multiple cartilaginous exostosis
Oculodentodigital dysplasia
Otopalatodigital syndrome
Rubinstein–Taybi syndrome
Silver syndrome
Thiemann disease
Trichorhinophalangeal syndrome (Giedion)

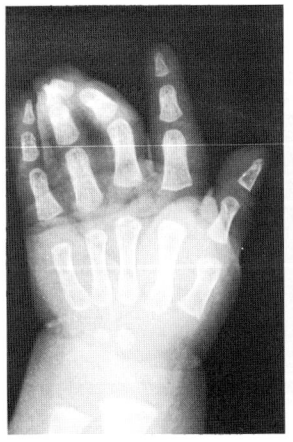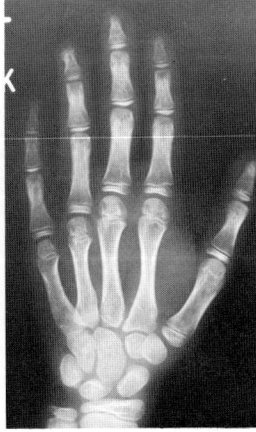

Fig. 12.1 Lateral deviation in the interphalangeal joints of the middle finger caused by distal bony fusion in a syndactyly case (left). Early separation has avoided any permanent deformity (result 9 years later; right).

adolescence (Pol 1921, Bell 1951). *Cone epiphyses* in numerous variations (Giedion 1966) are seen in otherwise normal individuals as well as in special pathological conditions (cleidocranial dysostosis, Ellis-van Creveld syndrome, trichorhinophalangeal syndrome, otopalatodigital syndrome). They are more common in females than in males and are located mostly in the distal phalanx of the thumb and the middle phalanx of the little finger. A very rare condition is *macrodactyly* which usually shows an enlargement of the articular structures without gross deformity. Barsky (1967) has introduced to the American literature the differentiation into a static and a progressive type which was described in the German literature by Wieland (1907) and Werthemann (1952). In the static, more localized type one may see excessive exostosis formation (Fig. 12.2) which necessitates surgical correction (mostly arthrodesis). Finally in this general description one should mention the lateral deviation of the distal phalanx—mainly in the thumb—by the eccentric insertion of the extensor and/or flexor tendon in cases of *duplication* or in *hypoplasia* of the thumb. Here again the correction should be performed early (preferably in the first 2 years of life), otherwise the damage to the articular surface can only be treated by arthrodesis.

CLINODACTYLY

Definition and anatomical findings

Lateral curvatures of digits are grouped under the term clinodactyly—'bent finger'. Since this name was introduced by Fort (1896) there have been different interpretations. Several authors including Fort himself have used this term for all deviations of the fingers including flexion contractures (camptodactyly). Nowadays we understand clinodactyly means only lateral deviations (to the radial or ulnar side) (Fig. 12.3). These occur mostly in the middle phalanx of the fingers or in the proximal thumb phalanx, less frequently in the proximal and middle phalanx of index and ring fingers. The causes are different: an oblique distal articular surface of a short middle phalanx (brachymesophalangy) with or without pseudoepiphysis, a more or less triangular shape of the phalanx with an abnormal epiphysis (delta phalanx), or an additional triangular ossicle (especially in the triphalangeal thumb). In cases of rectangular middle phalanx with a radially inclined distal joint surface, the length of the phalanx varies considerably; it ranges from normal to a complete absence, the so-called 'Assimilations-Hypophalangie' of Pol (1921). Generally it may be said: the more the shortness is present, the less it is a single deformity and the more it is combined with other malformations.

Incidence

Because there is no definition of the limits of normal, the incidence of clinodactyly is hard to determine. Reports range from 1% to 20% with a higher occurrence in males than in females. Cases of extreme clinodactyly (angle more than 30°) are rare. In Down's syndrome patients the presence of clinodactyly is reported to be between 11.1 and 78.8%. Clinodactyly caused by a delta phalanx occurs only infrequently (see below).

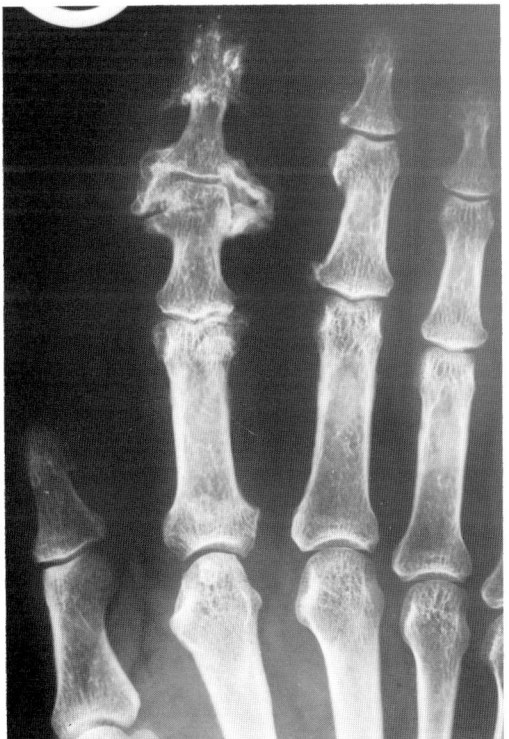

Fig. 12.2 Excessive exostosis formation in the static type of macrodactyly.

190 THE INTERPHALANGEAL JOINTS

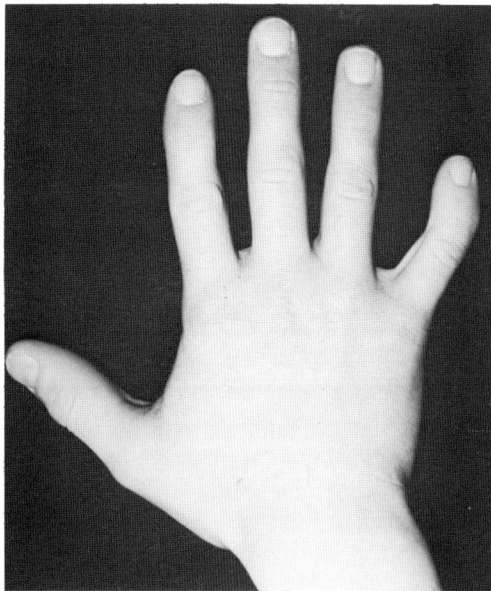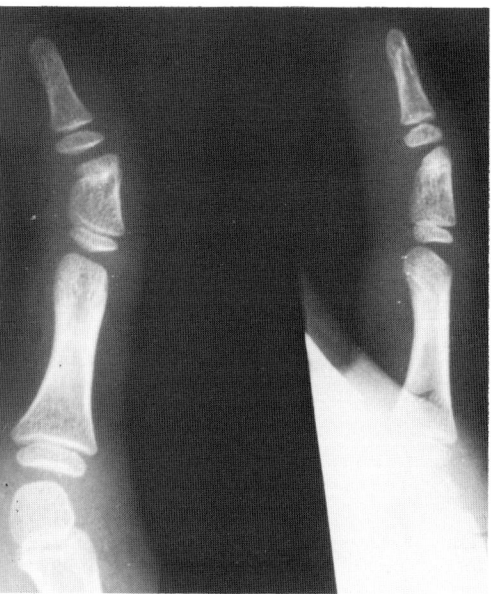

Fig. 12.3 Clinodactyly of the little finger of a 12-year-old boy caused by a short middle phalanx with radially inclined distal joint surface. Note the pseudoepiphysis (distally).

Treatment

Clinodactyly with an angle less than 15° does not need treatment—it is a physical sign, not a disease (Burke & Flatt 1979). If in cases of marked deviation a correction is desirable, there are three types of operative procedure: a closing, a reverse, and an opening wedge osteotomy (Fig. 12.4). The present author prefers the opening wedge osteotomy because it results in a lengthening (Fig. 12.5). It is technically easier than the reverse wedge osteotomy because in most cases it is possible to leave the cortical bone on the longer (convex) side intact which will avoid any malrotation and needs less bone fixation (bone suture and/or Kirschner wire), even if a bone graft is necessary. For the

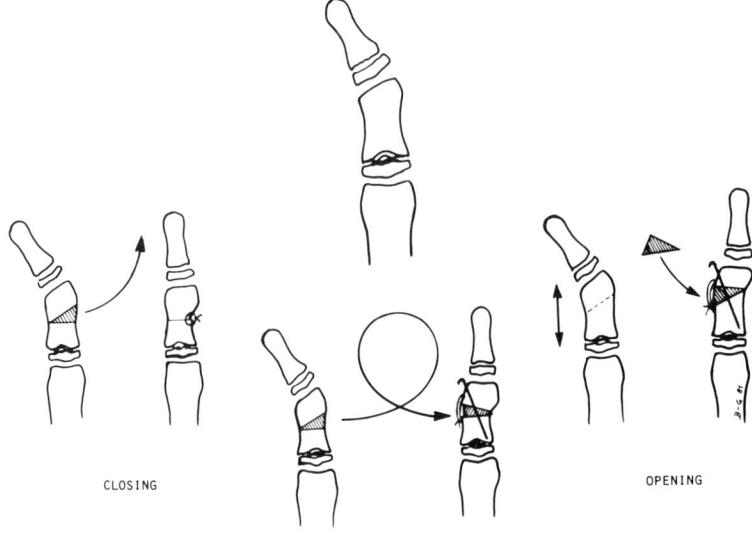

Fig. 12.4 Diagram of the different types of wedge osteotomy.

CONGENITAL AND DEVELOPMENTAL CONDITIONS 191

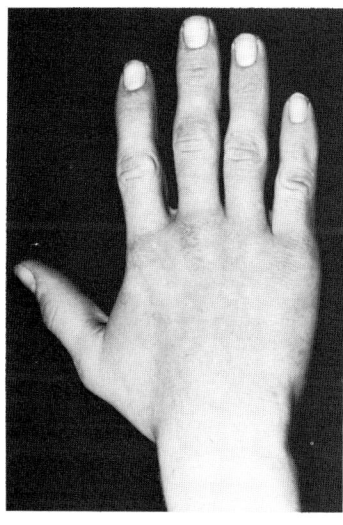
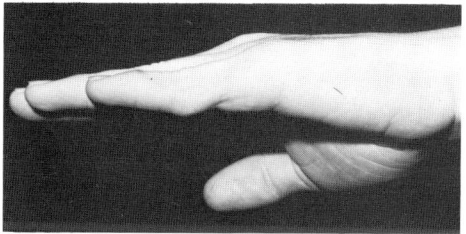
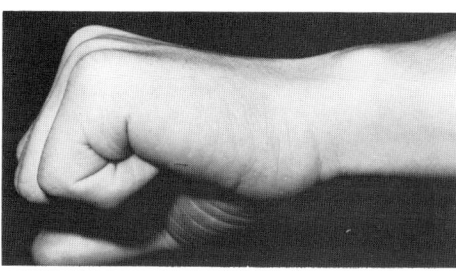
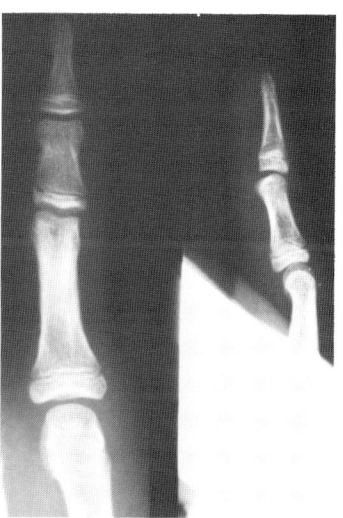

Fig. 12.5 Result of an opening wedge osteotomy in the case in Fig. 12.3, 4 years postoperatively with normal range of motion and straight axis of the lengthened middle phalanx.

release of skin tightness sometimes a local sliding flap has to be used. A closing wedge osteotomy will shorten the phalanx which is already short in most instances already short (Fig. 12.6). With good bone fixation external immobilization is necessary only for 2 or 3 weeks.

Complications

Only an insufficient operative technique will cause complications: division of the tendons which run directly adjacent to the bone, malrotation, damage to the epiphyseal plate and skin necrosis or dehiscence because of the tightness of the soft tissues.

Results

Usually the results are excellent in function as well as in appearance (see Fig. 12.5). Occasionally there is some limitation in the range of motion by tendon adhesions.

DELTA PHALANX

Definition and anatomical findings

The term 'delta phalanx' was introduced by Jones (1964) for a triangular-shaped bone which has a C-shaped continuous epiphysis running from the proximal to the distal end of the phalanx along the shortened side (Fig. 12.7). Because this deformity will occur also in metacarpals and metatarsals, Wood (Wood & Flatt 1977, Wood 1982) and Jaeger & Refior (1971) have recommended the term 'delta bone' or 'congenital triangular bone'. A triangular bone without a visible epiphyseal plate or with a normal looking epiphysis on the proximal end as it

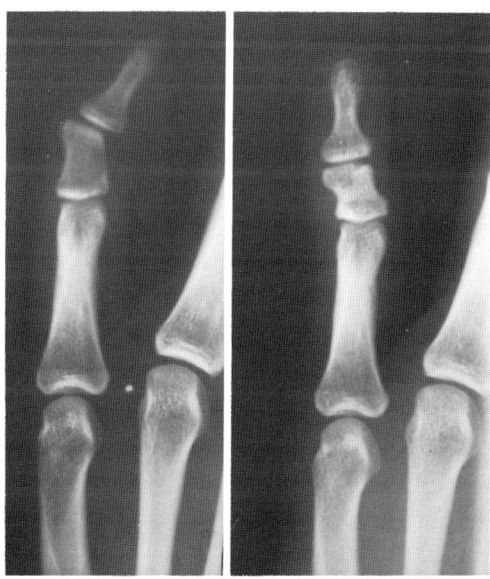

Fig. 12.6 Unsatisfactory result of a closing wedge osteotomy in clinodactyly, which has made the already short middle phalanx (left) shorter (right).

192 THE INTERPHALANGEAL JOINTS

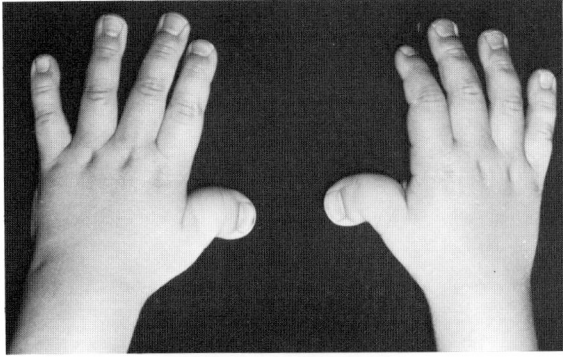

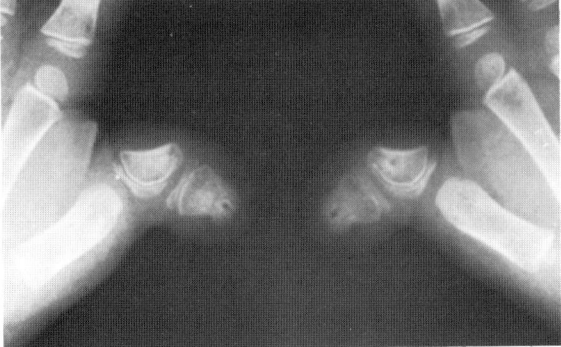

Fig. 12.7 Delta phalanx with typical angulations in a 4-year-old boy with bilateral broad thumbs (Rubinstein–Taybi syndrome).

is seen as ossicle in the brachymesophalangeal type of triphalangeal thumb (see Fig. 12.12) should not be named delta bone because there is no C-shaped epiphysis. Theander & Carstam (1974) have used the complicated term 'longitudinally bracketed diaphysis' to describe the same deformity.

A delta phalanx always causes a lateral deviation (clinodactyly), but in many cases additional palmar angulation occurs such that there is a clinical picture of a flexion contracture, especially in cases of central poly(syn)dactyly where the different shape and length of the bone will often result in contractures and deviations (Fig. 12.8). Delta phalanges occur in cases of polydactyly (Fig. 12.8), Apert's syndrome, Rubinstein-Taybi syndrome (Fig. 12.7), complex deformities such as oligosyndactyly (Fig. 12.9) or as a single deformity causing only clinodactyly. Wood & Flatt (1977) have given an excellent review, although they mixed the true delta phalanx with the triangular-shaped bone without continuous epiphysis. Delta phalanges occur most often in the proximal phalanges of the thumb and ring finger and in the middle phalanges (especially in the little finger). The distal phalanges are never involved.

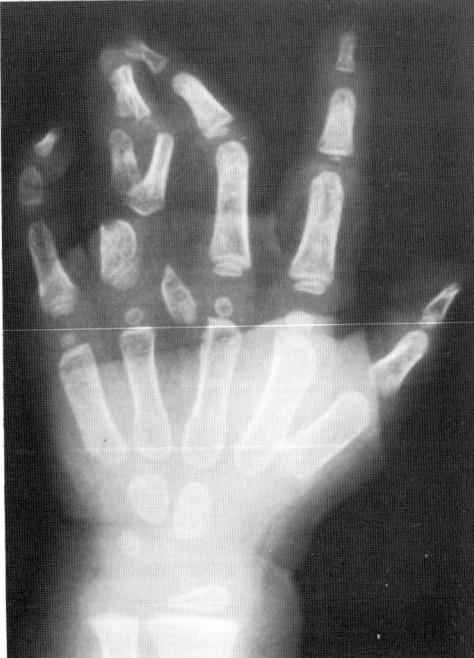
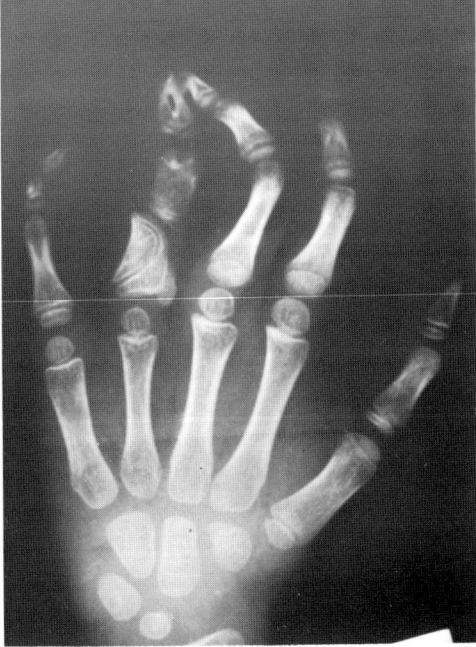

Fig. 12.8 Two cases of central polysyndactyly with contractures and deviations caused by delta phalanges and additional bone deformities.

CONGENITAL AND DEVELOPMENTAL CONDITIONS 193

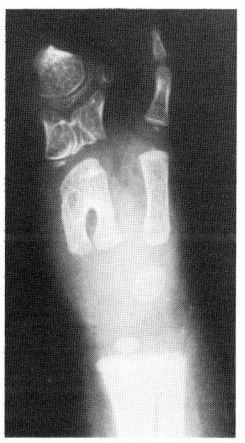
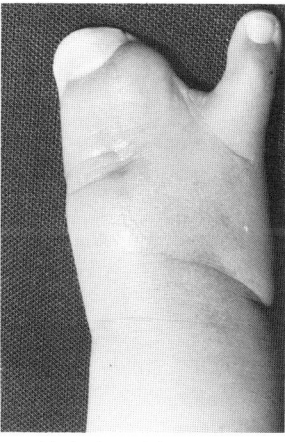

Fig. 12.9 Complex deformity with fusion of thumb and index finger with multiple delta phalanges and a two-phalangeal little finger (absence of middle and ring finger).

Incidence and heredity

Since not all triangular-shaped bones are delta phalanges, the correct incidence is hard to determine. Wood & Flatt (1977) report an incidence of 3.5% of their cases with congenital malformations in the upper extremity. Inheritance is often seen in the families of patients with delta phalanges.

Treatment

In a delta phalanx without additional bone deformity, usually the most appropriate operative procedure is an opening wedge osteotomy, using a bone graft from the iliac bone or other bone parts to be excised (Jones 1964, Watson & Boyes 1967, Wood & Flatt 1977). Carstam & Theander (1975) have recommended the reverse wedge osteotomy, while Smith (1977) has corrected the deviation by rotating the distal part of the osteotomized phalanx and using the resected bone piece as a graft. A different procedure was described by Vickers (1980, personal comment 1984) as 'physolysis' (resection of the middle part of the C-shaped epiphysis and filling the cavity with fat).

In cases of severe deformity of the involved digit, common in central polysyndactyly, a non-functioning finger results and amputation is the best treatment. In other cases arthrodesis may be the appropriate procedure, not only in adults (Fig. 12.10).

Complications

Complications can occur in the same way as in clinodactyly. Recurrence may lead to another osteotomy usually after finishing the growth period.

Results

Results are hard to classify because the conditions are so different. In a single delta phalanx the functional and cosmetic result is usually fair or good (Fig. 12.11), although a recurrence of the deviation has to be expected in many cases.

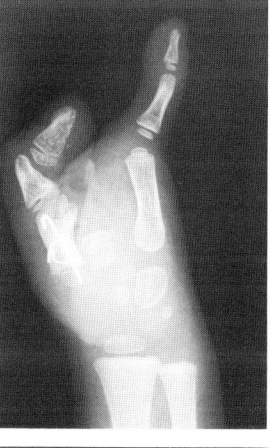
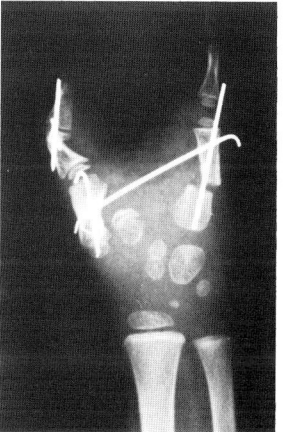
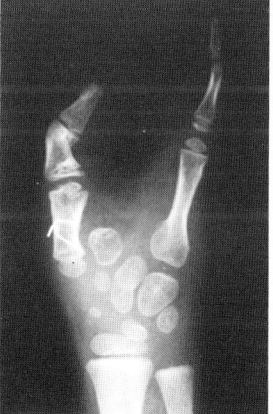
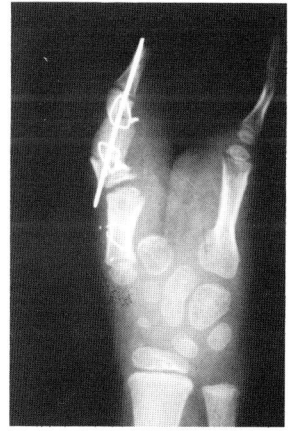

Fig. 12.10 Radiological phases of treatment of the same case as in Fig. 12.9: top left: following resection of the 'index finger' and rotational osteotomy of the first metacarpal (January 1981); top right: following rotational osteotomy of the ulnar metacarpal and interphalangeal joint fusion of the thumb with skin cover in the widened web space by local sliding flap (March 1983); bottom left: complete interphalangeal joint fusion of the thumb with intact growth plate (October 1984); bottom right: following lengthening of the proximal phalanx by iliac bone graft (January 1985). Clinically there is a span between the two digits of 5.5 cm with full pinch.

194 THE INTERPHALANGEAL JOINTS

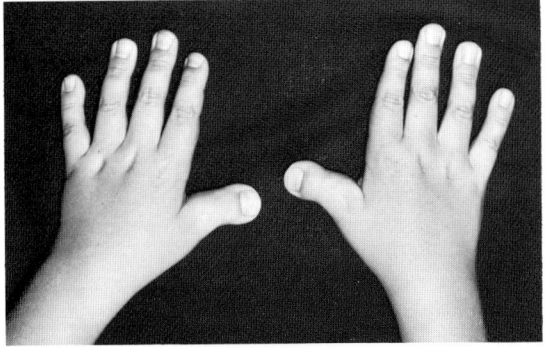

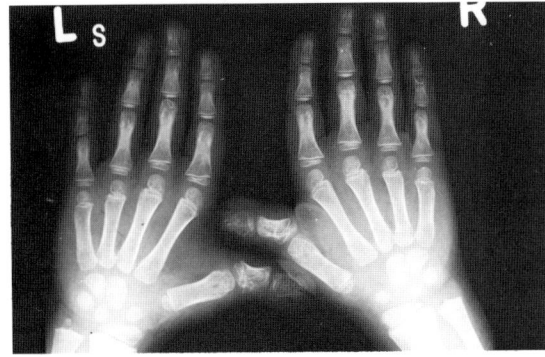

Fig. 12.11 Fair result of correction of the delta phalanx deviation of the case shown in Fig. 12.7 3 years after following an opening wedge osteotomy with rotation of the distal bone part according to Smith; a recurrence is to be expected.

TRIPHALANGEAL THUMB

Definition and anatomical findings

The occurrence of an additional phalanx in the thumb is an interesting deformity. Many papers over several centuries have argued the identity of the missing bone of the normally occurring biphalangeal thumb. Is it the metacarpal or the middle phalanx? Three different types of triphalangeal thumbs can be found. The *brachymesophalangeal type* (from the Greek: short middle phalanx) has a more or less marked lateral angulation caused by a small wedge-shaped middle phalanx (Fig. 12.12**a**). The deviation is usually directed to the ulnar side; only in very rare cases is the base of the triangular middle phalanx on the ulnar side, so that the distal part of the thumb deviates radially (Fig. 12.12**b**). The anatomy of the thumb is otherwise normal including thenar muscles and is therefore opposable. The first web space is of normal width and the thumb metacarpal has its

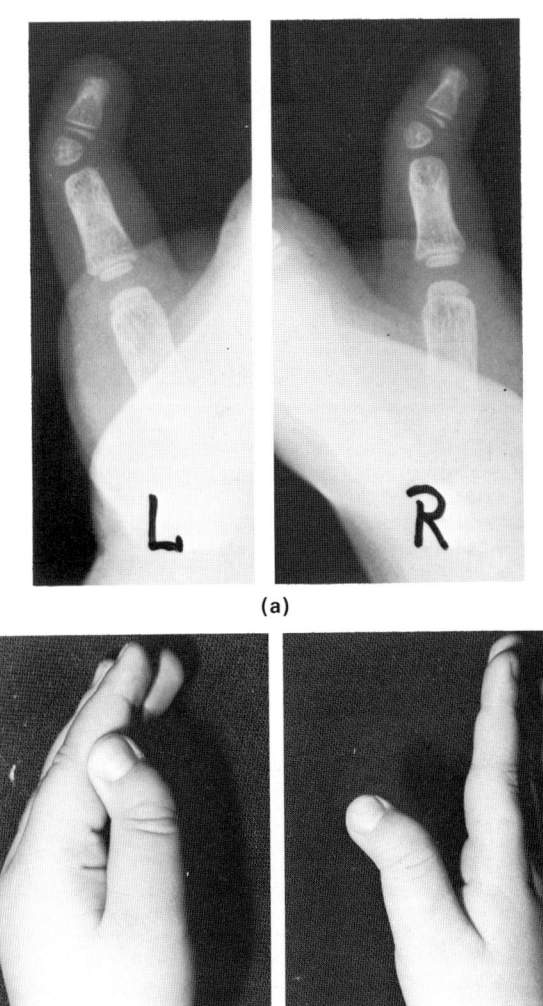

Fig. 12.12 Brachymesophalangeal type of triphalangeal thumb: The X-rays (**a**, posteroanterior view) show the triangular bone as the cause for the marked deviation (**b**), which is usually directed to the ulnar side (left thumb) and very rarely to the radial side (right thumb of the same girl).

epiphyseal plate at the base. In the *dolichophalangeal type* (Greek: dolichos means long) the thumb is like a regular finger with three phalanges of normal size (Fig. 12.13). It lies in the same plane as the other four fingers and is about the same length. The first web space is as narrow as the others and the metacarpal bone has its epiphyseal plate at its distal end or shows two epiphyseal plates, each on

CONGENITAL AND DEVELOPMENTAL CONDITIONS 195

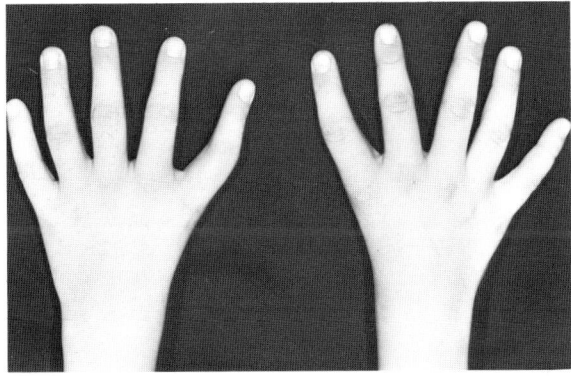
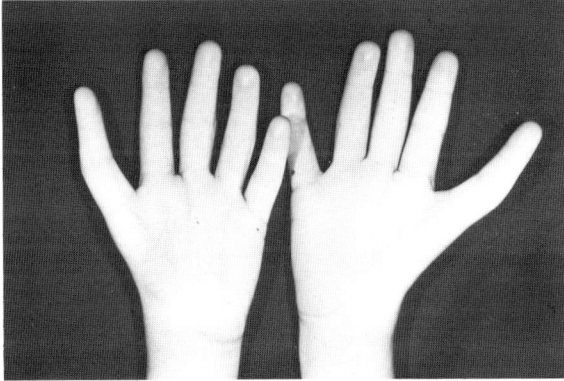
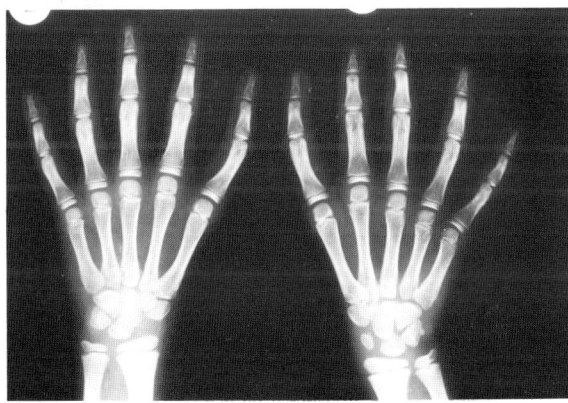

Fig. 12.13 Dolichophalangeal type of triphalangeal thumb: the thumb shows the anatomy similar to a finger with distal epiphyseal plate of the metacarpal, narrow web space and has no thenar muscles.

its proximal and distal end. The thenar muscles are missing and therefore this thumb is non-opposable. In many cases rudimentary adductor muscles can be found. This deformity is often called 'five fingered hand', although there is more evidence that the radial finger is a thumb and not an index finger duplication. The third type, an *intermediate type* or transient form (Fig. 12.14) is seen only in a few instances. The middle phalanx is rectangular or trapezoidal in shape, but significantly shorter than in the dolichophalangeal type. The first web space is wider, but not of normal width. The thumb lies not in the same plane as the other fingers, but is more rotated. Usually there are some hypoplastic thenar muscles, so that some opposition is possible. The metacarpal shows a proximal epiphyseal plate; sometimes at its distal end a pseudoepiphysis is seen.

This classification is necessary not only in regard to the different anatomical findings, but also for the different surgical treatments. It was described as early as 1907 by Hilgenreiner and mentioned in the English speaking literature by Swanson & Brown (1962), Miura (1976) and Wood (1976). Chan & Lamb (1983) have stressed the clinical and radiological features of differentiation. The terms, deriving from Greek words, were originated by Cocchi (1952).

Besides these three characteristic types, triphalangeal thumb can be found in combination with polydactyly (Wood 1978). Here all three above-mentioned types can be seen, but mixed with the anatomical structures of the duplicated thumb. Triphalangism of the thumb can be also associated with cleft hand and foot, congenital heart disease, syndactyly, anaemia and tibial aplasia.

Most patients with triphalangeal thumb have a bilateral deformity, even if the malformation is not the same in both hands. There is a high rate of inheritance, although most cases of unilateral occurrence of the brachymesophalangeal type of triphalangism are sporadic.

Incidence

It is again difficult to ascertain the true incidence of triphalangeal thumb because there are only a few reports of larger series. Wood (1976) has reported an incidence of about 3% of the upper extremity congenital deformities. In the present author's experience of patients with congenital malformations (about 1500) 73 patients are registered with triphalangeal thumbs: 13 of the brachymesophalangeal type, 7 of the intermediate type, 31 of the dolichophalangeal type, and 22 in association with polydactyly.

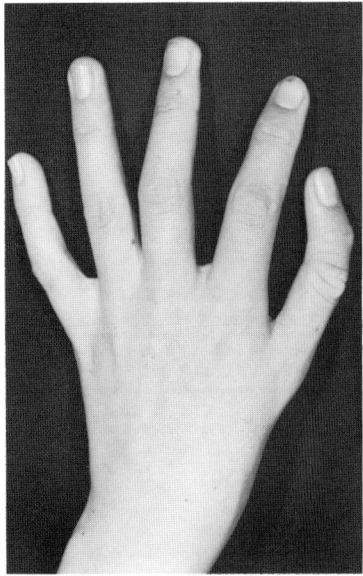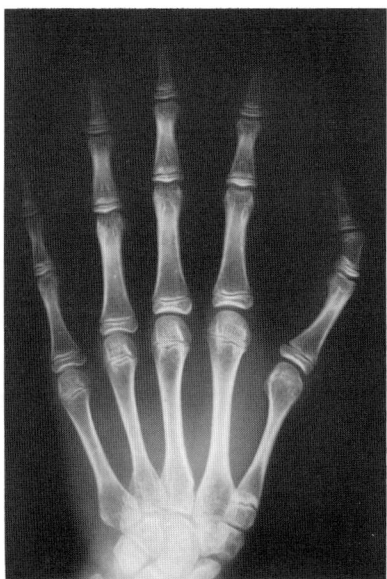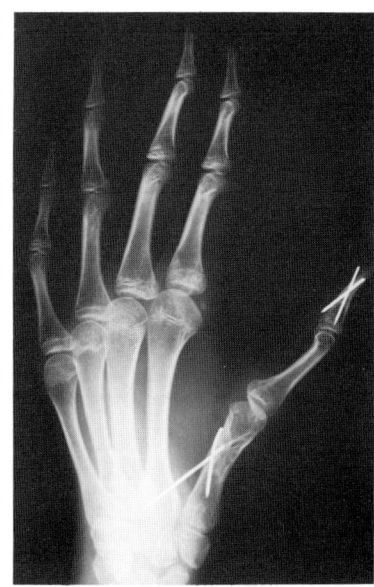

Fig. 12.14 Transient form of triphalangeal thumb with relatively short but rectangular middle phalanx, proximal epiphyseal plate of the metacarpal, more rotation of the ray, and presence of some thenar muscles. Right: postoperative X-ray.

Treatment

The surgical correction of the deformity is quite different in the three types of triphalangism and, in the type with a short middle phalanx, varies with the age of the patient.

Brachymesophalangeal type

The logical treatment is to excise the small wedge-shaped middle phalanx and to reconstruct the collateral ligament using parts of the two existing ligaments. The deviation is usually fully corrected by this procedure; if not, some cartilage shaving is necessary. Although the two joint surfaces are not congruous, remodelling usually occurs in the following years, so that the late result is a normal looking joint. This remodelling will occur only in a young child so that there is an age limit of about 6 years. If the patient is seen later, the angulation in the joint surface of the terminal phalanx is so marked that spontaneous remodelling is impossible (Figs. 12.15 and 12.16). In these cases the treatment consists of either a closing wedge osteotomy in the proximal phalanx (Fig. 12.15), or a resection and fusion of the oblique joint (Fig. 12.16). Both procedures will correct the lateral deviation and preserve joint mobility.

Dolichophalangeal type

The appropriate treatment is pollicization of the radialmost digit following the standardized principles for an index finger (Buck-Gramcko 1971, 1981).

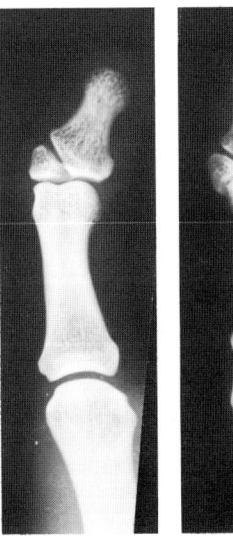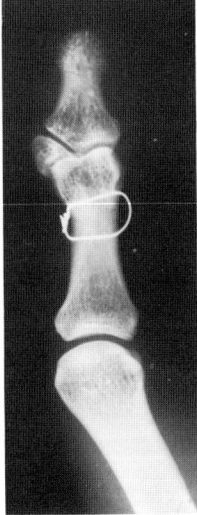

Fig. 12.15 Triphalangeal thumb with short triangular middle phalanx in a 17-year-old girl. Correction by closing wedge osteotomy.

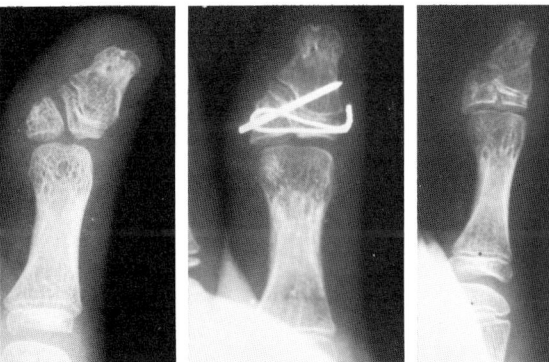

Fig. 12.16 Triphalangeal thumb with short triangular middle phalanx in a 10-year-old boy. Correction by wedge resection and fusion of the oblique joint.

Intermediate type

In these cases the middle phalanx is shorter than in the aforementioned type, often with an oblique distal joint surface, thus pollicization is not indicated. The appropriate treatment should comprise:

1. Resection of the distal joint and fusion of the two phalanges after adequate shortening
2. Shortening and rotation of the metacarpal by an osteotomy in its middle third
3. Detachment and more distal reattachment of the thenar muscles and the adductor muscle in regard to the skeletal shortening
4. Widening of the first web space by a Z-plasty
5. Opponens plasty with the flexor digitorum superficialis of the ring finger or the abductor digiti minimi

For triphalangism in association with polydactyly the treatment is adjusted to the type of polydactyly.

Complications

With the correct operative technique the number of complications is very low. Unstable joints or restriction of active motion may occur.

Results

The late results following the excision of a small triangular middle phalanx with collateral ligament reconstruction are usually excellent; appearance and function are like a normal thumb. The results of pollicization in the dolichophalangeal type are also very encouraging. In adolescence with wedge osteotomy of the proximal phalanx or arthrodesis of the oblique joint space, some broadening of the distal joint region may influence the cosmetic result, because the middle phalanx is not removed. In the intermediate type the thumb is usually slender with a relatively long terminal phalanx, but the total appearance of the hand is much improved as well as its function.

BIFID JOINTS IN POLYDACTYLY

Definition and anatomical findings

Polydactyly is a term under which all types of increased number of digits are united, varying from broad terminal phalanges in which only a hole shows the incomplete duplication (See Fig. 12.7) to duplications of phalanges or complete digits to mirror hands. Only those special forms of polydactyly in which the duplication starts in an interphalangeal joint are discussed here; this deformity is termed a 'bifid joint'.

This special type of duplication can occur in any digit (Fig. 12.17), but is most frequently seen in the thumb (Fig. 12.18). Although the bones are

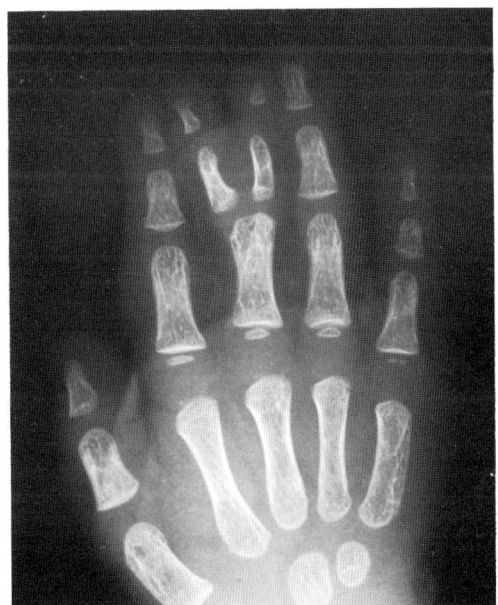

Fig. 12.17 Duplication of middle and end phalanx in a middle finger.

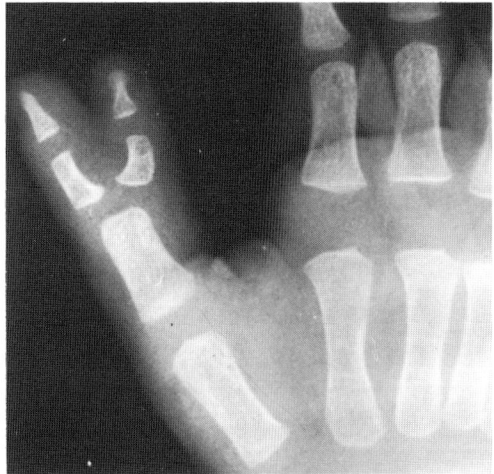

Fig. 12.18 Bifid joint in a triphalangeal thumb with duplicated distal parts.

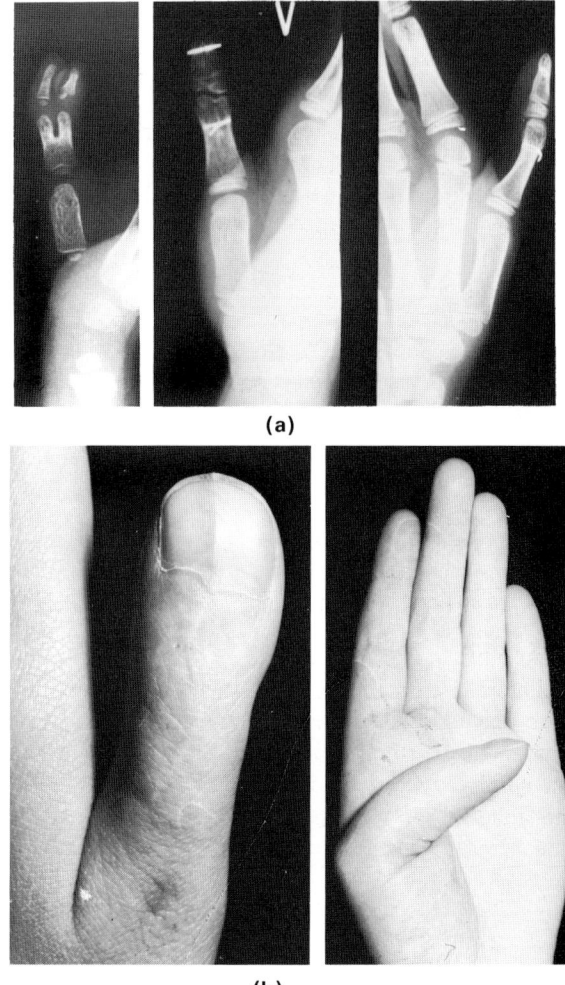

Fig. 12.19 Duplication of the left thumb. (**a**) Pre- and postoperative X-ray; (**b**) result 7 years postoperatively with good appearance and function in spite of restricted motion in the distal joint.

completely separated, usually there is only one palmar neurovascular bundle for each part: The flexor and extensor tendons bifurcate at the joint level and tend to insert eccentrically on the adjacent borders of the two phalanges. These are often different in size and shape, which makes the treatment more difficult. In most instances the head of the phalanx which forms the proximal part of the bifid joint is wider than normal; its articular surface is often angulated to one or to both sides. Collateral ligaments are present on only the two lateral parts of the conjoined joint, while the two distal bones frequently have a common cartilagenous base or sometimes a bony fusion. In cases of distal duplication in the ring finger, usually associated with syndactyly between the middle finger and the duplicated ring finger (so-called 'central polydactyly'), often a partial or sometimes a complete fusion between the bones of the distal phalanges of the duplicated ring finger is seen.

Incidence and heredity

These are not relevant here because the bifid joint is only one of many types of polydactyly.

Treatment

The operative procedure is either the resection of one part, if this is smaller than the partner, or the sharing method of Bilhaut-Cloquet. The first author described this procedure in 1890, while the bibliographic source of Cloquet has not yet been found (the name was introduced by Marc Iselin). The method consists of a wedge-shaped excision of about the middle third of the duplicated part and fusion of the two outer thirds including the bifurcated tendinous insertions. This will create a thumb of about usual size (Fig. 12.19). The disadvantage is the ridge in the nail, which can be prevented by using the modification of Miura (1976) which preserves the whole nail of one part and resects the other.

In the case of resection of the smaller part, which

is usually on the radial side, it is necessary to give the joint sufficient stability by reconstructing the collateral ligament. This is best done with a piece of extensor tendon from the deleted part which is sutured to the periosteum. It requires 6 weeks' immobilization by plaster or by a Kirschner wire. Often the head of the proximal phalanx is too broad and needs narrowing by excision of a small slice, either from the outer part of the head (under preservation or reattachment of the collateral ligament), or from the central part of the articular surface followed by compression of the two remaining parts with a screw or intraosseous wiring. Sometimes, in addition, a wedge osteotomy for the correction of an angulation is necessary as well as a relocation of eccentric insertions of flexor and/or extensor tendons.

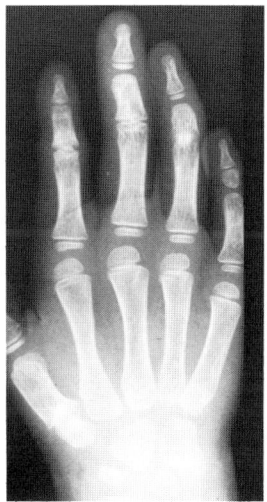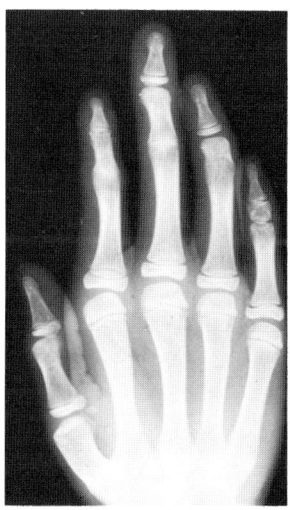

Fig. 12.20 Symphalangism with aplasia of the proximal interphalangeal joints in the right hand of a girl. Left: at the age of 4 years with open epiphyseal plates at the proximal interphalangeal joint level; right: at the age of 13 years.

Complications

Instability is seen in cases of missing or insufficient collateral ligament reconstruction; lateral deviation occurs if an eccentric tendon insertion is not corrected. In the Bilhaut wedge-shaped resection an epiphysiodesis can occur if the two parts will not match exactly, which may also cause a step in the articular surface with restriction of motion.

Results

The results of the operative treatment of bifid joints are satisfactory in most cases. The mentioned complications may cause more cosmetic than functional damage because a restriction of motion or a moderate lateral angulation must not interfere with an almost normal use of the thumb.

SYMPHALANGISM

Definition and anatomical findings

Symphalangism is a congenital aplasia of the proximal interphalangeal joint (Fig. 12.20). It is not found as an isolated digital anomaly in the distal joint or in the metacarpophalangeal joint; all published cases of distal interphalangeal joint fusion (Flatt & Wood 1975) belong to the group of symbrachydactyly. The term was introduced by Cushing (1916) in his description of a family with 84 involved persons among 313 examined. These exhibited a dominantly inherited deformity. This pedigree was up-dated by Strasburger et al (1965). Although very rare, symphalangism has the longest pedigree of any human genetic malformation; Drinkwater (1917) and later Elkington & Huntsman (1967) described the distribution of this deformity in the Talbot family beginning with John Talbot, the first Earl of Shrewsbury, who was killed in 1453. The condition is frequently associated with carpal (Fig. 12.20) and tarsal synostoses, and with conductive hearing loss.

Treatment

As a consequence of the rareness of symphalangism, few surgeons have experience with its treatment. In most cases no treatment is required because the patients usually adapt to the deformity. An angulatory osteotomy at the site of the proximal interphalangeal joint to give the digits a more flexed position is, therefore, often refused by the patient. Flatt & Wood (1975) have described the use of a silicone cap prosthesis to create a joint space, while Palmieri (1980) has performed a silicone rubber implant arthroplasty. Both proce-

CAMPTODACTYLY

Definition and anatomical findings

Camptodactyly is a descriptive term and means bent finger; it is a flexion contracture of the proximal interphalangeal joint of various degrees and usually occurs in the little finger (Fig. 12.21). The involvement of other fingers is relatively rare and the severity and the incidence of this deformity decrease from the ulnar to radial side. The pathogenesis is not clear and the only certain fact is that there are several different causes. Flatt (1977) described all the abnormalities which have been said to produce the deformity. Other important reviews have been given by Engber & Flatt (1977) and Smith & Kaplan (1968). Millesi (1968) has described a hypoplasia of the extensor apparatus, while Wilhelm & Kleinschmidt (1968) have seen anomalous insertions of the lumbrical muscle which were reported by McFarlane et al (1983) in *all* of their cases, in contrast to almost all other authors. Often it is difficult to differentiate between primary and secondary deformities. This is especially true in regard to the bone and joint deformities (Fig. 12.22).

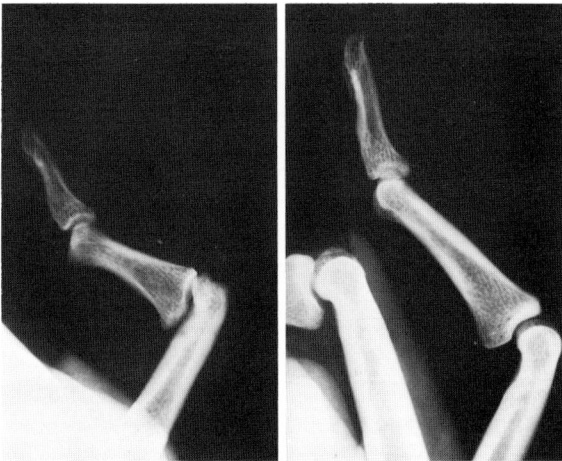

Fig. 12.22 Bone deformities in the proximal interphalangeal joints of little and ring fingers with flattened head of the proximal phalanx (left) and groove in the base of the middle phalanx (both fingers).

Incidence

It is impossible to give reliable numbers for the incidence because camptodactyly is a minor clinical sign which is often neglected by the patients if the flexion contracture is only 10–20° and not progressive.

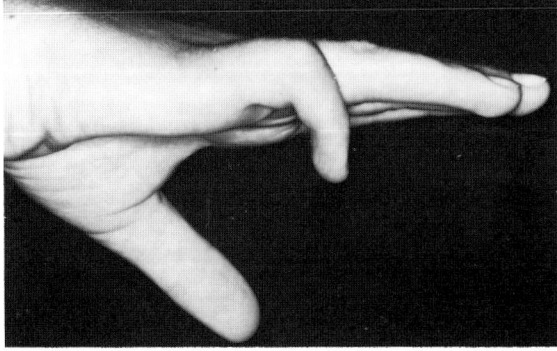

Fig. 12.21 Typical camptodactyly with flexion contracture in the proximal interphalangeal joint of the little finger.

Treatment

In most cases the patients will not want any treatment because the cosmetic appearance and function are not impaired. The surgeon should not persuade a patient to have an operative treatment, because the results are not consistently satisfactory. Only in cases of severe flexion deformity (70° or more) and in cases with progression may an operation be indicated. The procedure should consist of exploration of the lumbrical insertion and the tendon of the flexor digitorum superficialis. Any anomaly must be corrected, and in most cases combined with a soft tissue release (Z-plasty, skin graft), and arthrolysis. Postoperative Kirschner wire fixation of the proximal interphalangeal joint in extension is often necessary. If there are no anomalies, a transposition of the flexor digitorum superficialis to the extensor apparatus can improve the possible imbalance between flexors and extensors. Osteotomies and arthrodeses are indicated only in severe contractures (more than 90°). Considerable bone deformities are a contraindication to all soft tissue procedures.

Complications

A too extensive arthrolysis (capsulotomy) can cause a subluxation of the proximal interphalangeal joint. Scarring especially following secondary healing will make the flexion contracture usually worse than it was preoperatively.

Results

In general the results are only fair, and in many instances poor. Only the correction of a real anomalous lumbrical insertion and the arthrodesis have a good prognosis.

REFERENCES

Barsky A J 1967 Macrodactyly. Journal of Bone and Joint Surgery 49A: 1255–1266

Bell J 1951 On Brachydactyly and Symphalangism. In: Penrose L S (ed) The treasury of human inheritance, vol. V, part I. Cambridge University Press, Cambridge

Bilhaut 1890 Guérison d'un pouce bifide par un nouveau procédé opératoire. Congres Français de Chirurgie 4: 576–580

Buck-Gramcko D 1971 Pollicization of the index finger. Journal of Bone and Joint Surgery 53A: 1605–1617

Buck-Gramcko D 1981 Angeborene Fehlbildungen der Hand. In: Nigst H, Buck-Gramcko D, Millesi H (eds) Handchirurgie. Vol. I. Georg Thieme Verlag, Stuttgart, pp. 12.1–12.115

Burke F, Flatt A 1979 Clinodactyly. A review of a series of cases. Hand 11: 269–280

Carstam N, Theander G 1975 Surgical treatment of clinodactyly caused by longitudinally bracketed diaphyses (delta phalanx). Scandinavian Journal of Plastic and Reconstructive Surgery 9: 199–202

Chan K M, Lamb D W 1983 Triphalangeal thumb and five-fingered hand. Hand 15: 329–334

Cocchi U 1952 Erbschäden mit Knochenveränderungen. In: Schinz H R, Baensch W E, Friedl E, Uehlinger E (eds) Lehrbuch der Röntgendiagnostik. 5th edn, vol. I, part I. Georg Thieme Verlag, Stuttgart

Cushing H 1916 Hereditary anchylosis of the proximal phalangeal joints (symphalangism). Genetics 1: 90–106

Drinkwater H 1917 Phalangeal anarthrosis (synostosis, ankylosis) transmitted through fourteen generations. Proceedings of the Royal Society of Medicine 10: 60–68

Elkington S G, Huntsman R G 1967 The Talbot fingers: a study in symphalangism. British Medical Journal 1: 407–411

Engber W D, Flatt A E 1977 Camptodactyly: an analysis of sixty-six patients and twenty-four operations. Journal of Hand Surgery 2: 216–224

Flatt A E 1977 The care of congenital hand anomalies. C V Mosby, St Louis

Flatt A E, Wood V E 1975 Rigid digits or symphalangism. Hand 7: 197–214

Fort J-A 1869 Des difformités congénitales et acquises des doigts et des moyens d'y remédier. Thèse, A Delahaye, Paris

Giedion A 1966 Cone-shaped epiphyses of the hands and their diagnostic value. The tricho-rhino-phalangeal syndrome. Annals of Radiology 10: 322–329

Hilgenreiner H 1907 Ueber Hyperphalangie des Daumens. Beiträge zur Klinischen Chirurgie 54: 585–629

Jaeger M, Refior H J 1971 The congenital triangular deformity of the tubular bones of hand and foot. Clinical Orthopaedics 81: 139–150

Jones G B 1964 Delta phalanx. Journal of Bone and Joint Surgery 46B: 226–228

McFarlane R M, Curry G I, Evans H B 1983 Anomalies of the intrinsic muscles in camptodactyly. Journal of Hand Surgery 8: 531–544

Millesi H 1968 Zur Pathogenese und operativen Korrektur dem Kamptodaktylie. Chirurgia Plastica et Reconstructiva 5: 55–61

Miura T 1976 Triphalangeal thumb. Plastic and Reconstructive Surgery 58: 587–594

Palmieri T J 1980 The use of silicone rubber implant arthroplasty in treatment of true symphalangism. Journal of Hand Surgery 5: 242–244

Pol R 1921 'Brachydaktylie'—'Klinodaktylie'—Hyperphalangie und ihre Grundlagen: Form und Entstehung der meist unter dem Bild der Brachydaktylie auftretenden Varietäten, Missbildungen der Hand und des Fusses. Virchow's Archiv für Pathologische Anatomie und Physiologie 229: 388–530

Smith R J 1977 Osteotomy for 'delta-phalanx' deformity. Clinical Orthopaedics 123: 91–94

Smith R J, Kaplan E B 1968 Camptodactyly and similar atraumatic flexion deformities of the proximal interphalangeal joints of the fingers. Journal of Bone and Joint Surgery 50A: 1187–1204

Strasburger A K, Hawkins M R, Eldridge R, Hargrave R L, McKusick V A 1965 Symphalangism: genetic and clinical aspects. Bulletin of the Johns Hopkins Hospital 117: 108–127

Swanson A G, Brown K S 1962 Hereditary triphalangeal thumb. Journal of Heredity 53: 259–265

Theander G, Carstam N 1974 Longitudinal bracketed epiphysis. Annals of Radiology 17: 355–360

Vickers D W 1980 Premature incomplete fusion of the growth plate: causes and treatment by resection (physolysis) in fifteen cases. Australian and New Zealand Journal of Surgery 50: 393–401

Watson H K, Boyes J H 1967 Congenital angular deformity of the digits. Delta phalanx. Journal of Bone and Joint Surgery 49A: 333–338

Werthemann A 1952 Die Entwicklungsstörungen der Extremitäten. In: Lubarsch O, Henke F, Rössle R (eds) Handbuch der speziellen pathologischen Anatomie und Histologie. vol. 9. part 6. Springer, Berlin

Wieland E 1907 Zur Pathologie der dystrophischen Form des angeborenen partiellen Riesenwuchses. Jahrbuch der Kinderheilkunde 65, p 519–584

Wilhelm A, Kleinschmidt W 1968 Neue ätiologische und therapeutische Gesichtspunkte bei der Kamptodaktylie und Tendovaginitis stenosans. Chirurgia Plastica et Reconstructiva 5: 62–67

Wood V E 1976 Treatment of the triphalangeal thumb. Clinical Orthopaedics 120: 188–200

Wood V E 1978 Polydactyly and the triphalangeal thumb. Journal of Hand Surgery 3:436–444

Wood V E 1982 Delta phalanx. In: Green D P (ed) Operative hand surgery. Churchill Livingstone, New York

Wood V E, Flatt A E 1977 Congenital triangular bones in the hand. Journal of Hand Surgery 2:179–193

FURTHER READING

Kelikian H 1974 Congenital deformities of the hand and forearm. W B Saunders Co, Philadelphia

Poznanski A K 1984 The hand in radiological diagnosis, 2nd edn. W B Saunders Co, Philadelphia

J. P. W. Varian

13

Developmental conditions

Developmental conditions of the fingers include an assortment of tumorous conditions which can basically be divided into cystic lesions and solid lesions. The cystic lesions include mucous cysts of the terminal joint and ganglia of the proximal interphalangeal joint. The solid lesions include enchondroma and osteochondroma, both of which are often thought of as benign tumours but are in fact hamartomata (Aegerter & Kirkpatrick 1968), and the rare malignant tumours chondrosarcoma, osteosarcoma and fibrosarcoma. There are two other conditions which are currently thought to be inflammatory—pigmented villonodular synovitis and benign periostitis. Only those conditions that affect the interphalangeal joints directly will be covered in detail. Osteophytes, Heberden's nodes and similar lesions associated with degenerative joint disease, and gouty arthrosis have already been discussed in Chapter 9.

CYSTS

Ganglion

A ganglion is a benign cyst associated with a synovial cavity, most commonly the wrist joint or the flexor tendon sheath (Nelson et al 1972). Less commonly they can arise from an intercarpal joint and rarely are associated with the interphalangeal joints. There is no underlying joint degeneration. They are occasionally to be found arising from the proximal interphalangeal joint where they present as a swelling on the side of the finger just proximal to the flexor crease (Fig. 13.1). The reason for this presentation is that the extensor mechanism prevents their appearance dorsally and they must therefore track out from under the side of the lateral band, either proximal to the transverse retinacular ligament, or more distally from under the oblique retinacular ligament of Landsmeer. Like all ganglia, it is important that their connection with the underlying joint is removed, and in order to do this in these circumstances, it is often necessary to divide the retinacular ligament and reflect it volarly in order to reveal the neck of the ganglion arising from the proximal interphalangeal joint. Cysts arising from the terminal joint, usually in association with osteoarthritis of that joint are called mucous cysts (Fig. 13.2).

Mucous cyst

The mucous cyst of the terminal joint of the finger or thumb has been the source of controversy for many years with regard to its origins. Nasca & Gould (1983) describe a definite synovial lining as in a ganglion and are happy to call it a cyst, while Goldman et al (1977) could find no such lining and have called it a pseudocyst. It has also been termed a myxoid cyst in the belief that it was simply a localized degenerative process (Gross 1937). Previously it was thought that these cysts had no connection with the terminal joint as histologically none could be seen (Bourns & Sonerkin 1962), but it has now been conclusively established by pathological studies (King 1951) and by injection of the terminal joint with methylene blue that there is a connection between that joint and the cyst (Newmeyer et al 1974, Goldman et al 1977). As in the case of ganglia, the connection is more easily demonstrated by showing the passage of fluid from the joint into the cyst rather than vice versa. Other

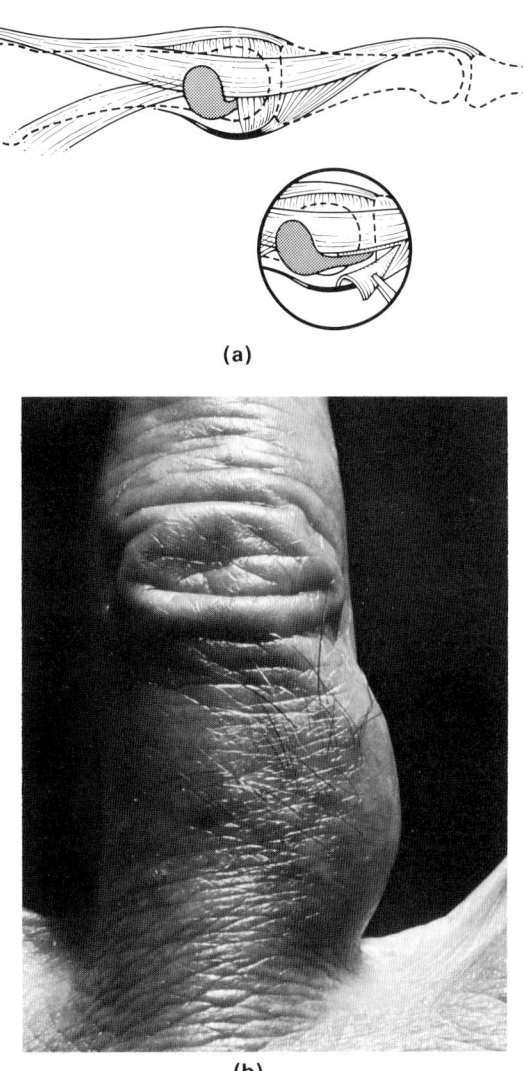

Fig. 13.1 (a) Illustration to show the appearance of a ganglion from behind the retinacular ligaments of a proximal interphalangeal joint. (b) Clinical appearance of such a ganglion.

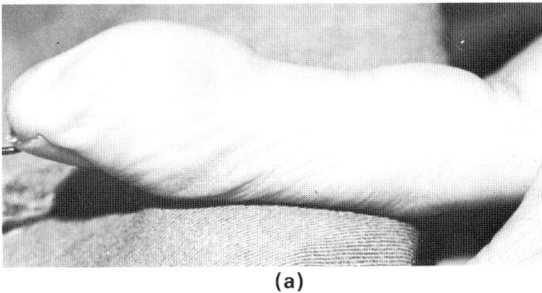

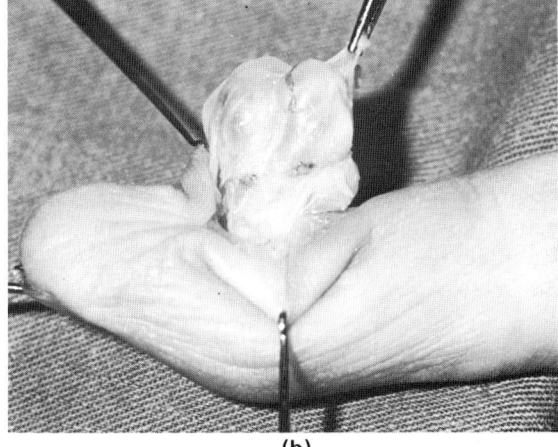

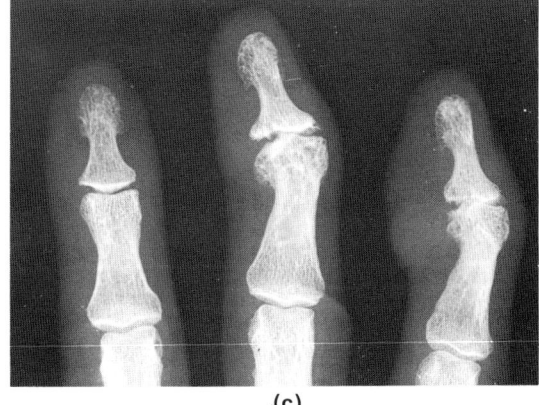

Fig. 13.2 (a) Cystic swelling on the flexor aspect of the terminal segment of a ring finger. (b) Ganglion or mucous cyst? (c) Degenerative change in the terminal joint makes the condition a mucous cyst.

authors (Kleinert et al 1972, Eaton et al 1973) have implicated the presence of osteophytes in the formation of these cysts, but it is the present author's belief that both the osteophytes and the cysts arise independently from a degenerative joint. One frequently observes this condition in a joint prior to the formation of osteophytes and one frequently sees a degenerative joint with quite large osteophytes wherein there is no mucous cyst.

Clinical presentation

The patient usually presents with a well formed cyst lying just under the dorsal skin between the terminal joint of the finger and the nail fold. The lesion is usually small, measuring about 4 mm in diameter. It arises from the joint between the extensor tendon and the collateral ligament and it presents as a swelling to one side at the back of the terminal segment of the finger. There may indeed be two such cysts, one on either side of the extensor tendon insertion (Fig. 13.3). As it develops the cyst tends to move distally and may come to lie right in the nail fold. When it lies on the edge of the germinal layer of the nail bed, it often causes a distinct groove running longitudinally down that side of the nail (Fig. 13.4). Indeed, this groove may be the first symptom that the patient will notice. As the cyst matures it appears to erode the dermis so that it becomes covered with a thin epidermal layer of skin which is almost transparent. This may burst either spontaneously or as the result of a knock and a clear jelly is then extruded. The lesion usually heals and then, over a period of weeks, recurs. Not infrequently a pattern of recurrence and discharge develops taking about a month for the cycle to repeat itself. The lesion is rarely painful although the patient may complain of intermittent low grade pain arising from the degenerative arthritis in the terminal joint. Advice and treatment

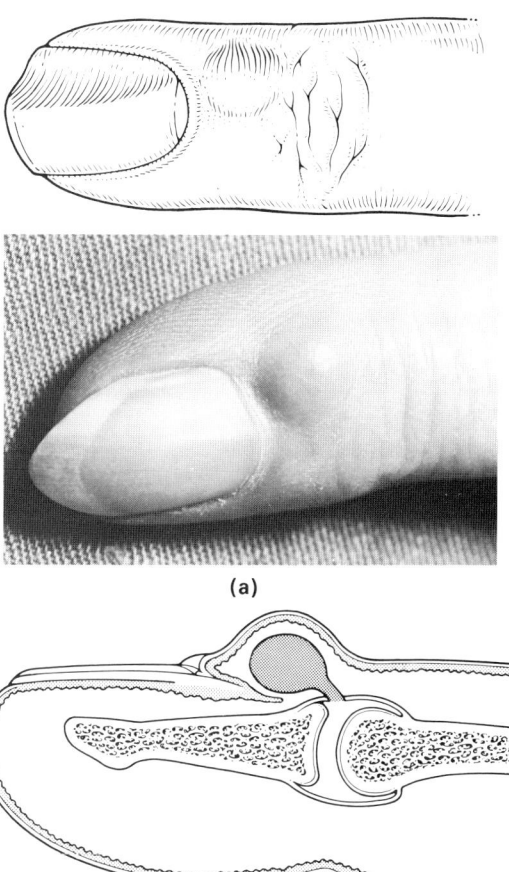

Fig. 13.4 (a) A mucous cyst that has migrated distally into the nail fold and is causing longitudinal grooving of the nail. **(b)** Illustration of such a cyst to show that it has a long neck connecting it to the terminal joint which must be removed at surgery.

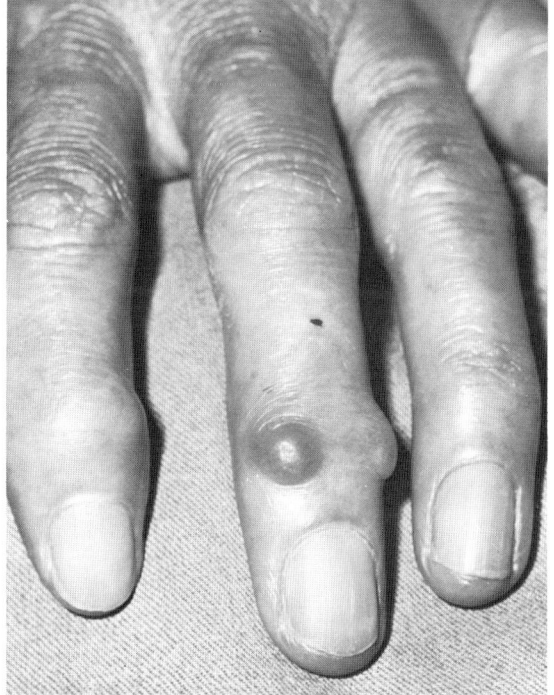

Fig. 13.3 Typical appearance of a mucous cyst on the back of the fingertip, in this case a double lesion. The typical clinical appearance of underlying osteoarthritis can be seen in the adjacent fingertips.

are usually sought for cosmetic reasons. Occasionally the lesion can be extremely large (Fig. 13.5). In these circumstances the clinician might understandably consider that the lesion was a ganglion, but an X-ray will reveal the underlying osteoarthrosis which is the hallmark of the mucous cyst. Occasionally when the cyst is hard and overlying the terminal joint it can be mistaken for a Heberden's node, but the two can easily be differentiated by transilluminating the lesion with a pencil torch.

Treatment

Treatment of these lesions has been the subject of some discussion in the literature. Some authors

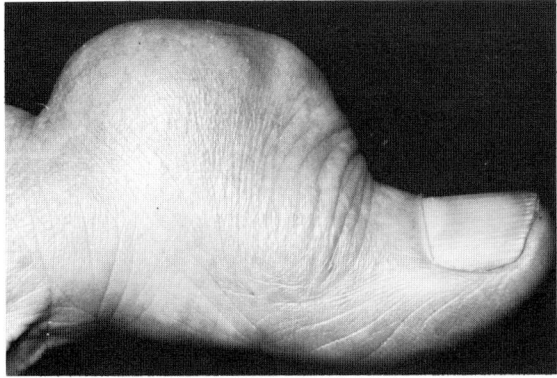

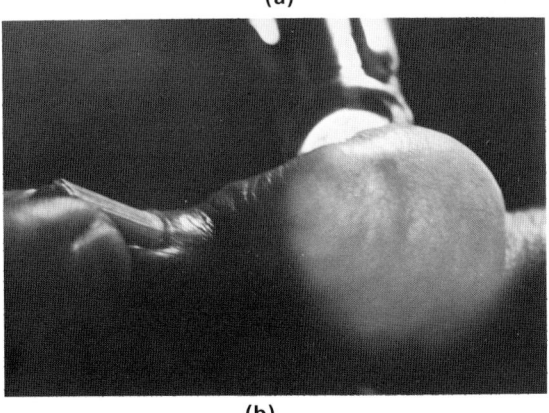

Fig. 13.5 (a) Mucous cysts can be large, here arising from the terminal joint of the thumb. **(b)** Transillumination can be an aid to diagnosis.

describe a high recurrence rate (Arner et al 1956) and others a low recurrence rate following surgery (Nasca & Gould 1983), and this would appear to depend very largely on whether or not care was taken to excise the connection between the cyst and the joint. Repeated puncture and expression of the cyst contents has been advised by some authors with success (Epstein 1979). Others believe that, having excised the cyst, it is necessary to close the resultant defect with either a full thickness or a partial thickness skin graft (Bourns & Sonerkin 1962, Constant et al 1969). The present author agrees with Nasca & Gould (1983) that it is usually possible to dissect the cyst away from the overlying epidermis and no skin grafting is necessary. Some authors, believing that the osteophytes play a part in the formation of these cysts, advise that the osteophytes be removed at the time of surgery (Kleinert et al 1972, Eaton et al 1973). In a case of severe degenerative osteoarthritis of the terminal joint it may be necessary to arthrodese that joint. It is important to warn the patient that the symptoms arising from the underlying osteoarthritis will not be affected by the simple removal of the cyst. Recurrence following inadequate surgery is usually rapid, developing within a month or two of the operation. Recurrence later is probably the development of another cyst from the persisting osteoarthritis.

PIGMENTED VILLONODULAR SYNOVITIS

This condition is known by a great many different names reflecting the uncertainty as to the aetiology of the lesion to this day. Fyfe and McFarlane (1980) list 15 different names that have been given to it since it was first described in 1852 by Chaissaignac. It is now most commonly known as giant cell tumour of tendon sheath, benign synovioma, and pigmented villonodular synovitis. Targett introduced the name of giant cell tumour of tendon sheath in 1897 from the histological appearance of a large number of giant cells in many of the lesions. For many years it was known as xanthoma or xanthogranuloma due to its yellow colour and de Santo and Wilson in 1939 suggested it was a disorder of lipid metabolism. Stewart in 1948 suggested that it was a benign tumour arising from the synovium and this view was supported by Wright in 1951 when he stated that the lesion 'must certainly be regarded as neoplastic'. Jaffe et al in 1941 considered that the lesion was a benign inflammatory response to an unknown agent. This view has subsequently been supported by other authors (Larmon 1965, Byers et al 1968, Granovitz et al 1976). This condition most commonly presents in the hand in its nodular form, usually arising from the flexor tendon sheath. It does, however, also arise from either of the interphalangeal joints and has been reported in its diffuse form in the distal interphalangeal joint (Crawford & Offerman 1980).

Clinical presentation

Villonodular synovitis usually presents as a painless lump in the hand or finger, gradually increasing in size. It most commonly arises from flexor sheath (Fig. 13.6) and occasionally pain or paraesthesia can be produced by pressure on a digital nerve. It may have been noticed by the patient over a period of months or years. Those arising from the interphalangeal joints may produce some slight limitation of movement by distending the joint from which it arises. The tumour tends to follow the path of least resistance when it is growing and so most commonly appears on the side of the joint between the flexor and extensor tendons. It may grow around the edge of the extensor tendon onto the dorsum of the finger (Fig. 13.7). Occasionally a tumour arising from the centre of the proximal interphalangeal joint will grow laterally in both directions producing a dumb-bell shaped lesion (Fig. 13.8). A lesion arising from the terminal joint can cause grooving of the nail (Fig. 13.9) as is commonly seen associated with a mucous cyst, and for this reason these two conditions can be confused.

X-ray appearance

The lesion can be seen on X-ray as a soft tissue shadow in the finger. There is no calcification in the lesion. It can also appear as a smooth erosion of the cortex of the phalanx from pressure on the bone and occasionally, it will penetrate into the bone and produce a localized radiolucent lesion suggestive of a bone cyst.

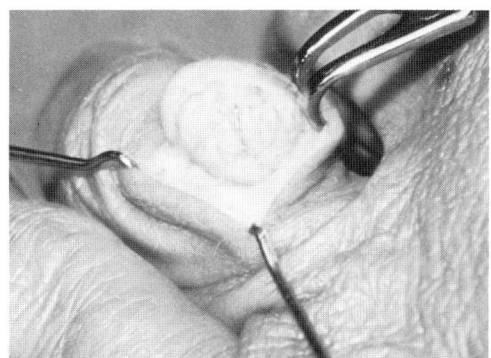

Fig. 13.7 Nodule of villonodular synovitis appearing on the back of a finger.

Pathological appearance

The localized nodular type of villonodular synovitis takes the form of a discreet multilobulated mass, the colour varying throughout the tumour between yellows and browns, depending on the amount of haemosiderin pigmentation, lipid deposition, and fibrous stroma. It is enclosed in a thin capsule and does not invade the surrounding tissues. It therefore separates easily on removal although it is usually firmly attached at its point of origin to either the fibrous flexor sheath or the capsule of a joint.

Microscopically the tumour consists of a fibrous stroma containing islands of cells which are mainly histiocytes, many containing haemosiderin pigment. Scattered throughout the cells are multinucleated giant cells and macrophages filled with lipoid material, commonly called foam cells. The histological picture varies according to the maturity of the lesion and in its active cellular phase mitoses are frequently seen. The details of the histological picture are well described by Jaffe et al (1941).

Treatment

Treatment is by complete excision of the lesion. A high recurrence rate in some series has been reported (Wright 1951, Fyfe & MacFarlane 1980), possibly where the lesion has been removed as an outpatient procedure under local anaesthesia. It is essential, if recurrence is to be avoided, that a careful and methodical excision be carried out

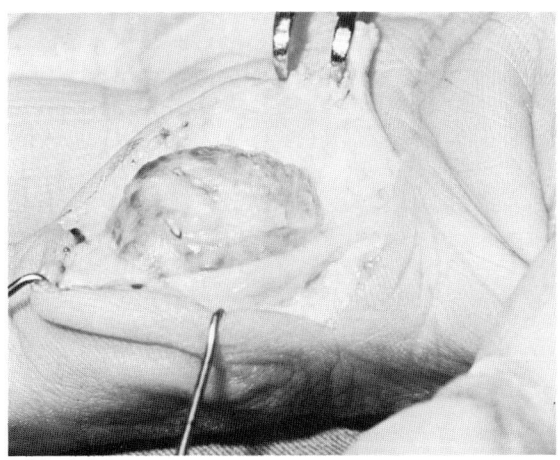

Fig. 13.6 Villonodular synovitis arising from the flexor tendon sheath in the proximal segment of an index finger.

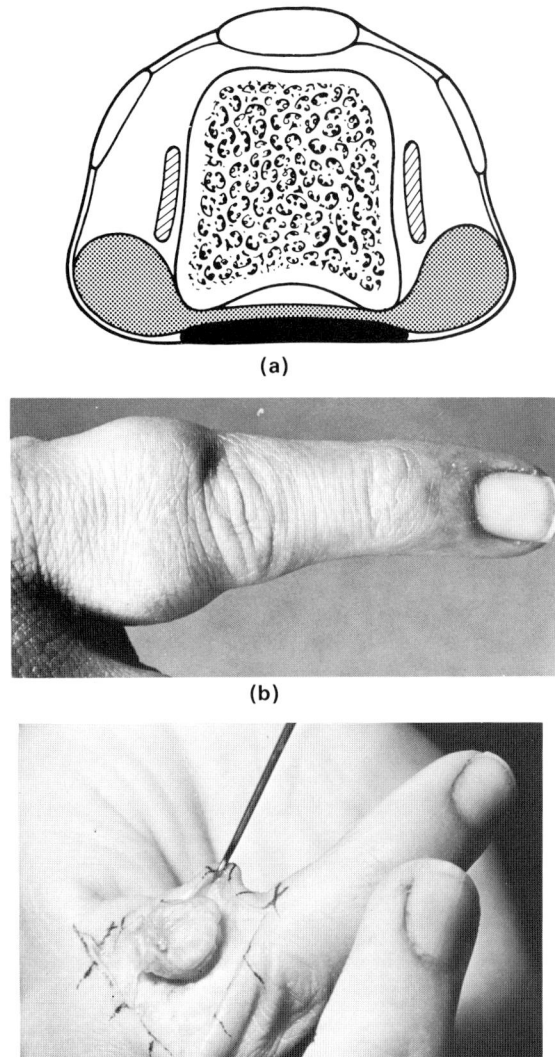

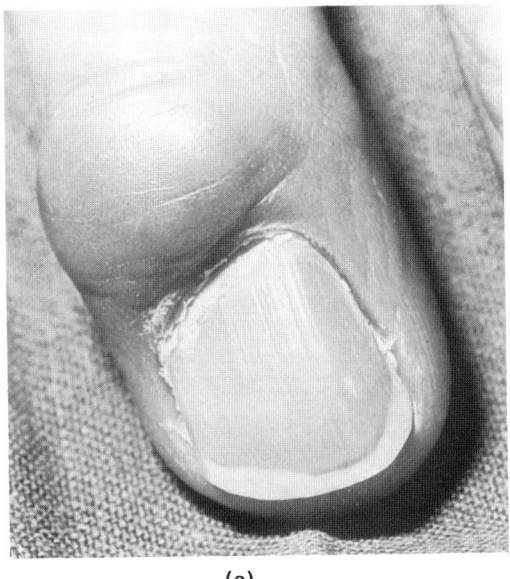

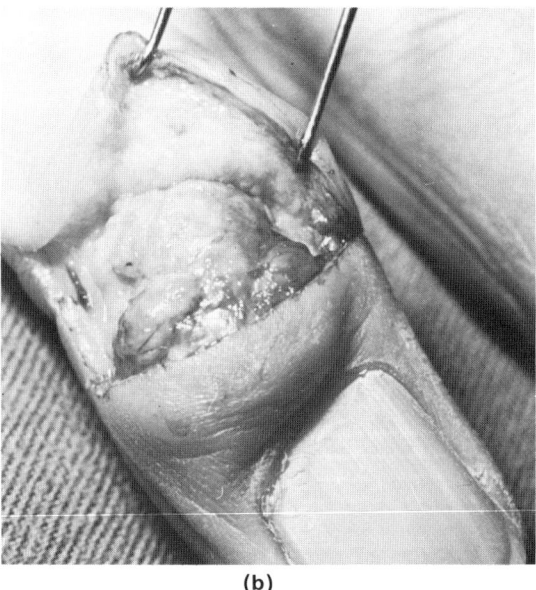

Fig. 13.8 (a) Villonodular synovitis arising from the proximal interphalangeal joint occasionally develops as a dumb-bell lesion protruding from either side of the joint. **(b)** Clinical appearance of such a lesion. **(c)** Ulnar mid-axial incision to approach one side of the lesion. A similar approach is used for the other side.

Fig. 13.9 (a) Villonodular synovitis arising from the terminal joint and causing grooving of the nail, mimicking the appearance of a mucous cyst. **(b)** Operative appearance of the lesion.

under a tourniquet. The lobulated nature of the condition and its tendency to extend along tissue plains and behind tendons and ligaments can easily result in a small piece being left behind which will grow on to produce a recurrence. There is usually no problem in obtaining a complete removal from the flexor sheath, but when excising it from the proximal interphalangeal joint it is often difficult to be certain that the lesion has been cleared in toto and two mid-axial incisions on either side of the joint may be necessary. Block dissection of the lesion is not necessary as it is not malignant.

TUMOURS

Solitary enchondroma is a common incidental finding in the X-rays of the hands of young people up to the age of skeletal maturity. They are occasionally responsible for pathological fractures of the fingers. They develop from islands of cartilage within the bone that have not undergone the normal process of ossification with bone growth. They do not arise from or affect the interphalangeal joints. They occasionally will perforate through the cortex of the side of the bone forming an osteochondroma (Aegerter & Kirkpatrick 1968). This latter condition has also been reported arising from the tuft or shaft of the terminal phalanx (Apfelberg et al 1979) but does not arise or affect either of the interphalangeal joints. Both these conditions will be dealt with in a later book in this series on tumours of the hand. Multiple enchondromatosis and multiple osteochondromatosis are both congenital conditions and will be discussed in a book on congenital conditions.

Sarcomas are rare malignant tumours in the hand. The commonest of these is the chondrosarcoma. Eighty-four cases have now been published in the literature (Popovici 1934, Allendale 1936, Cruickshank 1945, Coley & Higginbotham 1954, Gottschalk & Smith 1963, Dahlin & Salvador 1974, Patel et al 1977, Roberts & Price 1977, Armino et al 1978, Granberry & Bryan 1978, Trias et al 1978, Pierce 1979, Wu et al 1980, Justis & Dart 1983, Wu et al 1983, Palmieri 1984). The vast majority arise on either side of the metacarpophalangeal joint and a few have been reported arising from either the middle phalanx or the distal phalanx. There is, as yet, no reported case arising from the interphalangeal joints and it is remarkable how these tumours, arising within the bone, do not seem to invade the joint directly. Osteosarcoma is a much rarer tumour in the hand than chondrosarcoma and also arises within the bones of the hand rather than the joints. These tumours will be dealt with in the book in this series on tumours of the hand.

REFERENCES

Aegerter E, Kirkpatrick J A 1968 Orthopaedic diseases. W B Saunders Co, Philadelphia, pp 569–576

Allendale G 1936 Osteocondroma de la tibia y condrosarcoma de los dedos. Revista de Orthopedia y Traumatolgia 6:71–81

Apfelberg D B, Druker D, Maser M R, Lash H 1979 Subungual osteochondroma. Archives of Dermatology 115:472–473

Armino J A, Ashley P F, Herrera L O 1978 Chondrosarcoma of the hand. Delaware Medical Journal 50:383–385

Arner O, Lindholm A, Romanus R 1956 Mucous cysts of the fingers, report of 26 cases. Acta Chirurgica Scandinavica 111:314–321

Bourns H I, Sonerkin N G 1962 Mucoid lesion (mucoid cysts) of the fingers and toes. Clinical features and pathogenesis. British Journal of Surgery 50:860

Byers P D, Cotton R E, Deacon O W et al 1968 The diagnosis and treatment of pigmented villonodular synovitis. Journal of Bone and Joint Surgery 50B:290–305

Chaissaignac C M E 1852 Cancer de la gaine des tendons. Gazette des Hospitaux Civils et Militaires 47:185–186

Coley B L, Higginbotham N L 1954 Secondary chondrosarcoma. Annals of Surgery 139:547–559

Constant E, Roger J R, Pollard R J, Larsen R D, Posch J L 1969 Mucous cysts of the fingers. Plastic and Reconstruction Surgery 43:241

Crawford G P, Offerman R J 1980 Pigmented villonodular synovitis in the hand. The Hand 12:282–287

Cruickshank A H 1945 Chondrosarcoma of a phalanx with cutaneous metastases. Journal of Pathology and Bacteriology 57:144–145

Dahlin D C, Salvador A H 1974 Chondrosarcoma of bones of the hands and feet—a study of thirty cases. Cancer 34:755–760

de Santo D A, Wilson P D 1939 Xanthomatous tumours of joints. Journal of Bone and Joint Surgery 21:531–558

Eaton R G, Dobranski A I, Littler J W 1973 Marginal osteophyte excision in the treatment of mucous cysts. Journal of Bone and Joint Surgery 55A:570–574

Epstein E 1979 A simple technique for managing digital mucous cysts. Archives of Dermatology 115:1315–1316

Fyfe I S, MacFarlane A 1980 Pigmented villonodular synovitis of the hand. The Hand 12:179–188

Goldman J A, Goldman L, Jaffe M S, Richfield D F 1977 Digital mucinous pseudocysts. Arthritis and Rheumatism 20:997–1002

Gottschalk R G, Smith R T 1963 Chondrosarcoma of the hand. Journal of Bone and Joint Surgery 45A:141–150

Granberry W M, Bryan W 1978 Chondrosarcoma of the trapezius: a case report. Journal of Hand Surgery 3:277–279

Granovitz S P, D'Antonio J, Mankin H L 1976 The pathogenesis and long-term end results of pigmented villonodular synovitis. Clinical and Orthopaedic Related Research 114:335–351

Gross R E 1937 Recurring myxomatous, cutaneous cysts of the fingers and toes. Surgery of Gynaecology and Obstetrics 65:289–302

Jaffe H L, Lichtenstein L, Sutro C J 1941 Pigmented villonodular synovitis, bursitis and tenosynovitis. A discussion of the synovial and bursal equivalents of the tenosynovial lesion commonly denoted as xanthoma, xanthogranuloma, giant-cell tumour or myeloplaxoma of the tendon sheath, with some consideration of this tendon sheath itself. Archives of Pathology 31 : 731–765

Justis E J, Dart R C 1983 Chondrosarcoma of the hand with metastasis : a review of the literature and case report. Journal of Hand Surgery 8 : 320–324

King E S J 1951 Mucous cysts of the fingers. Australian and New Zealand Journal of Surgery 21 : 121–129

Kleinert H E, Kutz J E, Fishman J H 1972 Etiology and treatment of the so-called mucous cyst of the finger. Journal of Bone and Joint Surgery 54A : 1455–1458

Larmon W A 1965 Pigmented villonodular synovitis. The Medical Clinics of North America 49 : 141–150

Nasca R J, Gould J S 1983 Mucous cysts of the digits. Southern Medical Journal 76 : 1142–1144

Nelson C L, Sawmiller S, Phelen G S 1972 Ganglions of the wrist and hand. Journal of Bone and Joint Surgery 54A : 1459–1464

Newmeyer W C, Kilgore E S Jr, Graham W P 1974 Mucous cysts : the dorsal distal interphalangeal joint ganglion. Plastic and Reconstruction Surgery 53 : 313–315

Palmieri T J 1984 Chondrosarcoma of the hand. Journal of Hand Surgery 9A : 332–338

Patel M R, Pearlman H S, Engler J, Wollowick B S 1977 Chondrosarcoma of the proximal phalanx of the finger. Journal of Bone and Joint Surgery 59A : 401–403

Pierce R O 1979 A case report—soft tissue chondrosarcoma of the hand. Journal of Indiana State Medical Association 72 : 124–125

Popovici A 1934 Chondrosarcomatoza bilaterala a manilor, metastaze multiple. Revista de Chirurgie (Bucuresti) 37 : 756–760

Roberts P H, Price C H G 1977 Chondrosarcoma of the bones of the hand. Journal of Bone and Joint Surgery 59B : 213–221

Stewart M J 1948 Benign giant-cell synovioma and its relation to 'xanthoma'. Journal of Bone and Joint Surgery 30B : 522–527

Targett J H 1897 Giant-celled tumours of the integuments. Transactions of the Pathological Society of London 48 : 230–235

Trias A, Basora J, Sanchez G, Madarnas P 1978 Chondrosarcoma of the hand. Clinical Orthopaedics 134 : 297–301

Wright C J E 1951 Benign giant-cell synovioma. An investigation of 85 cases. British Journal of Surgery 38 : 257–271

Wu K K, Collon D J, Buise E R 1980 Extra-osseous chondrosarcoma. Journal of Bone and Joint Surgery 62A : 189–194

Wu K K, Frost H M, Guise E E 1983 A chondrosarcoma of the hand arising from an asymptomatic benign solitary enchondroma of 40 years duration. Journal of Hand Surgery 8 : 317–319

SECTION 5

Rehabilitation

14

Therapeutic management of the proximal interphalangeal joint

M. S. Carter

INTRODUCTION

Rehabilitation of the proximal interphalangeal joints following injury, disease or surgery involves careful assessment, meticulous recording of progress (Adamson 1970), an individualized therapy programme and intensive patient education.

Problems at the interphalangeal level can occur from a multitude of causative factors and involve any or all of the structures of the hand including soft tissues, bones, joints, periarticular and vascular systems (Watson et al 1979, Bowers et al 1980, Bowers 1980). Despite the original causative factor, the major complication encountered is a stiff joint. Limited motion with pain, swelling and occasional instability are the most common sequelae presenting to the therapist.

Most authors writing on the subject of joint stiffness emphasize that prevention should be the primary consideration (Curtis 1964, McCormack 1964, Arem 1981, Laseter 1983). They agree that acute stiffness of the joint is expected following many types of trauma or surgery, but that this condition is temporary and responds well to appropriate conservative measures (Sprague 1975, Bowers 1983). Since prevention is the primary goal, the ideal situation is to begin the patient's therapy as soon as possible (McCormack 1964).

Post injury/operative management does seem to have a 'golden period' during which initiation of treatment can help to ensure the best results. The earlier the patient is started on a structured programme, the better are the chances to avoid complications (Adamson 1970).

There are several common elements in both evaluation and treatment of acute or chronic interphalangeal joint disorders. The major difference lies in the emphasis on prevention in the acute stage and alleviation of established complications in the chronic stage (McEntee 1984).

EVALUATION

Previous chapters have emphasized the necessity and described the procedure for physical examination and viewing of X-rays. For effective resolution of the stiff interphalangeal joint, the therapist *must* obtain a copy of the patient's medical records and surgical reports, review the X-rays with the physician and be able to communicate closely with him concerning the goals and progress of treatment. In addition, the therapist must perform a separate physical examination to assess the current status of the joint.

Oedema

Most stiff joints evidence swelling whether the condition is acute or chronic. In early cases, the joint will be tender and possess a 'soft' oedema that can be depressed by touch (Fig. 14.1). In a chronic case, the oedema will be 'brawny' with a putty-type feel to it. If the swelling is primarily within the joint, there will be a visual fullness that can be indented by pressure. If periarticular tissues are also involved, the joint will have a 'boggy' feel that extends both proximally and distally with little definition (Fig. 14.2).

Objective measures of the oedema include circumferential measurements of the joint itself or assessment of the entire hand utilizing the volu-

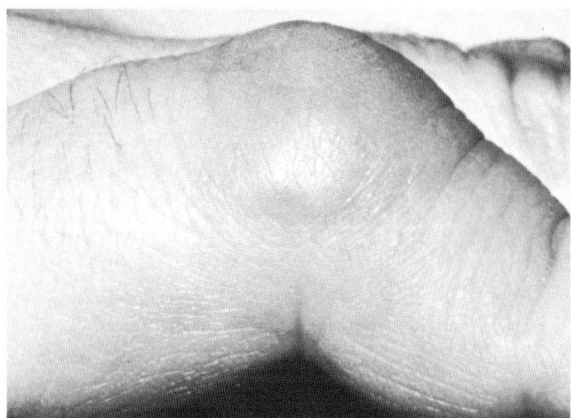

Fig. 14.1 Acute PIP oedema that can be depressed by touch.

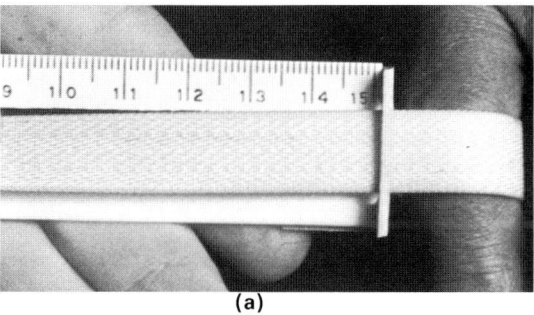
(a)

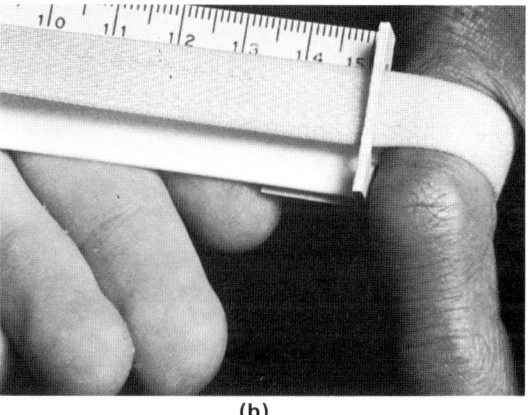
(b)

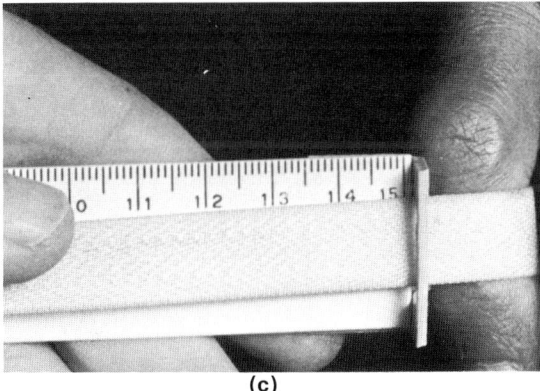
(c)

Fig. 14.3 Circumferential measurements for a PIP disorder should include (**a**) the PIP joint, (**b**) proximal phalanx and (**c**) the middle phalanx.

meter (Brand & Wood 1974). If the swelling is localized in the area of the proximal interphalangeal (PIP) joint, circumferential measurements are more accurate. Measurements should be made around the proximal phalanx, the PIP joint itself, and the middle phalanx (Fig 14.3). Comparisons are taken on the same digit of the uninvolved hand using exact anatomical landmarks or distance measurements to ensure precision.

Pain

Interphalangeal joint pain, especially at the PIP joint, is a major contributor to limitation of motion. Pain that occurs with joint motion elicits a protective mechanism that further immobilizes the digit (Watson et al 1979). The patient must be advised to expect 'normal' discomfort; however, for optimal treatment, pain must be closely monitored and minimized as quickly as possible. If joint pain is disproportional to the injury with proximal radiation and vasomotor changes, the therapist must be alert to the possibility of a single finger dystrophy.

To maintain a subjective record of the patient's

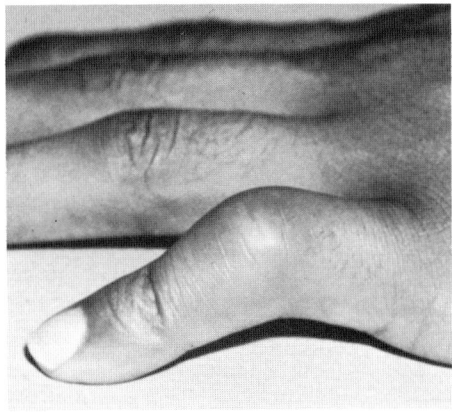

Fig. 14.2 Chronic PIP oedema that is diffuse in nature with little definition.

pain, he may be asked before and after each treatment to give his pain a number rating from 0 to 10. A 0 represents no pain and a 10 equals severe pain. A more objective assessment (Richards et al 1982) records measures such as posturing, verbal, and non-verbal expressions of pain (Fig. 14.4).

Active/passive range of motion

When dealing with immobility of the interphalangeal joint, individual goniometric readings, as established by the American Academy of Orthopedic Surgeons (1965) are more useful to the clinician than total digit measurements (Fig. 14.5). While total active and passive range of motion give a clear picture of the complete digit, they cannot demonstrate the often minute changes occurring specifically at the joint in question. Even if the injury or surgery is confined to one interphalangeal joint, all joints of the upper extremity including the shoulder should be checked for abnormality. Measures of active and passive range of motion of the involved and the non-involved hand help to monitor changes. Differences between active and passive motion can be significant in determining the possible need for surgical intervention (Weeks & Wray 1978).

Intrinsic and extrinsic tests for musculotendinous tightness complete the total picture of range of motion. To test for tight intrinsic muscles, the examiner attempts to flex passively the proximal and distal interphalangeal joint with the metacarpophalangeal (MP) joint held in extension. If the intrinsic muscles are tight, the interphalangeal

PATIENT:		Upper extremity pain behaviour scale				
		I	II	III	IV	
1. Vocal complaints verbal:	None	0	0	0	0	0
	Occasional	$\frac{1}{2}$	$\frac{1}{2}$	$\frac{1}{2}$	$\frac{1}{2}$	$\frac{1}{2}$
	Frequent	1	1	1	1	1
2. Vocal complaints non-verbal:	None	0	0	0	0	0
(moans, groans, gasps, etc)	Occasional	$\frac{1}{2}$	$\frac{1}{2}$	$\frac{1}{2}$	$\frac{1}{2}$	$\frac{1}{2}$
	Frequent	1	1	1	1	1
3. Down-time:	None	0	0	0	0	0
(Time lying down per day	0–60 min	$\frac{1}{2}$	$\frac{1}{2}$	$\frac{1}{2}$	$\frac{1}{2}$	$\frac{1}{2}$
because of pain)	60 min	1	1	1	1	1
4. Facial grimaces	None	0	0	0	0	0
	Mild and/or infrequent	$\frac{1}{2}$	$\frac{1}{2}$	$\frac{1}{2}$	$\frac{1}{2}$	$\frac{1}{2}$
	Severe and/or frequent	1	1	1	1	1
5. Posture of involved arm:	Normal	0	0	0	0	0
	Mildly impaired	$\frac{1}{2}$	$\frac{1}{2}$	$\frac{1}{2}$	$\frac{1}{2}$	$\frac{1}{2}$
	Distorted	1	1	1	1	1
6. Mobility of involved arm:	No visible impairment	0	0	0	0	0
	Mildly impaired	$\frac{1}{2}$	$\frac{1}{2}$	$\frac{1}{2}$	$\frac{1}{2}$	$\frac{1}{2}$
	Marked limitation	1	1	1	1	1
7. Body language:	None	0	0	0	0	0
(clutching, rubbing site)	Occasional	$\frac{1}{2}$	$\frac{1}{2}$	$\frac{1}{2}$	$\frac{1}{2}$	$\frac{1}{2}$
	Frequent	1	1	1	1	1
8. Visible support:	None	0	0	0	0	0
(splint, pillow, furniture,	Occasional	$\frac{1}{2}$	$\frac{1}{2}$	$\frac{1}{2}$	$\frac{1}{2}$	$\frac{1}{2}$
other upper extremity)	Dependent; constant use	1	1	1	1	1
9. Body movement:	Sits or stands still	0	0	0	0	0
	Occasional shifts of position	$\frac{1}{2}$	$\frac{1}{2}$	$\frac{1}{2}$	$\frac{1}{2}$	$\frac{1}{2}$
	Constant movement, position shifts	1	1	1	1	1
10. Medication:	None	0	0	0	0	0
	As prescribed	$\frac{1}{2}$	$\frac{1}{2}$	$\frac{1}{2}$	$\frac{1}{2}$	$\frac{1}{2}$
	Increased frequency	1	1	1	1	1

Based on the UAB pain behaviour scale

Date of measurement	I	II	III	IV
Total				

Fig. 14.4 An adapted version of the University of Alabama pain scale records measures such as posturing, and verbal and non-verbal expressions of pain.

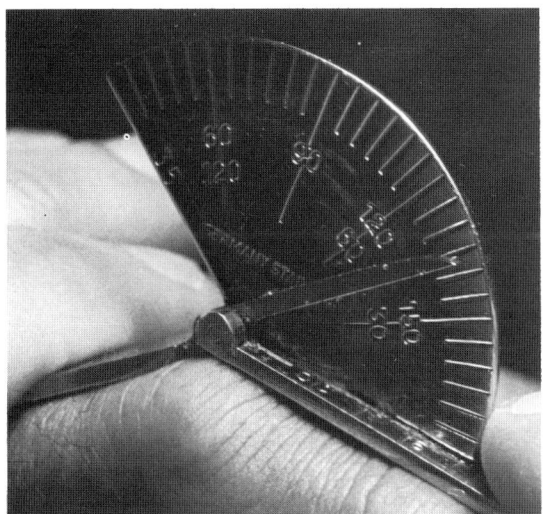

Fig. 14.5 Precise goniometric measurements of each individual joint can demonstrate even minute changes.

joints will not fully flex in this position (Fig. 14.6). However, if the MP joint is held in flexion, the interphalangeal joints can then be fully flexed passively.

To test for tight extrinsic extensors on the dorsum of the hand, the MP joints are held in flexion and then extension while attempting to flex passively the interphalangeal (IP) joints. If the test is positive, the IP joints will not flex with the MP joints held in flexion (Fig. 14.7). For tight extrinsic flexors, the interphalangeal joints will extend passively with the MP joint flexed, but not when the MP joint is then extended (Fig. 14.8).

Palpation/visual inspection

Palpation of the interphalangeal joint helps to identify instability and to localize points of tenderness (Redler 1967). Additional visual observation, such as unilateral swelling of the joint, can help to identify the specific problem such as a collateral ligament tear. Both factors will require immediate and careful attention in planning a course of treatment.

Grip/pinch measurements

Pulp, tip, key pinch and gross grasp as described by the American Society for Surgery of the Hand (1978) are taken on both extremities depending on the time since injury or surgery (Fig. 14.9). In acute cases, it is not appropriate to take the measurements until resistance can be applied to the injured or repaired structures. In a chronic case, pain often limits the patient's ability to apply his potential pressure on either the dynamometer or the pinch meter (Watson 1982).

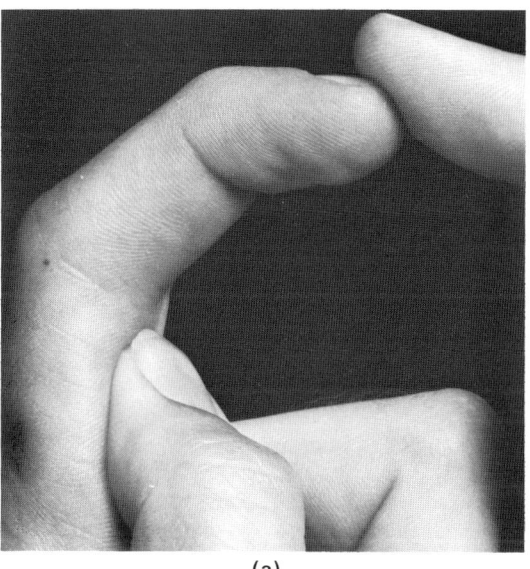

(a)

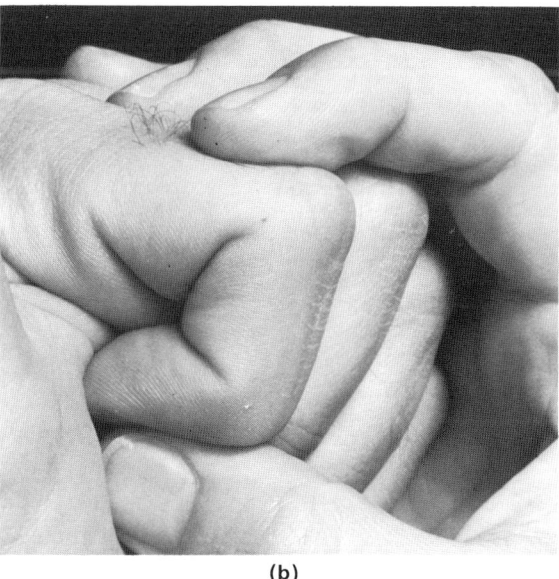

(b)

Fig. 14.6 (a) If the intrinsics are tight, the IP joints will not passively flex completely with the MP joint in extension. (b) But when the MP is flexed, the IPs can then be fully passively flexed.

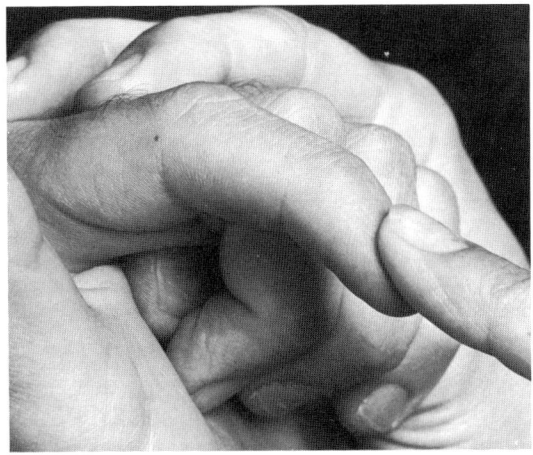

Fig. 14.7 In testing for tight extrinsic extensors on the dorsum of the hand, the test is positive if the IP joints will not flex with the MP joints held in flexion.

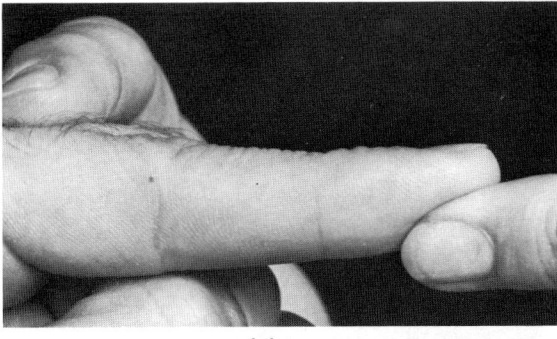

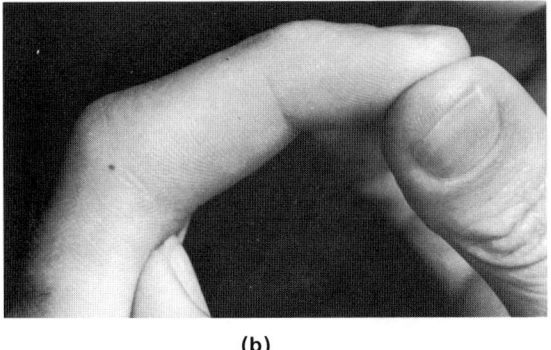

Fig. 14.8 With tight extrinsic flexors (**a**) the IP joints will passively extend with the MP joint flexed (**b**) but not when the MP joint is extended.

Sensibility

If sensibility is altered, testing includes vibration, moving and constant touch, cutaneous sensibility testing, moving two-point, static two-point discrimination and Tinel's sign. Compromise of digital nerve function may occur with massive oedema, but should subside as the condition lessens. Continued sensory changes may indicate actual damage to the nerve.

Functional testing

With IP joint problems, two of the most common functional complaints are pain on motion and the fact that the involved finger gets in the way when attempting to perform an activity (Sprague 1976).

The Jebson Hand Function Test (Fig. 14.10) helps to define areas of difficulty in performing home-care activities (McEntee 1984, Reynolds 1984). Combined with a self-care evaluation, difficulties in personal care, communication skills and object manipulation can be identified.

Other standardized tests such as the Crawford Bennett tool board, Pennsylvania bimanual test, Perdue pegboard, and the Minnesota rate of manipulation can record coordination and dexterity deficits (Fig. 14.11).

The upper extremity Valpar work samples, actual simulated tasks and the BTE work simulator can be utilized for assessment of job related skills (Fig. 14.12).

TREATMENT

Treatment concepts can be divided into the preventative or acute phase and the remedial or chronic phase (McCormack 1964). In both instances, control of oedema and pain, restoration of motion and patient education are the key components. Modalities, procedures and splinting are an integral part of each individualized programme, but will vary with the nature, timing and extent of the presenting condition.

Previous chapters have addressed the anatomy, repair and reconstruction of a wide variety of PIP disorders. Basic anatomical considerations, principles and objectives must also be understood by

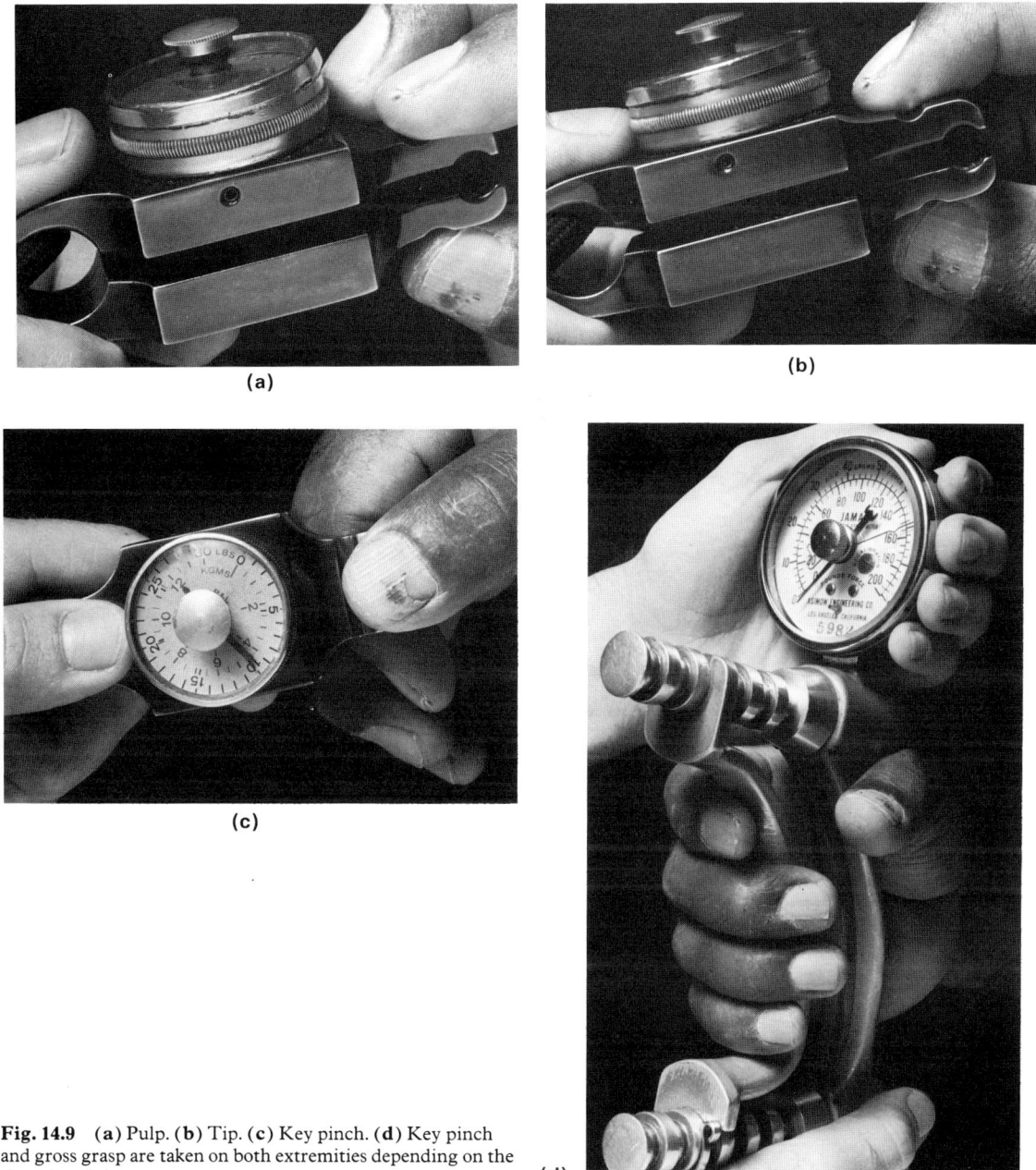

Fig. 14.9 (a) Pulp. (b) Tip. (c) Key pinch. (d) Key pinch and gross grasp are taken on both extremities depending on the time since injury or surgery.

the therapist involved in the patient's rehabilitation. Specific treatment guidelines for several of the more common acute and chronic conditions of the PIP joint follow. The emphasis is on precluding complications. A later discussion will deal with the remedial or chronic phase of rehabilitation.

SPECIFIC TREATMENT GUIDELINES

PIP collateral ligament injury

Collateral ligament injuries are common and may vary from a mild sprain to a complete rupture. They are frequently regarded as a trivial injury

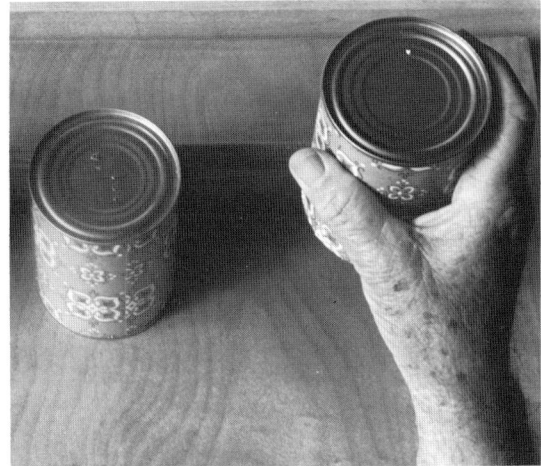

Fig. 14.10 The Jebson hand function test helps to define areas of difficulty in performing home care activities.

despite the fact that they can seriously restrict hand function and result in long-term or permanent disability of the injured finger (Redler 1967).

In treatment, the primary emphasis is on mobilizing the joint, preventing a flexion contracture and guarding against reinjury. Without an early appropriate therapeutic programme, complications often seen are fixed flexion contractures, insufficient active flexion, pain, weakness of pinch and grip, and chronic swelling (Redler 1967).

Stable ligament sprains are immobilized until the initial discomfort subsides which is about 3–10 d (Bowers 1983, Wilson & Carter 1984b). Partial to almost complete disruptions may require immobilization for up to 3 weeks (Bowers 1983, Wilson & Carter 1984b). Lateral dislocations are usually held for 3 weeks whether reduced with splinting or surgically repaired. An additional form of protective splinting continues for another 3–4 weeks (Bowers 1983, Wilson & Carter 1984b).

Specific treatment programme (Table 14.1)

Since oedema is one of the major contributors to immobility at the PIP joint, control must be immediate and continuous. Elevation and retrograde massage can be practised in both the clinic and at home by the patient (Fig. 14.13). Various forms of compression such as individual finger Coban wrapping, finger stalls, elasticized gloves or use of the Jobst intermittent compression unit (Curtis 1984) can be effective for persistent swelling (Fig. 14.14).

To prevent protective posturing of the joint, which produces stiffness, pain must be alleviated as soon as possible. Specific points of tenderness may benefit from a course of iontophoresis using a steroid compound as an alternative to a periarticular injection (Glass et al 1980, Case 1984). Iontophoresis administers a water soluble anti-inflammatory medication through an ion exchange at the medication site (Langley 1984) (Fig. 14.15). A recent study by Glass et al (1980) found that iontophoresis using dexamethasone was able to penetrate the tissues to a depth of 1.7 cm.

Decadron 4% in a 1:2 ratio with xylocaine is commonly used in the upper extremity. A recom-

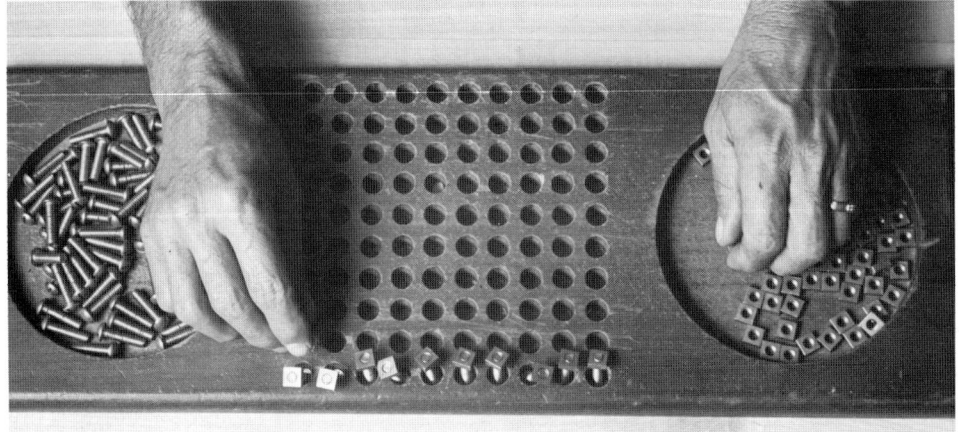

Fig. 14.11 Standardized tests such as the Pennsylvania bimanual test can record coordination and dexterity deficits.

THERAPEUTIC MANAGEMENT OF THE PROXIMAL INTERPHALANGEAL JOINT

Table 14.1 Treatment programme for PIP collateral ligament injury

Diagnosis	Primary objectives	Timing factor to begin motion	Resistance
PIP collateral ligament injury	1. Functional, pain-free motion 2. Prevent flexion contracture 3. Protect against re-injury	1. Stable sprains 3–10 d 2. Partial to complete tears 3 weeks 3. Lateral dislocation 3 weeks 4. No grip or pinch measurements until resistance is allowed	1. Stable sprain 4.5–6 weeks 2. Partial tear/dislocation 6–8 weeks

Specific treatment procedures	Complications	Splinting
1. Patient education; to prevent re-injury, emphasize long healing time, necessity for adherence to directed exercise programme 2. Passive stretching of joint, intrinsics and ORL 3. *No forceful, painful manipulation* 4. Directed exercise: *active*, isolated motions of intrinsics, long flexors and extensors 5. Pain control: ice/heat, TENS and iontophoresis 6. Joint mobilization when appropriate 7. Oedema control 8. Exacting, frequent reassessment of oedema and range of movement	1. Fixed flexion contracture 2. Pain 3. Weakness 4. Chronic oedema 5. Incomplete motion 6. Finger 'in the way' for function 7. Decreased range of movement of adjacent digits	1. Buddy taping for protection 2. Night extension splinting 3. When stable: alternate dynamic flexion and extension as necessary

mended course of treatment is three applications spread over an 8–10 d period. Each treatment session is 20 min in duration. Treatment is discontinued if relief is not achieved after the trial period.

Transcutaneous electrical nerve stimulation (TENS) can be used both in the clinic and at home to help relieve pain with movement (Mullins-Taylor & Cannon 1984, Reynolds 1984). To avoid limiting motion, one electrode can be placed around the proximal phalanx such that it does not encroach on the joint crease. The second electrode can be placed more proximally in the hand or at the wrist (Fig. 14.16). The patient is encouraged to use the TENS during exercise and activity.

Ice massage or moist heat in elevation can be used for comfort and reduction of oedema and pain depending on its effect on the individual patient (Fig. 14.17). High voltage electrical stimulation can also help to reduce swelling and produce a local

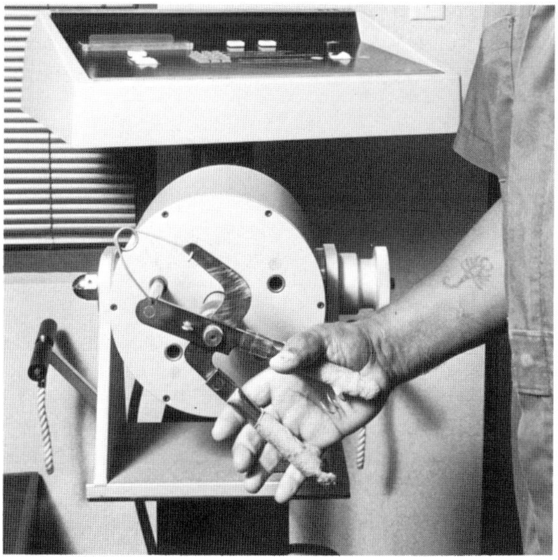

Fig. 14.12 The BTE work simulator is utilized for assessment of job related skills.

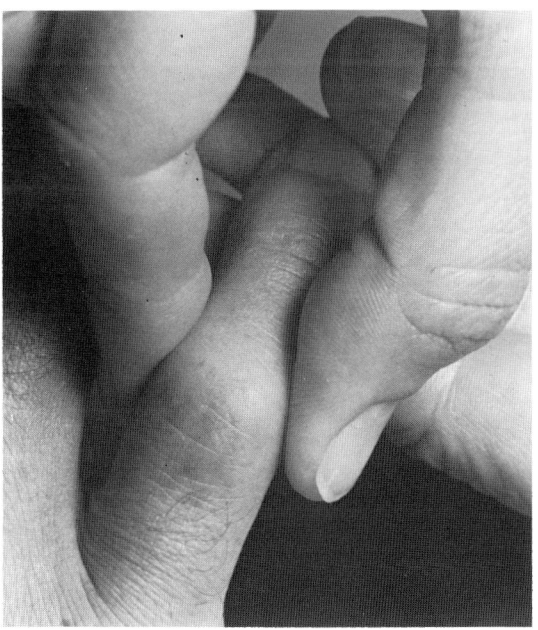

Fig. 14.13 Retrograde massage done in elevation, can be practised both in the clinic and at home to reduce oedema.

220 THE INTERPHALANGEAL JOINTS

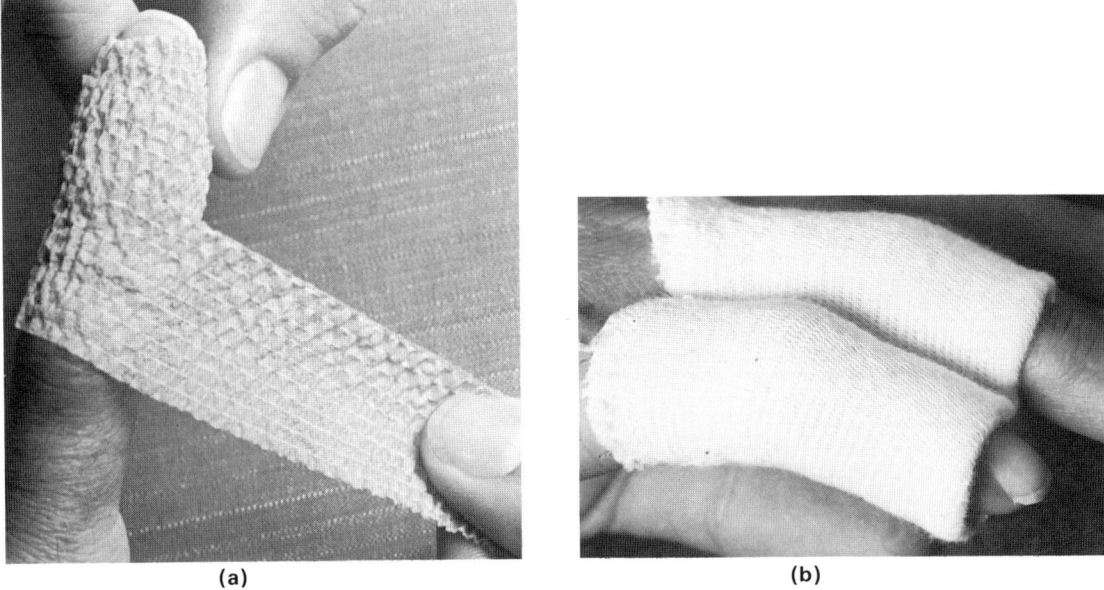

Fig. 14.14 (a) Individual finger Coban wrapping or (b) elastic finger stalls are effective means of applying compression for persistent swelling.

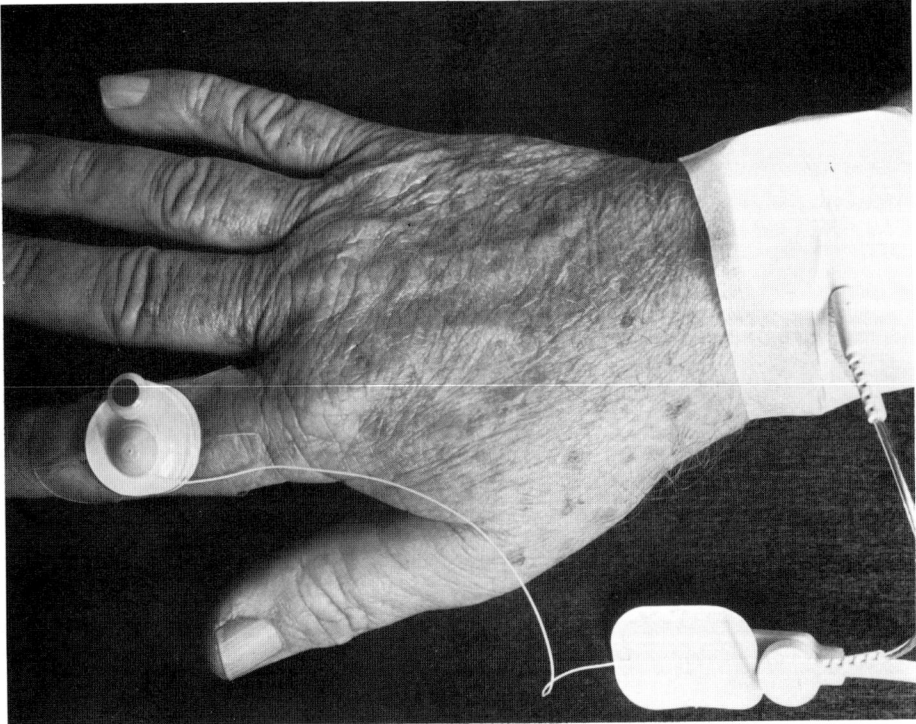

Fig. 14.15 Iontophoresis administers a water soluble anti-inflammatory medication through an ion exchange at the medication site.

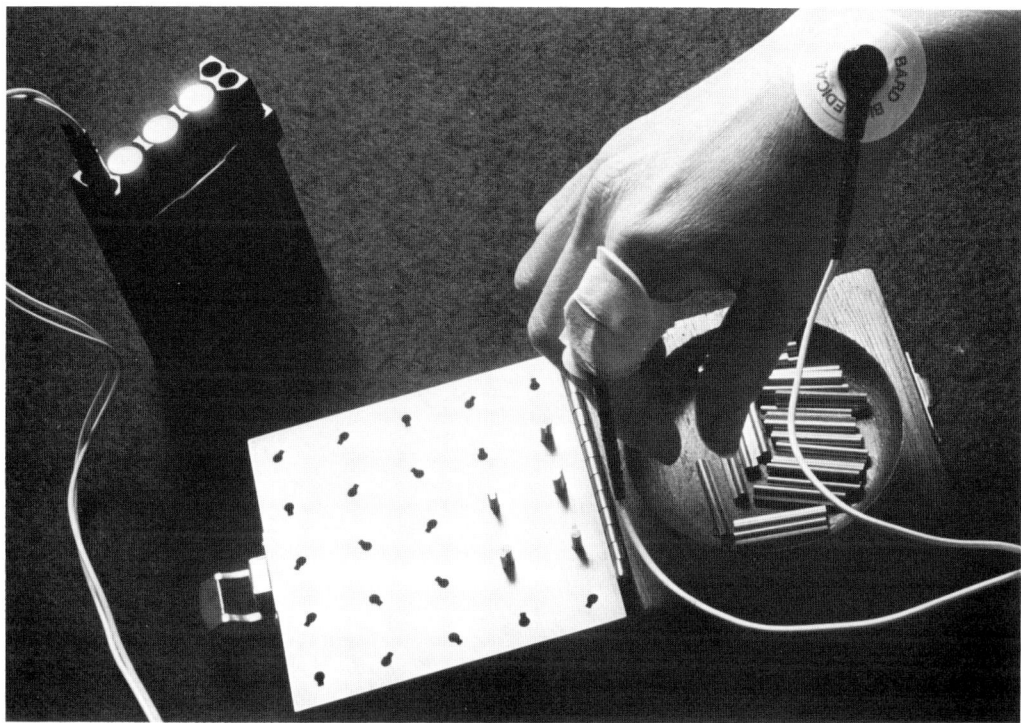

Fig. 14.16 Placement of TENS electrodes should not encroach on the joint crease, limiting motion.

analgesia (Mullins-Taylor & Cannon 1984, Reynolds 1984) (Fig. 14.18).

The primary emphasis in exercise, activity and splinting is the *avoidance of lateral stress at the PIP level*. The possibility of reinjury and the slow time for ligamentous healing have to be stressed to the

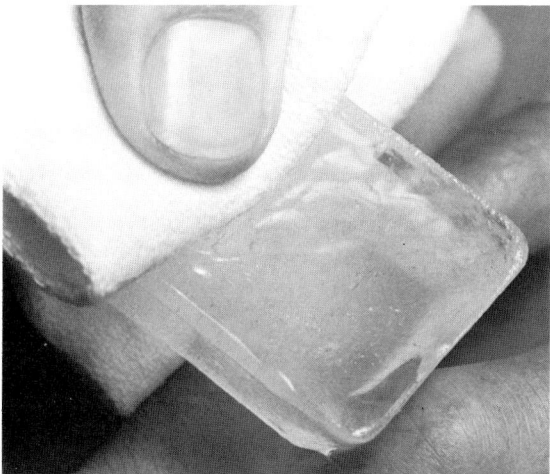

Fig. 14.17 Ice massage can help to reduce oedema and pain in a localized area.

patient from the beginning and reinforced frequently (Bowers 1983, Wilson & Carter 1984) (Fig. 14.19). Because ligament injuries are often passed off as insignificant, the patient has to be counselled as to the potential seriousness of the injury. For the best result, he must understand that protection, oedema control and a specific exercise regimen will be necessary for months and sometimes for up to a year before complete healing occurs.

Since a ligament injury can produce adhesions to the adjacent lateral bands or to the oblique retinacular ligament (ORL), exercises to prevent either condition should begin early (Hamilton 1966). The intrinsic muscles are stretched by holding the MP joint in extension, while passively flexing the interphalangeal joints. The oblique retinacular ligament is put on a maximum stretch by maintaining the PIP joint in full extension and having the patient actively flex the distal interphalangeal joint (Fig. 14.20). If active flexion is not possible, then the distal interphalangeal joint should be gently taken passively into flexion. Great care must be taken to perform all passive range of

222 THE INTERPHALANGEAL JOINTS

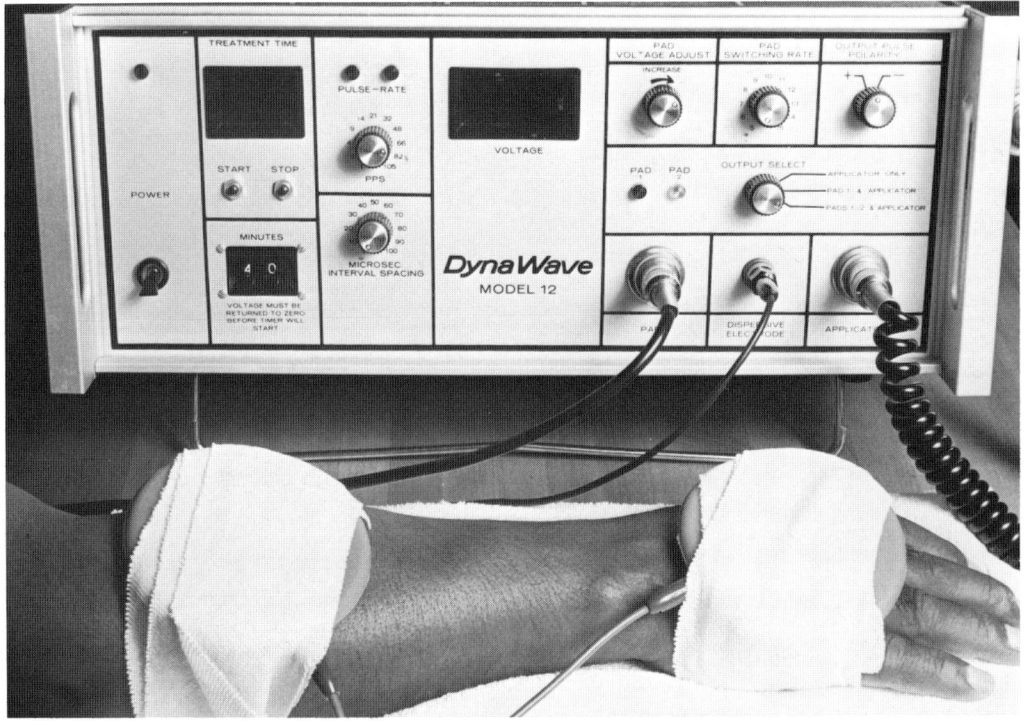

Fig. 14.18 High voltage electrical stimulation can produce a local analgesia in areas of pain.

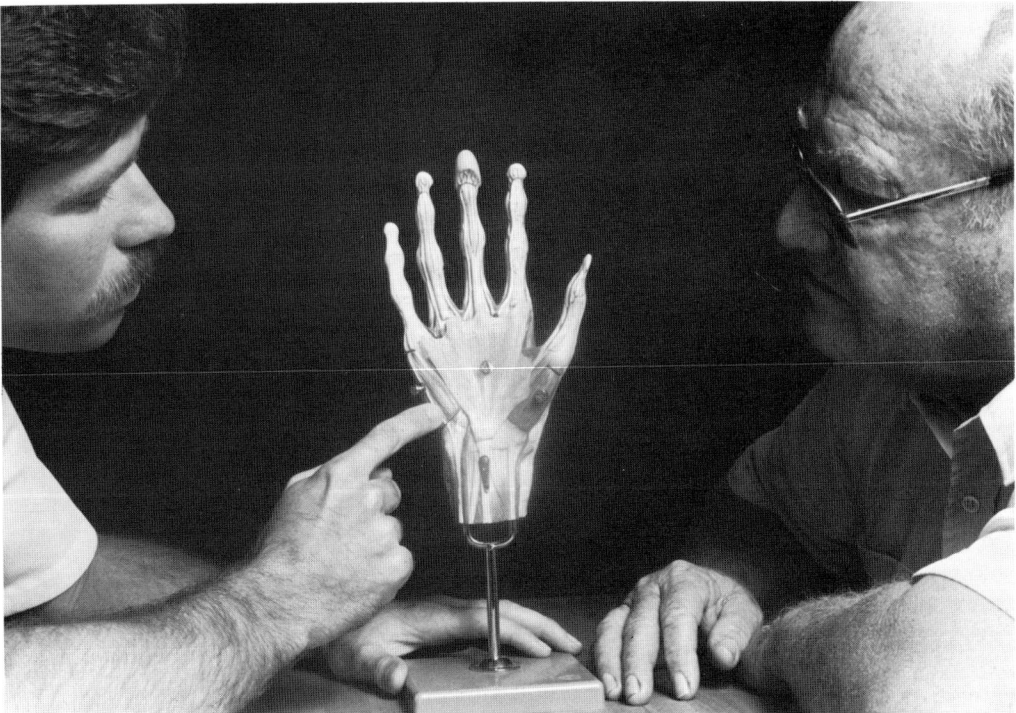

Fig. 14.19 Patient education needs to be stressed to the patient from the beginning of treatment and reinforced frequently.

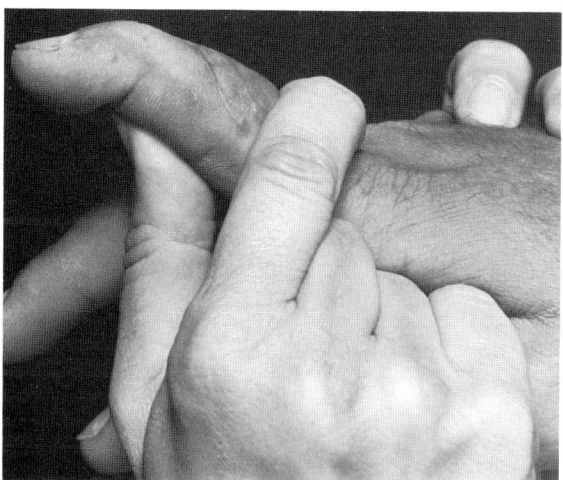

Fig. 14.20 The oblique retinacular ligament is put on a maximum stretch by maintaining the PIP joint in full extension and the patient actively flexing the DIP joint.

motion slowly and not beyond the point of pain. There must be *no forceful passive range of motion* (Arem 1981, Tubiana 1985). When appropriate, joint mobilization may be initiated (see Ch. 16).

In addition to passive stretching, a directed exercise programme needs to include active isolated abduction and adduction of the digits for gliding of the intrinsics; blocking of the IP joints for active isolated motion of the flexor digitorum profundus and flexor digitorum sublimis; isolated active motion of the long extrinsic extensors and the intrinsic extensors crossing the joint; and lastly, full active motion of all other joints of the hand to prevent stiffness in the adjacent digits (Fig. 14.21). To prevent oedema, exercise periods should be brief (3–5 min) but repeated frequently throughout the day.

A stable ligament sprain should not begin resistance for at least 4.5–6 weeks, while a partial tear or dislocation should wait 6–8 weeks. Since grip and pinch strength are usually weakened by a ligament injury (Watson 1982), a progressive resistive programme can be initiated beginning with resistance directed at non-involved areas of the extremities such as wrist flexion and extension. The affected joint is not allowed to bear weight during the exercise period. For example, in performing wrist extension exercises, the arm is pronated, and the hand held weight does not exert pressure against the joint (Fig. 14.22). Gradually,

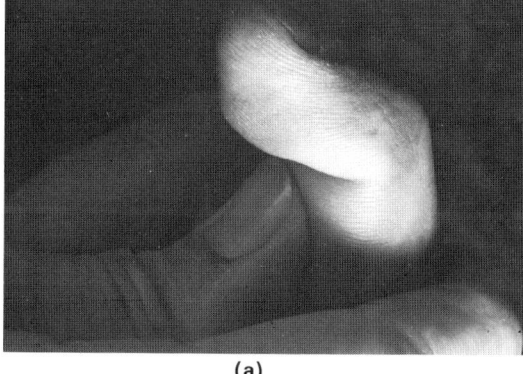

(a)

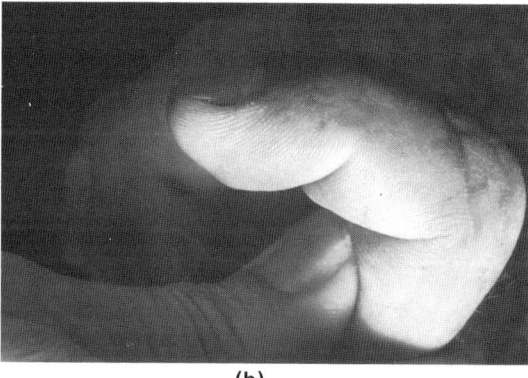

(b)

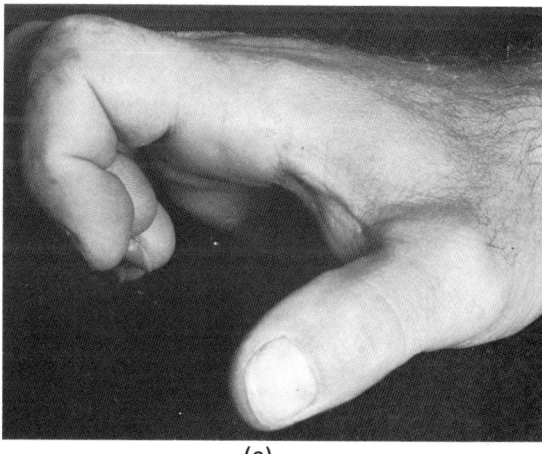

(c)

Fig. 14.21 A directed exercise programme needs to include (**a**) blocked active motion of the FDP and (**b**) the FDS and (**c**) a clawing motion to isolate the long extrinsic extensors.

as resistance is allowed at the injured joint, specific attention can be given slowly to building strength and endurance. Theraputty and hand helper exercises can be issued for home use. Pinch and grip measurements are considered resistive and should *not* be taken until the joint is again stable.

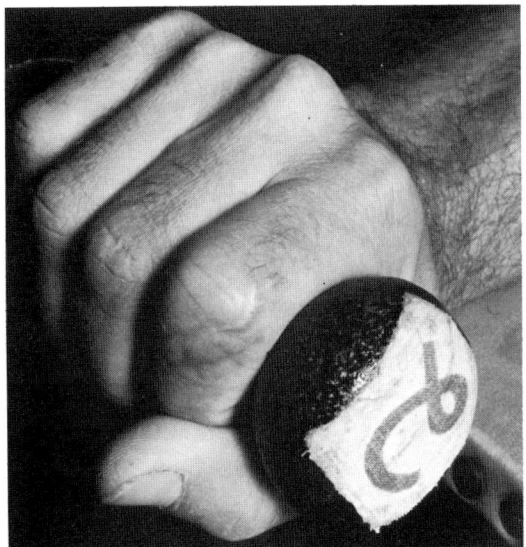

Fig. 14.22 Resistance at the wrist is performed with the arm in pronation to prevent stress against the small finger joints.

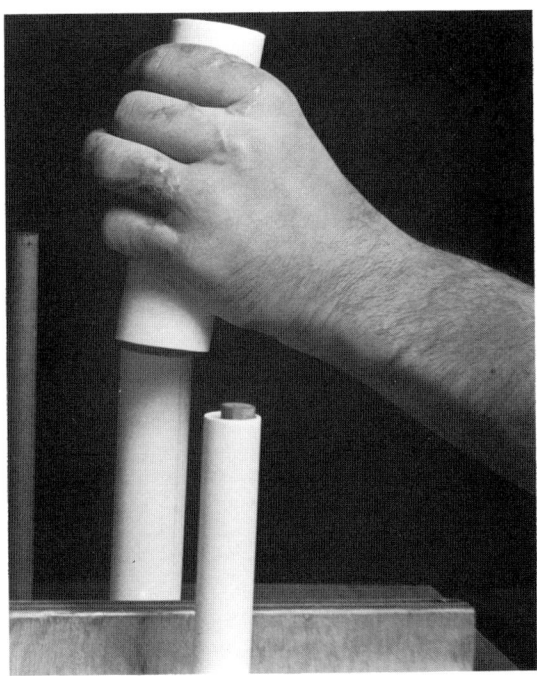

Fig. 14.23 Early activities should be light, avoid lateral stress and be designed to encourage active normal hand motion, increase endurance and re-establish coordination and dexterity.

Forceful manipulative activities must be avoided after ligament injuries. A good result is best achieved through gentle active motion. Early activities should be light, avoid lateral stress and be designed to encourage active, normal hand motion, increase endurance and re-establish coordination and dexterity. Activities such as the Minnesota rate of manipulation or the Crawford test worked by hand rather than with tools would meet these criteria (Fig. 14.23).

The goals of splinting are to provide protection, prevent flexion or extension contractures and restore active motion. After the initial period of immobilization, ligament injuries are protected by buddy taping the injured finger to the adjacent digit with tape or Velcro loops (Bowers 1983, Wilson & Carter 1984b) (Fig. 14.24). A special step-off design can be fabricated for the ring and little fingers because of their disparity in length (Fig. 14.25). If a flexion contracture is impending, the taping can be alternated with dynamic extension splinting after stability has been determined.

At night, serial extension splinting with circumferential plaster casting (Bell 1984) or spring metal will rest the finger in the desired position (Fig. 14.26). Often, despite the tendency for a flexion contracture to develop, full active flexion is also limited. In such cases, one must carefully alternate

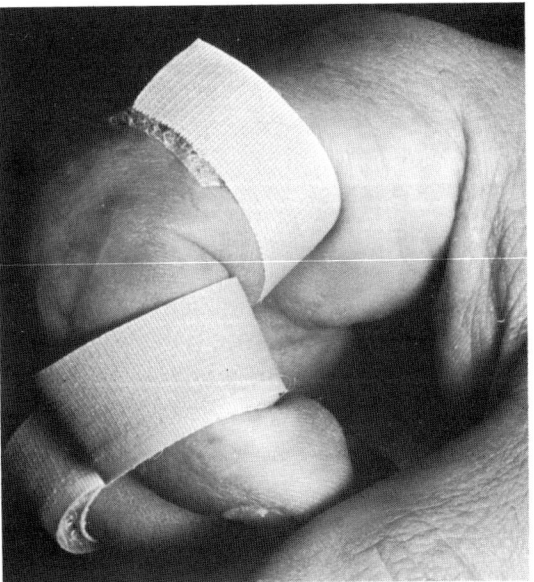

Fig. 14.24 After the initial immobilization, ligament injuries are protected by buddy taping the injured finger to the adjacent digit with tape or Velcro loops.

THERAPEUTIC MANAGEMENT OF THE PROXIMAL INTERPHALANGEAL JOINT

flexion and extension splinting to achieve full active motion (Fig. 14.27). Range of motion and circumferential measurements must be taken frequently to monitor closely gain or loss of even small numbers of degrees, or swelling. Splinting and exercises are adjusted to accommodate the changes.

Dorsal dislocation, unstable, no fracture, treated in dorsal splint

Dorsal displacement of the PIP joint is the most common dislocation. One treatment approach is to apply a dorsal extension block splint which prevents dislocation, but allows motion into flexion (Fig. 14.28).

Therapy for a dorsal dislocation that is treated in a dorsal block splint is viewed in two stages. The first stage is with the splint in place and the second is upon removal of the splint. Inappropriate treatment can result in flexion contractures of the PIP joint, incomplete active flexion, pain and recurrence of dislocation.

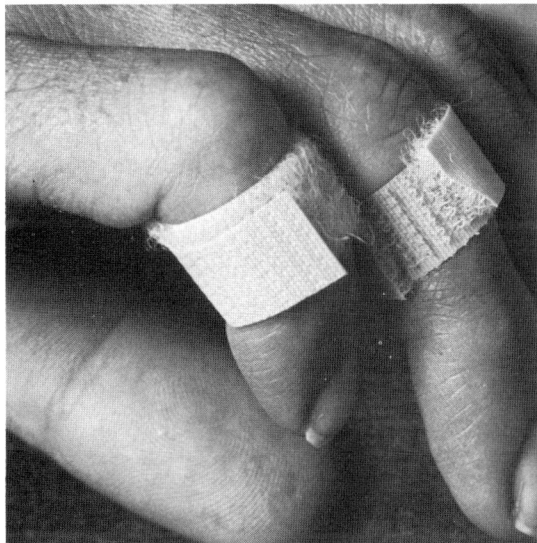

Fig. 14.25 A special step-off design of buddy loops can be fabricated for the ring and little fingers to take into account their disparity in length.

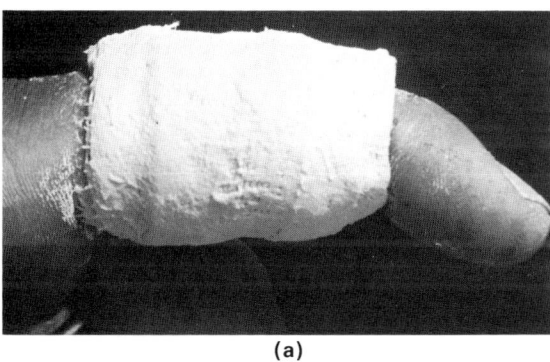
(a)

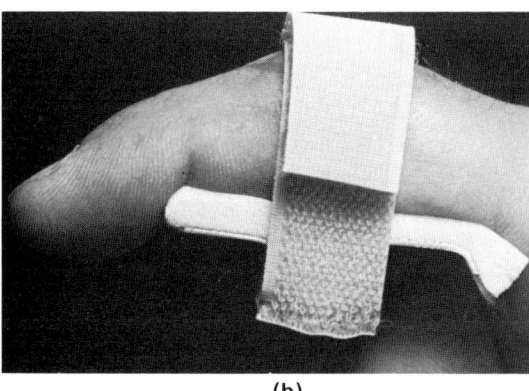
(b)

Fig. 14.26 Night splinting can include (a) serial extension splinting with circumferential plaster casting or (b) I-beam metal splint to rest the finger in the desired position of extension.

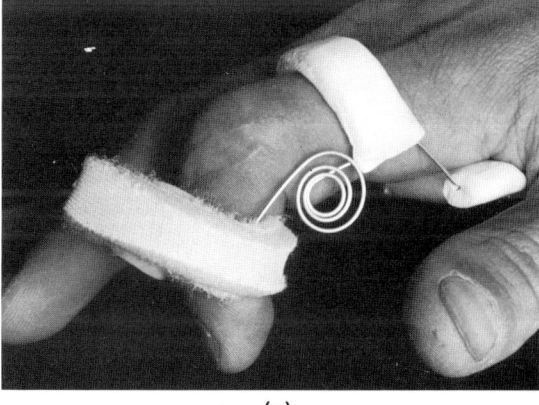
(a)

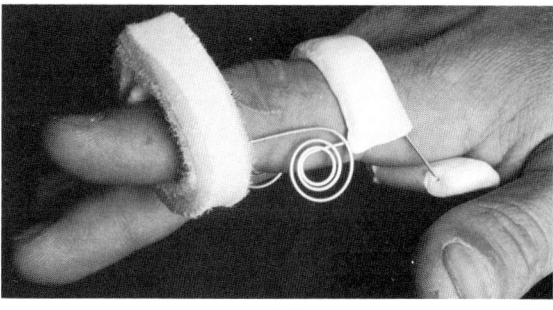
(b)

Fig. 14.27 The Capener splint allows (a) flexion and (b) extension while providing lateral protection.

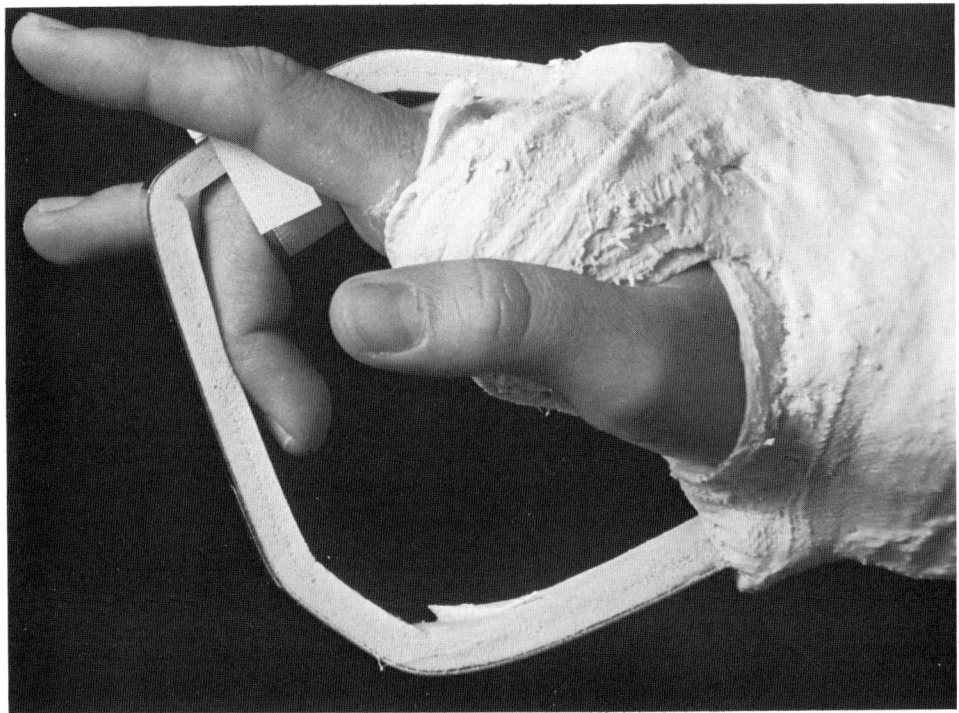

Fig. 14.28 The dorsal block splint limits extension but allows motion into flexion.

Phase one: in the splint

In the first stage, the goals are to achieve full active and passive flexion of the digits, to maintain active extension to the limit of the block, to prevent a flexion contracture and to maintain normal active and passive range of motion of the adjacent fingers.

If the PIP joint is unstable without a fracture, it is treated with a dorsal block splint for 3–5 weeks with active and passive flexion allowed within the limits of the splint (McElfresh et al 1972, Eaton & Dray 1982, Wilson & Carter 1984a).

Specific treatment guidelines. (Table 14.2) Initially while in the dorsal block splint, an exercise programme will include full active and passive flexion of the digit. With the finger stabilized against the dorsal block, blocking exercises are performed to isolate the flexor digitorum profundus (FDP) and flexor digitorum sublimis (FDS) (Fig. 14.29). Extension exercises are limited to the extent of the block. This is usually at 25° short of the point of demonstrated instability. The block is diminished 5–10° a week and is discontinued at approximately 15° short of full extension (McElfresh et al 1972, Eaton & Dray 1982). During the time period in the splint, there are several priorities.

The first is to be aware and guard against the patient's tendency to flex his digit away from the block and then fully extend his PIP joint in an intrinsic positive posture (Fig. 14.30).

The next priority is to help control oedema. This can be initiated through a retrograde massage. The therapist should stabilize the affected digit against the dorsal block and apply the massage to all digits to help increase circulation and decrease oedema in the entire hand (Fig. 14.31). Adjacent fingers can also be individually wrapped with compressive dressings if they demonstrate abnormal swelling.

To avoid frustration, the patient needs to understand the length of time required to achieve stability of the joint, the necessity for protecting the digit from reinjury when the splint is removed, and the fact that the active range of motion achieved within the splint can appear to be more complete than it really is when the splint is removed.

Each time the patient is seen in the clinic, the tape holding his digit to the dorsal splint should be

Table 14.2 Treatment programme for dorsal dislocation, unstable, no fracture

Diagnosis	Primary objectives	Timing factor to begin motion	Resistance
Dorsal dislocation unstable, no fracture	1. Achieve full active motion 2. Prevent flexion contracture 3. Prevent recurrence of dislocation	Dorsal block splint 3–4 weeks	7–8 weeks

Specific treatment procedures	Complications	Splinting

A. Phase I: in dorsal block splint
  1. Full active and passive flexion. Block for FDP and FDS
  2. Active extension to limits of block
  3. Oedema control through retrograde massage and compressive wrapping
  4. Patient education to prevent recurrence
  5. Skin care under tape
  6. Maintain full motion in all other digits
B. Phase II: after splint removal
  1. Active, assistive flexion
  2. Active extension
  3. Blocking for FDP, FDS, long extensors, stretch intrinsics
  4. Ice massage, heat, iontophoresis or TENS for pain and oedema
	1. Flexion contracture PIP
	2. Incomplete flexion or extension
	3. Pain
	4. Recurrence of dislocation
		A. Phase I:
		  1. Extension block splint (75°, brought out weekly about 15° to 10–15° of flexion upon removal)
		B. Phase II:
		  1. Figure-of-eight splint limiting extension by 10–15°, but allowing full flexion
		  2. Dynamic extension splinting at about 2–3 weeks following removal of dorsal block splint.

removed and the skin checked for maceration and fresh tape applied. All non-involved digits including the thumb should be placed through active and passive range of motion. The intrinsic tendons should be passively stretched and the thumb web space closely watched for contracture.

Phase two: splint removal

After the dorsal block splint is removed, the goals are to achieve full flexion, slowly regain full PIP extension, alleviate any flexion contracture, protect the joint from reinjury and mobilize the entire hand.

Emphasis is placed on gentle mobilization of the joint to regain extension. Active assistive exercise will be required to achieve full flexion. Intrinsic stretching will be necessary for all digits, especially the involved finger and its two adjoining digits.

No restriction is placed on full active flexion and extension exercises. Blocking of each joint for isolated motions of the individual long flexors and extensors will assist in tendon gliding.

Ice massage, heat in elevation and TENS could be beneficial if the patient is experiencing pain or oedema.

Following removal of the dorsal block splint, the patient is fitted with a figure-of-eight (swan-neck) splint to prevent hyperextension injury to the joint (Fig. 14.32). The splint blocks the last 10–15° of PIP extension while allowing full flexion, and is worn at all times except when exercising. Dynamic extension splinting is not usually instituted until an additional 2–3 weeks after removal of the splint.

Dorsal dislocation with comminuted fracture treated by volar plate advancement

In an unstable, displaced fracture where multiple, small fragments are present, these are excised and the volar plate is advanced into the defect with a pull-out wire. The volar plate advancement prevents redislocation.

The goals of treatment are to prevent contracture, restore motion and prevent attenuation of the volar plate. The digit is immobilized for 2–3 weeks.

Specific treatment guidelines (Table 14.3)

Active and active assistive flexion exercises can begin after immobilization with the digit protected in a dorsal extension block splint. Dynamic flexion splinting can start at 3–5 weeks, but dynamic extension splinting is not initiated until after 5–7 weeks (Eaton & Dray 1982, Wilson & Carter 1984b). If the physician believes a mild flexion contracture will prevent redislocation, a figure-of-

228   THE INTERPHALANGEAL JOINTS

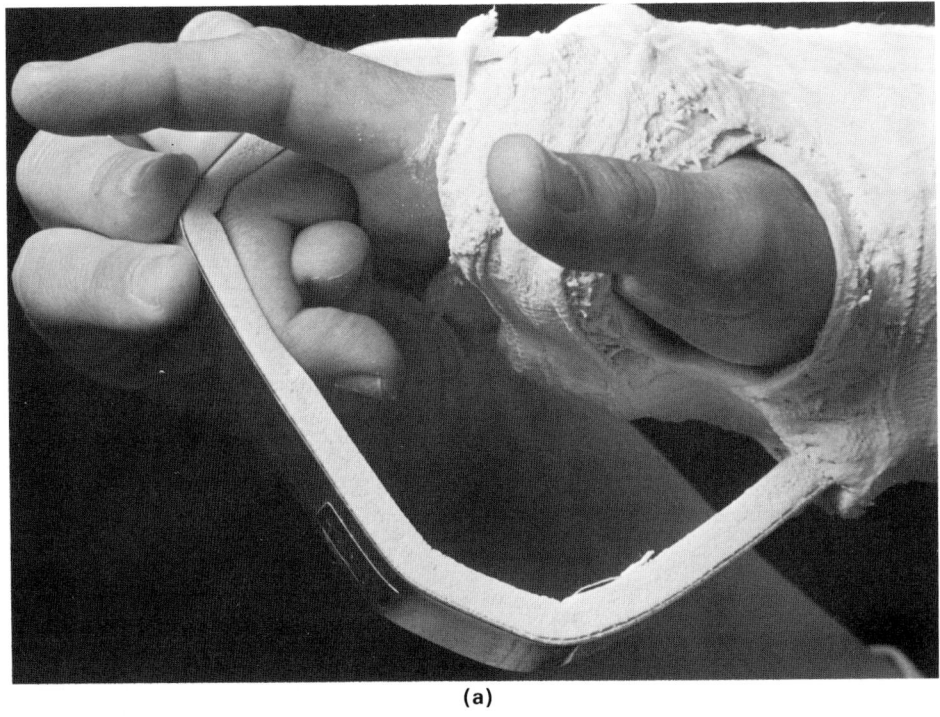

(a)

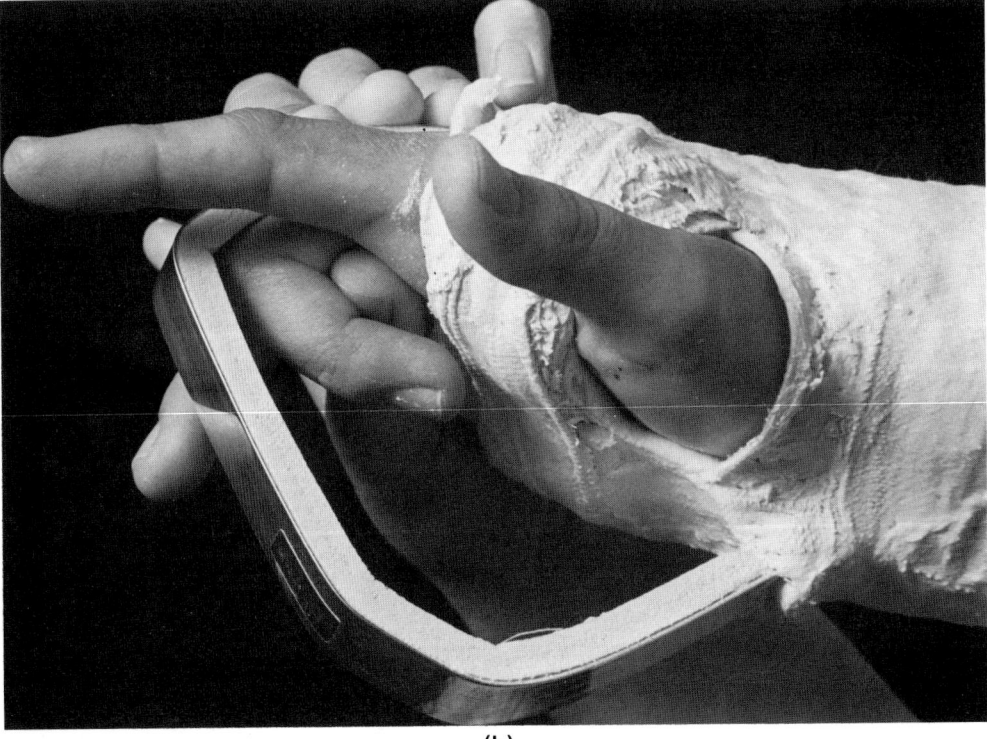

(b)

Fig. 14.29 With the digit stabilized against the dorsal block, blocking exercises are performed to isolate (**a**) the FDP and (**b**) the FDS.

THERAPEUTIC MANAGEMENT OF THE PROXIMAL INTERPHALANGEAL JOINT

Table 14.3 Treatment programme for dorsal dislocation with comminuted fracture

Diagnosis	Primary objectives	Timing factor to begin motion	Resistance
Dorsal dislocation with comminuted fracture and volar plate advancement	1. Prevent flexion contracture of PIP 2. Restore motion 3. Prevent attenuation of volar plate	Immobilized 2–3 weeks	7–8 weeks

Specific treatment procedures	Complications	Splinting
1. Active, active assistive flexion after immobilization 2. Gradual extension (may want to maintain small flexion contracture of 10–15° 3. Patient education not to stretch out volar plate advancement	1. Fixed flexion contracture of PIP 2. Attenuation of volar plate	1. Dorsal block splint or figure-of-eight in 10–15° of PIP flexion for protection after immobilization 2. Dynamic flexion 5 weeks 3. Dynamic extension 6–7 weeks If slight flexion contracture is desired figure-of eight in 10–15° of flexion

eight splint can be worn until the desired position is achieved (usually 10–15°). The patient must be educated to the possibility of attenuating the volar plate advancement through forceful extension of the digit in exercise or activity.

Proximal phalanx fracture

Fractures of the proximal and middle phalanx are more difficult to treat than metacarpal or distal phalanx fractures because of the frequent association of tendon and skin injuries, as well as instability due to the lack of soft tissue support. The complex anatomy of the PIP joint is most often affected by the fracture due to its proximity to the injury.

The primary emphasis in treatment of proximal phalanx fractures is preserving motion at the PIP joint while preventing a flexion contracture.

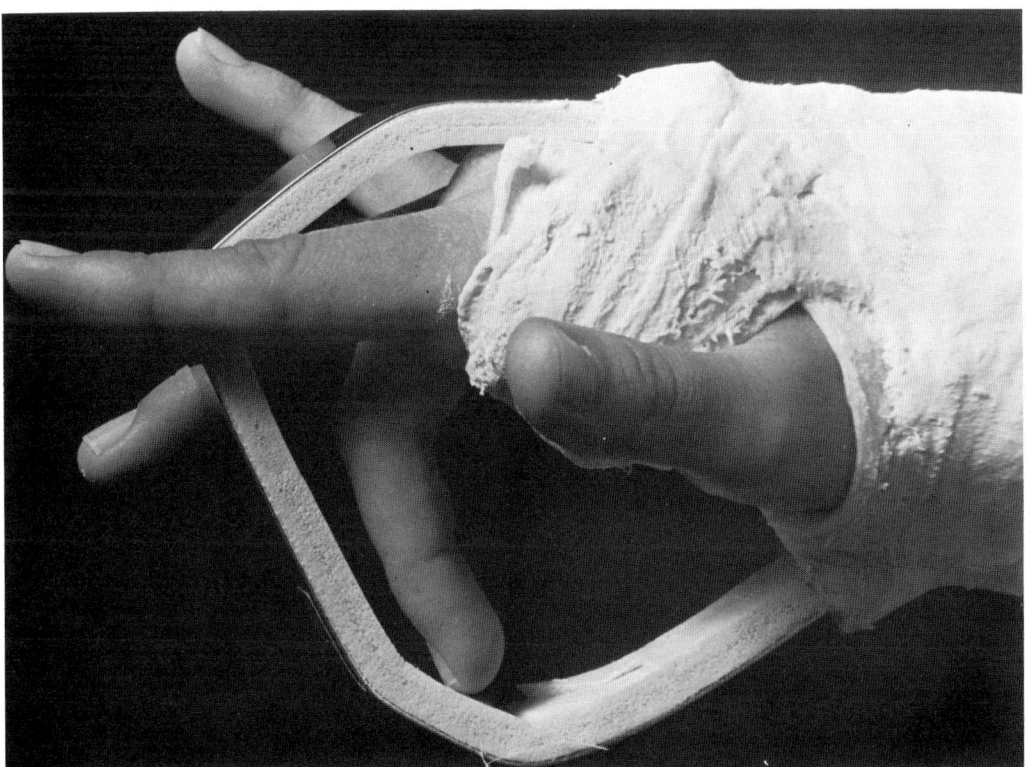

Fig. 14.30 The therapist must guard against the patient's tendency to drop his digit away from the block and extending his PIP joint in an intrinsic positive posture.

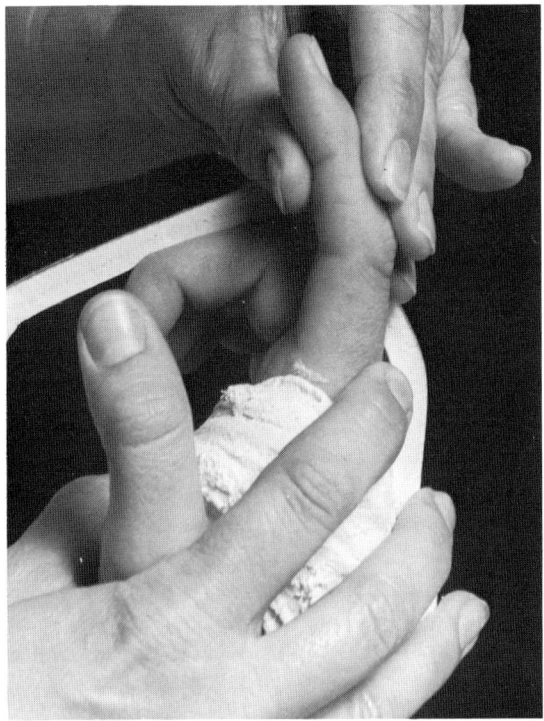

Fig. 14.31 Retrograde massage can be performed to the affected digit while in the splint if it is stabilized against the block. All other unaffected digits should be included in the massage.

Most stable, closed non-displaced fractures can begin motion within the first 21 days. Fractures of the midshaft region of the proximal phalanx require protective splinting for 5–7 weeks. Protected motion can be initiated at 3 weeks (Wilson & Carter 1984b).

Specific treatment guidelines (Table 14.4)

Patients are started on an immediate programme of elevation both day and night that continues until oedema subsides. If the swelling is diffuse throughout the hand, volumetric readings, in addition to circumferential measurements, will prove useful in gauging fluid changes (Fig. 14.33). If pins are present and extend externally, the volumeter should not be used. Coban wrapping and elastic gloves can be employed along with the elevation programme. The Jobst intermittent pressure unit can be used with stable fractures, but is contraindicated with any question in the stability of reduction (Fig. 14.34).

If pins are protruding, the patient is instructed in a daily pin care programme which includes cleaning around the pins with an application stick soaked in alcohol. The patient is warned not to get the pin area wet and is instructed to be alert for any signs of infection.

During passive exercise in the acute phase of treatment, the therapist must firmly support the fracture site while gently applying a passive stretch at the PIP joint and to the intrinsics (Fig. 14.35). Joint mobilization can be instituted when resistance is allowed (see Ch. 16).

During active exercise, manual support is again applied to the fracture site for performance of blocking exercises to isolate the FDP and FDS. Care must be taken to prevent an extensor lag at the PIP joint through attenuation of the extensor mechanism or intrinsic tendon adherence.

Early, light activities should stress reincorporation of the involved digit in normal prehension patterns. When the fracture has consolidated, dynamic splinting and resistive exercise can begin.

If a fracture is longitudinal and stable, early protected motion can usually begin at 3–5 d. The involved digit can be buddy taped to the adjacent finger for active protected motion (Wilson & Carter 1984b). If the patient is involved in heavy activity, a metal or plastic splint can be used for protection.

In more complex proximal phalanx fractures, the primary emphasis of splinting is on protection and prevention of flexion contractures of the PIP joint. This can best be achieved with functional positional splinting (Arem 1981) in an intrinsic positive position (with the wrist in 30–60° of extension, the MPs at 60–70° of flexion and the IPs as close to neutral as possible (Kuczynski 1968, Arem 1981, Wilson & Carter 1984b) (Fig. 14.36). Because of oedema and pain, it may take several days of serial splinting to reach the desired position (Tubiana 1985). The splint is worn for the first 5 weeks during the day between exercise periods and at night. If only one digit is involved, the digit can be splinted with the adjacent finger leaving the others free (Fig. 14.37). For maximum protection and maintenance of correct position, a volar/dorsal splint is most effective. After the fracture is considered solid, dynamic extension and flexion splinting can be alternated to restore full PIP joint motion.

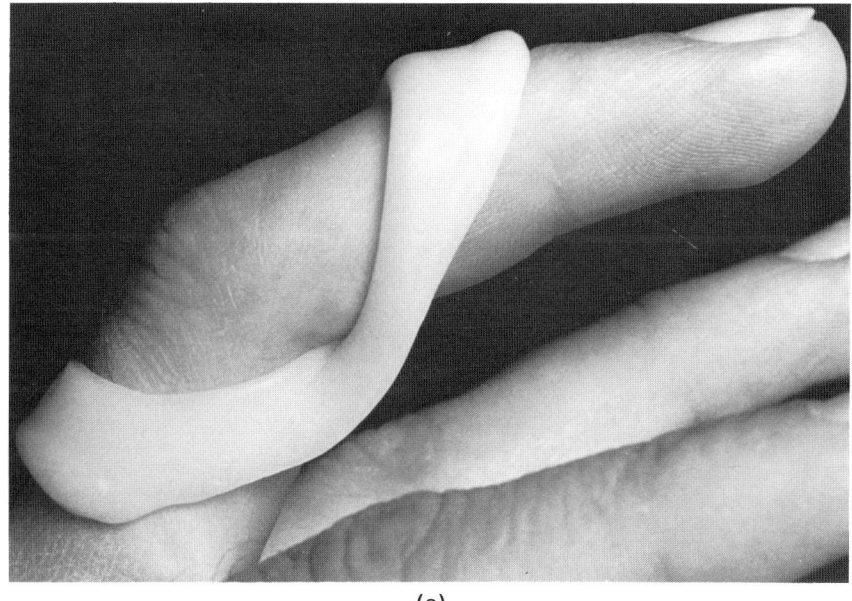

Fig. 14.32 Following removal of the dorsal block splint, the patient is fitted with a figure-of-eight splint that (**a**) prevents hyperextension of the joint (**b**) while allowing flexion.

Intra-articular fractures of the PIP joint (see Table 14.4)

The treatment programme for intra-articular fractures must concentrate on maintaining the gliding of the joint surfaces. The general programme is similar to that for a proximal phalanx fracture, but might include the use of a continuous passive motion device or the splinting procedure of Agee (Ågee 1978, Salter & Harris 1979).

Important considerations for use of continuous passive motion (CPM) would be a stable reduction of the fracture, careful placement of finger tape to prevent rotation (Kuczynski 1975) or painful extremes of motion. If the patient appears to be a good candidate for CPM, the device is fitted for a

232 THE INTERPHALANGEAL JOINTS

Table 14.4 Treatment programme for proximal phalanx fracture and PIP articular fracture

Diagnosis	Primary objectives	Timing factor to begin motion	Resistance
Proximal phalanx fracture	1. Prevention flexion contracture PIP 2. Achieve full motion 3. Prevent stiffness in adjacent digits 4. Promote tendon gliding over fracture site	1. Stable, closed, non-displaced—begin motion at 21 days 2. Midshaft fracture—protected motion at 3 weeks 3. Longitudinal, stable—3–5 days when pain subsides	When fracture has consolidated

Specific treatment procedures	Complications	Splinting
Initial: 1. Continuous elevation until oedema subsides, compressive wraps 2. Patient education in pin care 3. Stabilized, gentle passive stretch of joints and intrinsics 4. Active flexion and extension 5. Light prehension activities 6. Wrist exercises 7. Blocking active exercise for FDP, FDS, extensors and intrinsics Late: 1. Joint mobilization 2. Iontophoresis 3. CPM	1. Intrinsic contracture 2. Flexion contracture of PIP 3. Stiff hand 4. Tendon adherence at fracture site 5. Extension lag	1. Stable, longitudinal—buddy taped for protected active motion and protective metal or plaster splint when driving or doing heavy activity 2. Midshaft—protective functional position splint (wrist in 30–60° of extension, MPs in 60–70° of flexion and interphalangeal joints in neutral 5–7 weeks) 3. Complex fracture—functional position for 5 weeks except when exercising

Diagnosis	Specific treatment procedures
PIP articular fracture (same as proximal phalanx fracture)	CPM *or* Agee splinting technique may be applicable

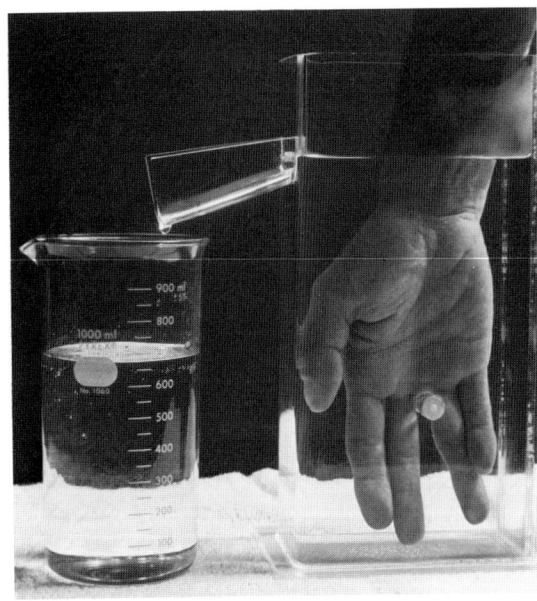

Fig. 14.33 The volumeter can accurately assess diffuse swelling in the hand.

1–2 h per day trial session under direct supervision in therapy for at least a week prior to renting a home unit (Fig. 14.38). Careful measurements of pain, oedema, and range of motion are recorded. Ideally, if a home unit is provided, the patient can eventually tolerate 6–8 h per day of use. When CPM is introduced into a patient's programme, it is essential to continue all other aspects of a fracture programme as well. CPM should only be considered as an adjunct to the normal programme for fractures involving the PIP joint.

A new and provocative method of treatment for this difficult problem has been presented by Agee (1978). He applies a small splint constructed from three Kirschner wires and activated by a rubber band (Fig. 14.39). The splint allows full early active flexion and extension while preventing dislocation (Fig. 14.40).

Therapy starts immediately after placement of the splint. While active flexion and extension are encouraged, the therapist needs to guard against regaining full extension too rapidly.

If this occurs, a metal splint is placed over the dorsum of the PIP joint to block full extension

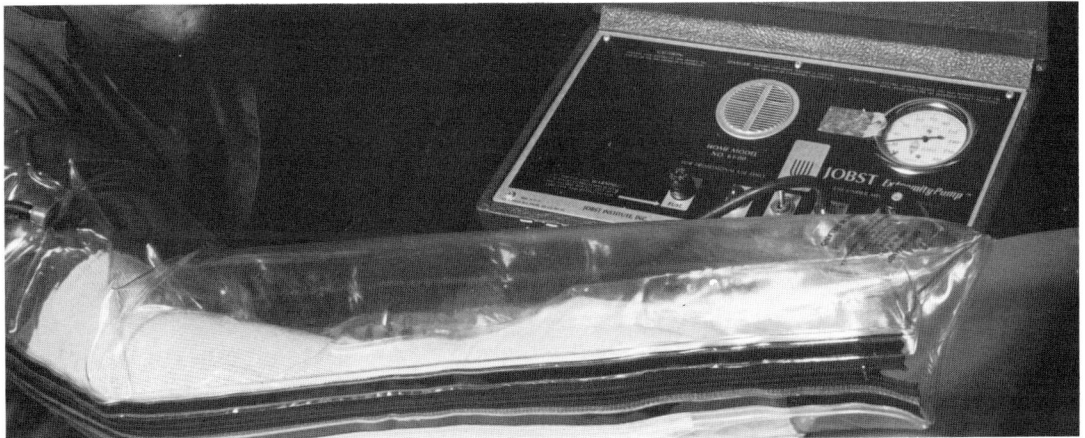

Fig. 14.34 The Jobst intermittent pressure unit can be used with stable fractures, but is contraindicated with any question in the stability of reduction.

(Fig. 14.41). The metal splint may have to have a hole placed in it to fit over any protruding part of the splint itself.

While the patient is wearing the splint, he is instructed in pin care and closely supervised during the 4–6 weeks that the device is in place. After the splint is removed, the injured finger is buddy taped to the adjacent finger for protection for another 1–2 weeks. Dynamic splinting to regain full flexion or extension can be introduced at 7–8 weeks.

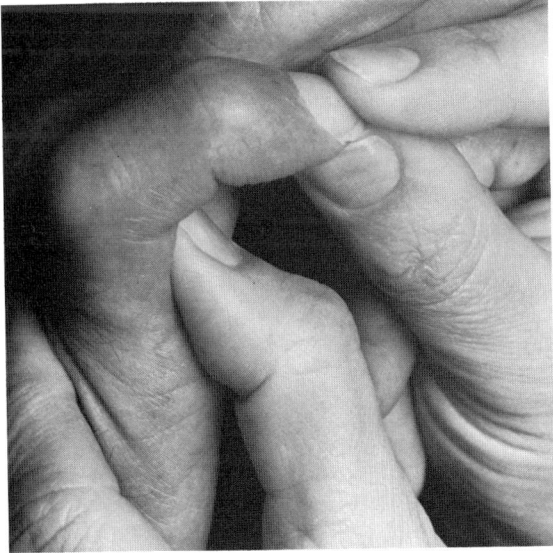

Fig. 14.35 The fracture site must be firmly stabilized by the therapist while applying a gentle stretch to the intrinsic muscles.

Extensor tendon injury over the PIP joint (central slip injury)

An injury over the PIP joint is the most critical of all extensor tendon injuries. Closed injuries are treated with the PIP joint held in extension by splinting for 4–6 weeks with the distal interphalangeal joint (DIP) left free to flex (Lovett & McCalla 1983, Evans 1985). A metal, thermoplastic or finger cast can be used, but they must rest the PIP joint in full (0°) extension to prevent an extensor lag (Fig. 14.42) (Rosenthal 1985). Gentle PIP joint motion begins at 4–6 weeks depending on evidence of extensor lag. If surgery is required for an open wound or an established boutonnière deformity, the entire digit is generally immobilized in extension for 6 weeks postsurgery (Fig. 14.43).

Specific treatment guidelines (Table 14.5)

A closed injury or disease, with avulsion or attenuation of the central slip creates a classic boutonnière deformity if left untreated. After a period of time, the deformity becomes fixed requiring a therapy programme prior to reconstruction. (The therapist should consider that closed management of the classic boutonnière deformity may, if successful, exceed in functional quality any series of operative results.) Stiff PIP and DIP joints must be mobilized along with stretching of the oblique retinacular ligament (Rosenthal 1978). A 3–5 mm excursion of the

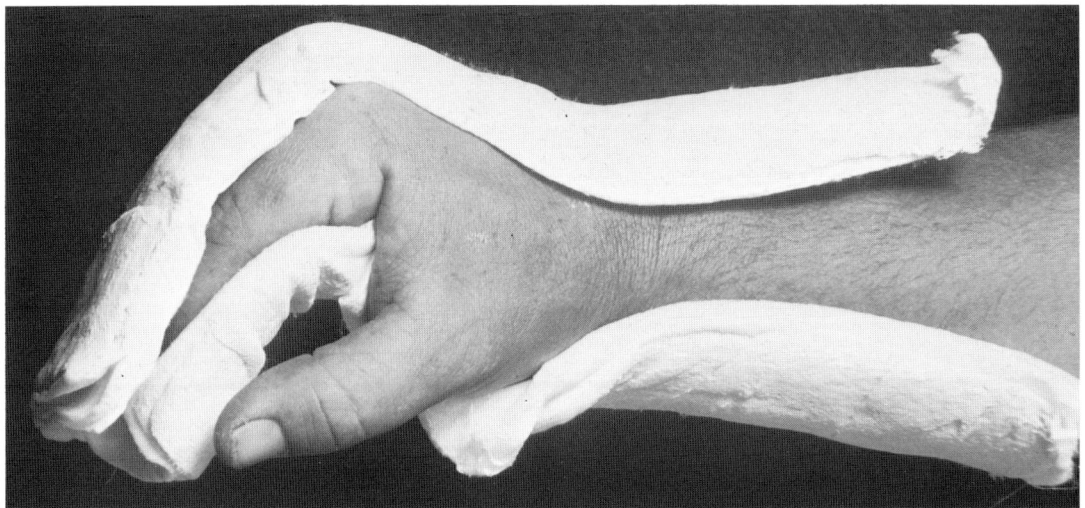

Fig. 14.36 Splinting in the functional position provides protection and prevents flexion contractures of the PIP joint (wrist in 30–60° of extension, MPs in 60–70° of flexion, IPs as close to neutral as possible).

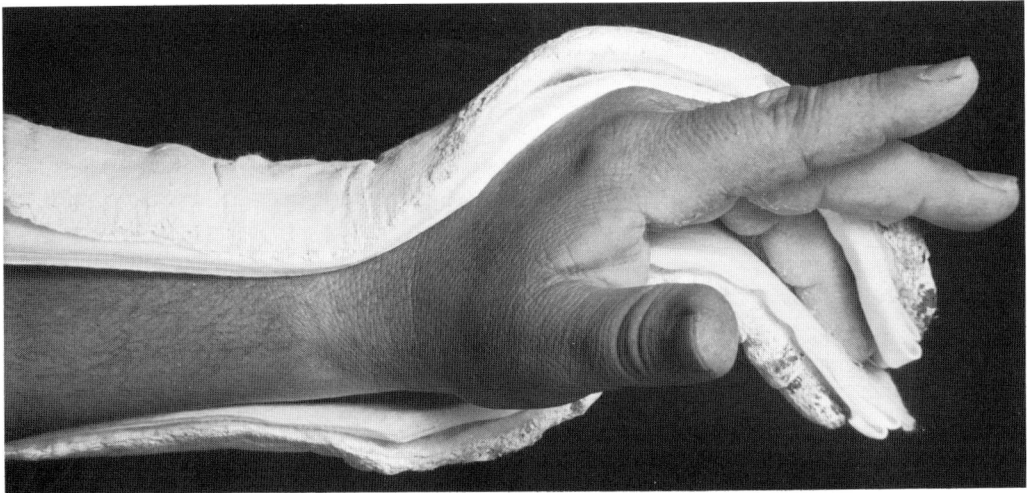

Fig. 14.37 If only one digit is involved, it can be splinted with the adjacent finger leaving the others free.

central slip is normal in this area (Rosenthal 1985). A congealed mass of scar over the PIP joint and a fixed deformity allows no tendon amplitude. Re-establishment of the gliding of the central slip is the major challenge following reconstruction.

An open injury with laceration of the extensor tendon over the PIP joint is treated by a primary repair. Both a closed boutonnière deformity requiring reconstruction and the open tendon laceration can be managed with a similar postoperative programme. The position of immobilization is with both the DIP and PIP joints in neutral. If only the central slip is involved, without lateral band repair, the therapist may remove the splint in therapy at about 10–14 d to begin movement of *only* the DIP joint to stretch the oblique retinacular ligament. In doing the exercise, the PIP joint is maintained in neutral while the DIP joint is flexed and extended (Fig. 14.44). The purpose is to have the lateral bands glide without disturbing the healing central slip.

The period of immobilization for the PIP joint

THERAPEUTIC MANAGEMENT OF THE PROXIMAL INTERPHALANGEAL JOINT

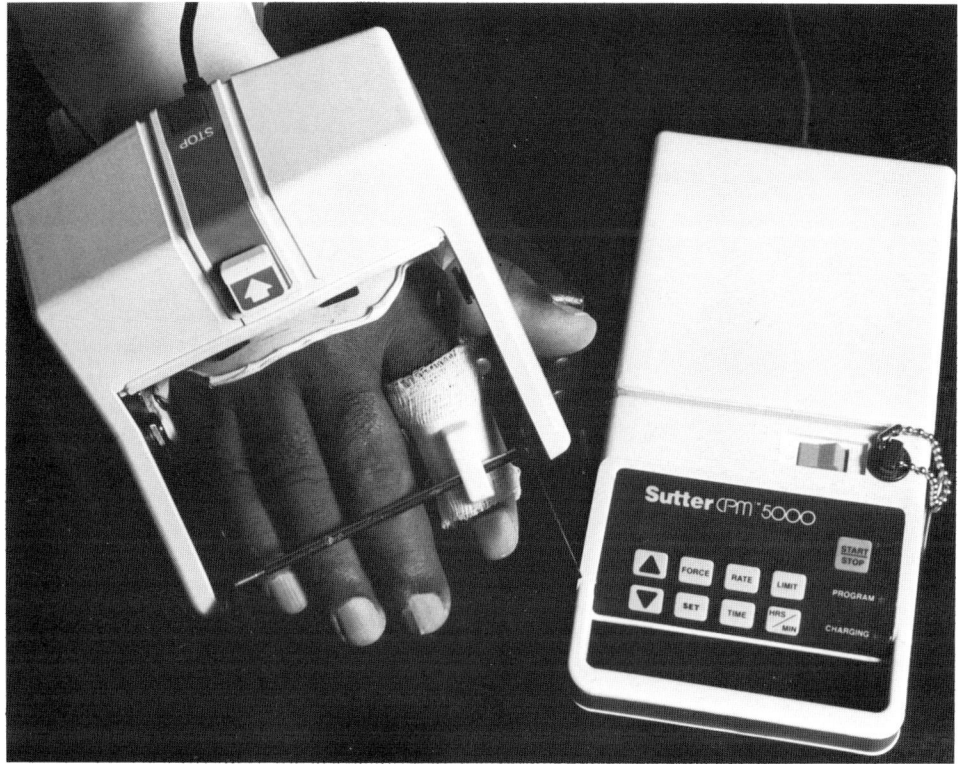

Fig. 14.38 Important considerations for use of CPM for an intra-articular fracture include stable reduction of the fracture, careful placement of finger tape to prevent rotation or painful extremes of motion.

Table 14.5 Treatment programme for extensor tendon injury over PIP joint

Diagnosis	Primary objectives	Timing factor to begin motion	Resistance
Extensor tendon injury over PIP joint (central slip injury)	1. To achieve full active and passive flexion and extension of PIP 2. To prevent extensor lag at PIP	1. Closed injuries—begin PIP motion at 4 weeks 2. Open wound with repair or reconstruction—begin motion at PIP and DIP 6 weeks 3. If only central slip repaired—begin DIP motion at 10–14 days, keeping PIP at neutral for 4–6 weeks	Active, assistive motion at 6–8 weeks depending on presence of extensor lag

Specific treatment procedures	Complications	Splinting
1. Closed injury—stretch ORL and promote gliding of central slip 2. Reconstruction or primary repair (after 4–6 weeks immobilization) flexion of MP with extension of PIP 3. Central slip repair only—immobilize PIP at 0° and at 10–14 days begin active flexion and extension of DIP only 4. In all injuries emphasis on gaining flexion, but always being alert to development of extensor lag	1. Extensor lag 2. Flexion contracture of PIP 3. Hyperextension contracture of DIP	1. PIP in absolute neutral during immobilization 2. Rest splinting in extension 8 weeks or longer if lag persists 3. Serial cast with DIP traction if DIP stiff in hyperextension

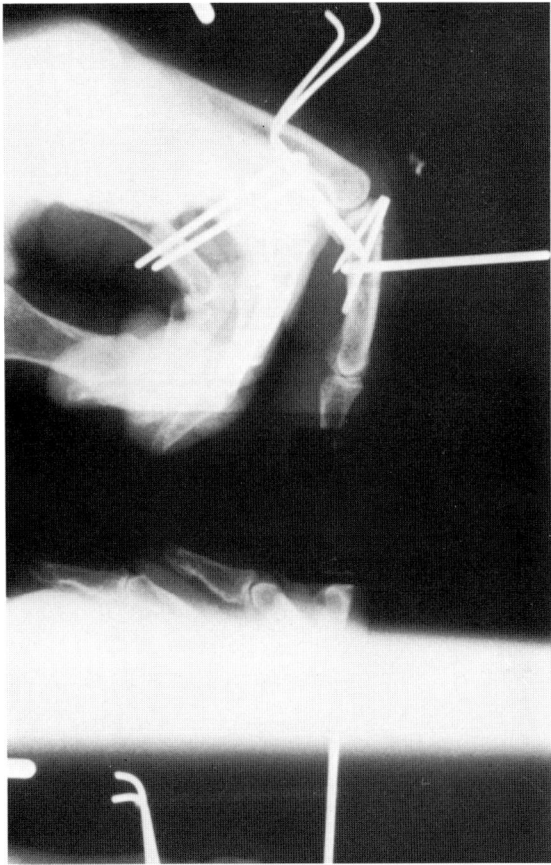

Fig. 14.39 Agee's splint is constructed from three Kirschner wires and is activated by a rubber band.

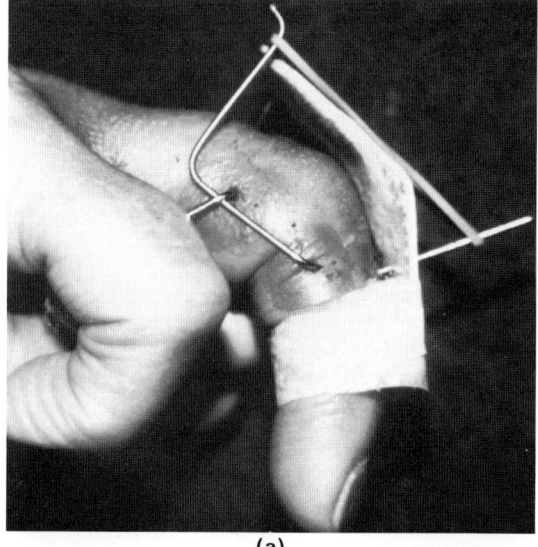

Fig. 14.40 The splint allows (**a**) full early flexion and (**b**) extension while preventing dislocation.

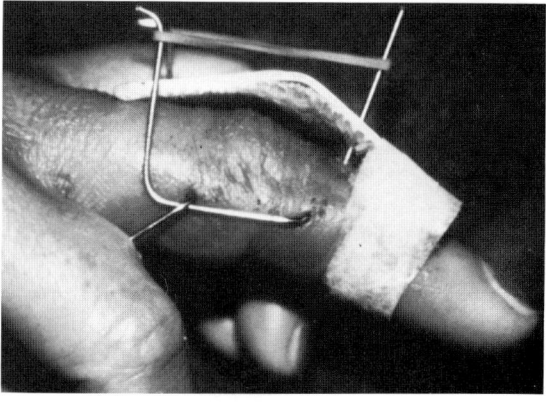

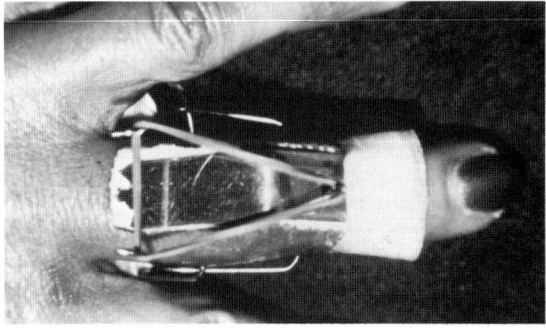

Fig. 14.41 A small metal splint can be placed over the dorsum of the PIP joint to prevent regaining full extension too rapidly.

itself is 4–6 weeks with gentle motion beginning at that time. The patient is taught to extend the PIP joint with the MP joint in flexion to promote action of both the long extensors and the intrinsics (Fig. 14.45). Exercise can be more vigorous with the tendon repair than with complex tendon reconstruction.

At 6 weeks, increased active and active assistive exercise can commence. Rest splinting in extension is applied between exercise and at night for 8 weeks. If the DIP joint is limited in flexion and rests in slight hyperextension, gentle rubber band traction can be applied to assist in gaining increased flexion of the joint (Evans 1985). The traction must be gentle and applied periodically throughout the day to prevent nailbed damage (Evans 1985) (Fig. 14.46). Resistance and dynamic splinting can usually be introduced at 8 weeks if there is no lag

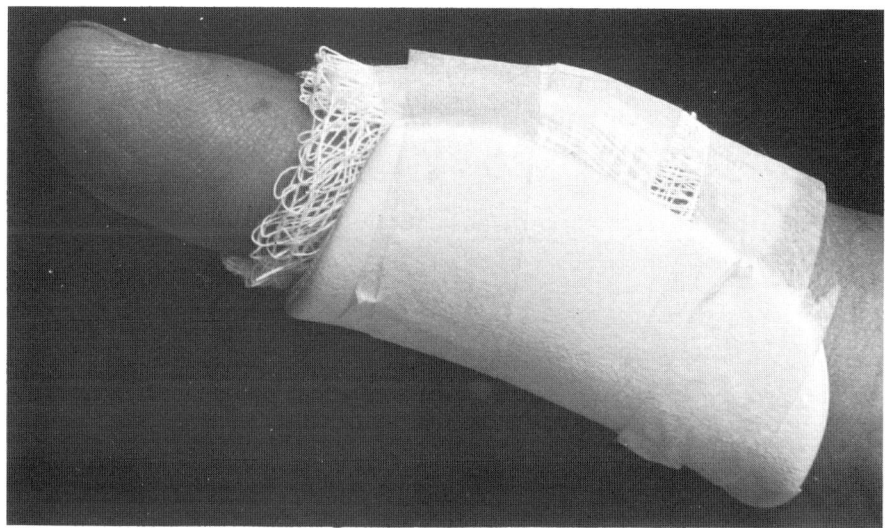

Fig. 14.42 A metal, thermoplastic or finger cast can be used to hold the PIP joint in full extension with the DIP left free to flex.

in extension. Should a lag persist, rest splinting will have to continue as long as necessary to overcome the problem—often several months. Muscle re-education exercises performed for injuries distal to the MP joint are most effective if extension is performed in mass, so that both intrinsic and extrinsic muscles are utilized.

INTERPHALANGEAL JOINT IN RHEUMATOID ARTHRITIS

Management of problems at the interphalangeal joints in rheumatoid arthritis is more difficult than at the more proximal joints because of the delicate balance of the extensor mechanism in the fingers, as well as the critical functional position occupied by the PIP joint (Swanson & Swanson 1973, Welsh & Hastings 1977). The postoperative care required at the PIP joint depends on the type of deformity present. Surgery may be required for reconstruction of the swan-neck deformity or boutonnière deformity (Swanson et al 1984). Depending on the stage of the deformity, conservative treatment may be more appropriate.

Swan-neck deformity (Table 14.6)

Swan-neck deformities vary from the mobile stage to a fixed extension contracture (Wilson 1981, Colditz 1984a). In the early swan-neck deformity, the PIP joint is mobile in all positions with no intrinsic tightness. Joint injections may be indicated as well as use of the figure-of-eight (or swan-neck) splints. The splint prevents hyperextension of the PIP joint, but allows full flexion (Fig. 14.47).

An intermediate swan-neck deformity is characterized by some limitation of PIP joint flexion, especially when the MP joint is stabilized in extension and is associated with intrinsic tightness. X-rays may show early erosion or joint space narrowing and intrinsic release may be indicated (Heywood 1979). As a conservative measure, the

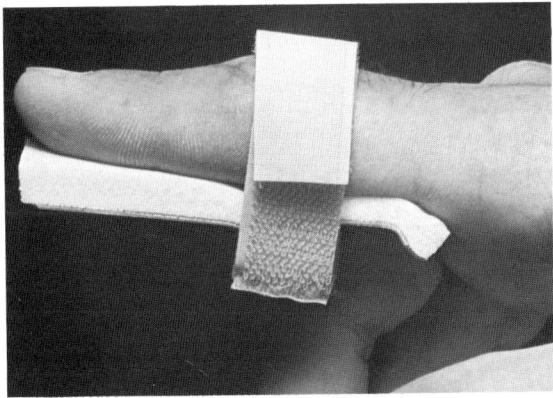

Fig. 14.43 Following surgery, for an open wound or reconstruction of a boutonnière deformity, the entire digit may have to be immobilized in extension for 6 weeks postsurgery.

Table 14.6 Treatment programme for swan-neck deformity

Diagnosis	Characterized by	Non-operative/operative treatment
Swan neck I (mobile)	1. PIP mobile in all positions 2. No tight intrinsics	1. Joint injections 2. Figure-of-eight splinting (prevents hyperextension PIP, but allows full flexion)
Swan neck II (intermediate)	1. Limitation of PIP flexion with MP in extension 2. Intrinsic tightness 3. Early joint space narrowed	1. Intrinsic release may be indicated
Swan neck III (established)	1. PIP motion limited with MP volar subluxation	1. Surgical treatment may include MP joint implant arthroplasty, intrinsic resection and manipulation of PIPs 2. Therapy: active PIP flexion and intrinsic stretching
Swan neck IV (end stage)	1. Marked erosion on X-ray 2. Loss of joint space 3. Absence PIP flexion	1. Surgical treatment may be implant arthroplasty with tendon lengthening 2. Therapy: dorsal PIP splint blocking extension (10–20° of flexion) 3. May need to splint DIP in extension, or splint MP in extension with PIP flexion

patient needs to be placed on an intrinsic stretching programme to help prevent an increase in the deformity.

With an established swan-neck deformity, the PIP joint motion is limited and the MP joint develops volar subluxation. Surgical treatment may necessitate an MP implant arthroplasty, intrinsic tendon resection and manipulation of the PIP joints to 80° of flexion (Nalebuff & Millender 1975a). In order to maintain flexion after surgery, the exercise programme must emphasize active flexion and intrinsic stretching. The patient's interphalangeal joints can be held in flexion by paper tape or a soft velfoam wrap (Fig. 14.48). This has proved to be a comfortable and effective means of maintaining range of motion gained in surgery.

In end stage swan-neck deformity, X-rays show marked erosion, loss of joint space correlated with an absence of PIP joint flexion. Treatment alternatives for the physician include arthrodesis or arthroplasty. If an implant arthroplasty at the PIP joint has been done for a swan-neck deformity in association with tendon lengthening, a padded taped on aluminium splint is placed on the digit after the postoperative oedema has subsided.

The splint maintains the PIP joint in 10–20° of flexion and is worn until a 10–20° flexion contracture is established in order to prevent recurrent hyperextension (Fig. 14.49). A figure-of-eight

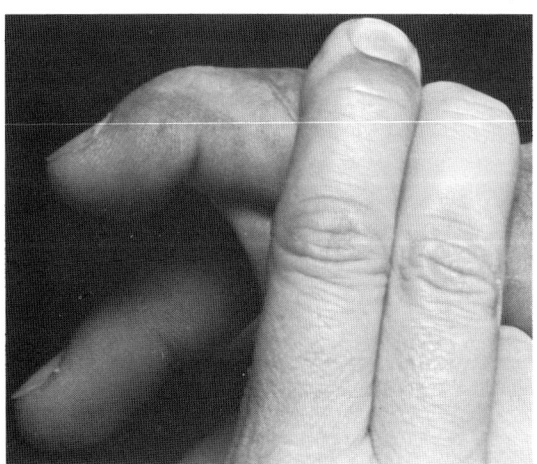

Fig. 14.44 If only the central slip is involved, the splint may be removed after 10–14 days to begin motion of the DIP only.

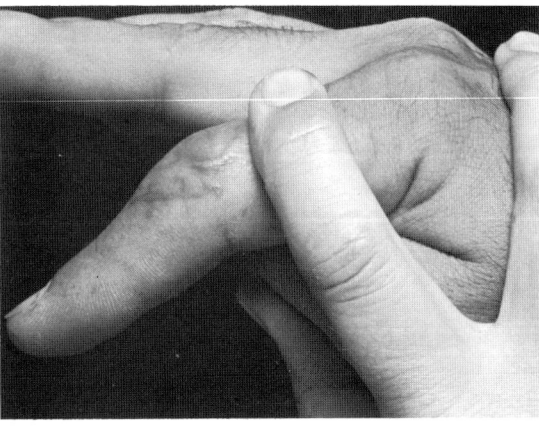

Fig. 14.45 The patient is taught to extend the PIP joint with the MP joint in flexion to promote action of both the long extensors and the intrinsics.

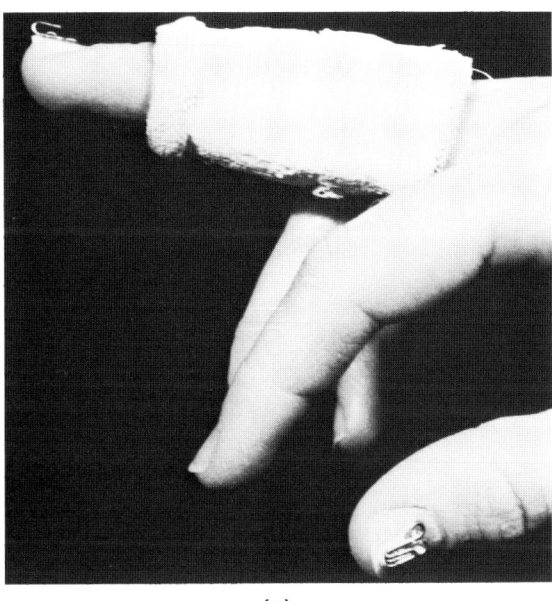

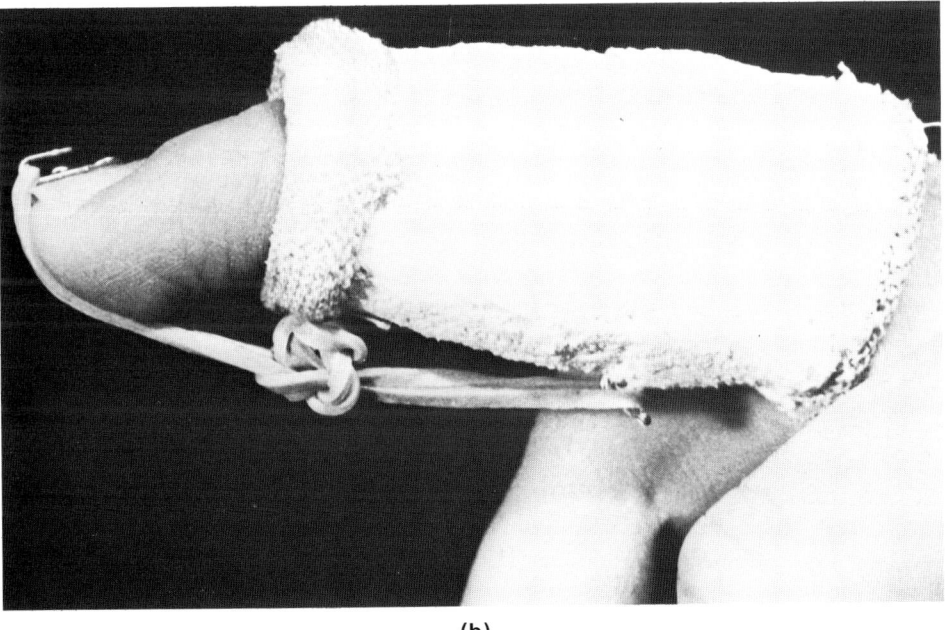

Fig. 14.46 If the DIP is limited in (**a**) flexion and rest in slight hyperextension (**b**) gentle rubber band traction can be applied to assist in gaining increased flexion of the joint.

splint usually cannot fit over the IP joints postsurgically, but may be used after the oedema has subsided. Active exercises to achieve flexion are started as soon as pain subsides and are performed with the splint in place. Care must be taken that the DIP joint does not remain in a marked flexed position. If so, the DIP joint must be splinted in extension.

The therapist also must be aware of the position of the MP joint and may find it necessary to fabricate a dorsal splint to combine MP extension with IP splinting to maintain tendon balance.

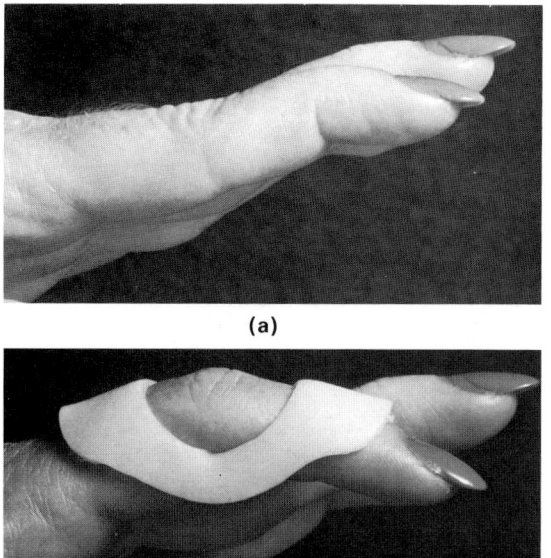

Fig. 14.47 (a) A mobile swan neck deformity can be splinted with (b) a figure-of-eight splint to prevent hyperextension, yet allow full flexion (see Fig. 14.32b).

Boutonnière deformity (Table 14.7)

The boutonnière deformity is the reciprocal of the swan-neck deformity demonstrating PIP joint flexion and hyperextension at both the distal and metacarpophalangeal joints. The boutonnière is classified by the degree of deformity (Colditz 1984a), the ability to correct passively the joint and status of the joint surface (Nalebuff & Millender 1975b).

One must distinguish between a true boutonnière deformity and other causes of PIP joint stiffness such as capsule contracture and flexor tenosynovitis. Despite the obvious deformity, finger function may be relatively good early in the disease. The patient in the early or preboutonnière stage with proliferative PIP synovitis is a candidate for surgical synovectomy before destruction of the extensor mechanism. More frequently, the therapist will see the patient with a slowly progressive PIP joint contracture, a boutonnière deformity and dry synovitis. Surgery may only aggravate this condition leading to further joint stiffness. The treatment of choice is a therapy programme that

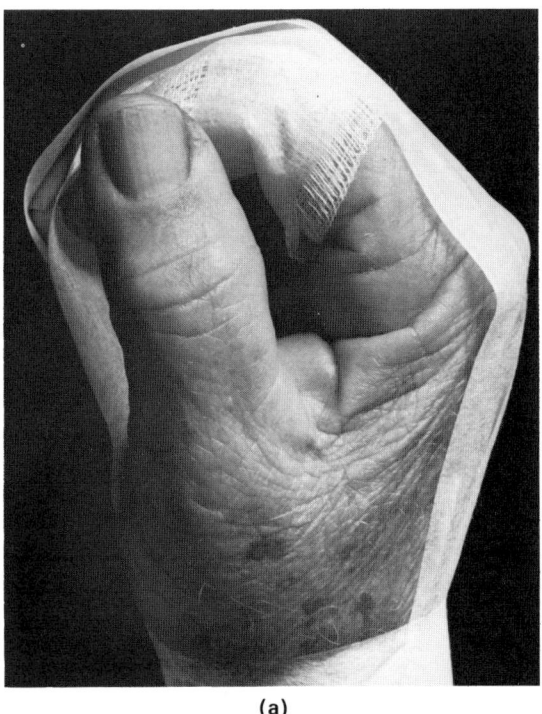

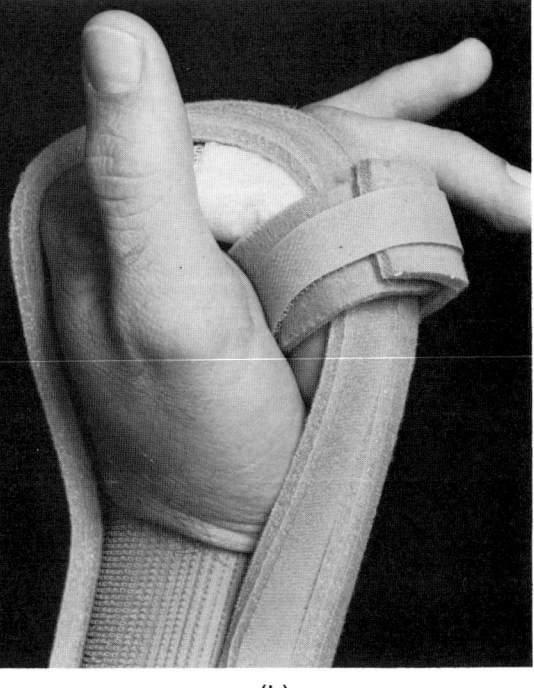

Fig. 14.48 Following surgery, the patient's IP joints can be held in flexion by (a) paper tape or (b) a velfoam flexion wrap.

THERAPEUTIC MANAGEMENT OF THE PROXIMAL INTERPHALANGEAL JOINT 241

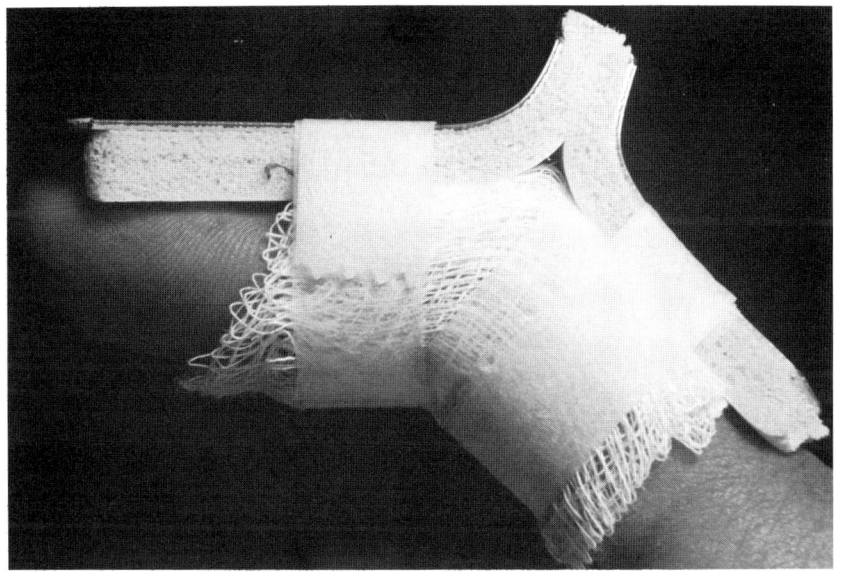

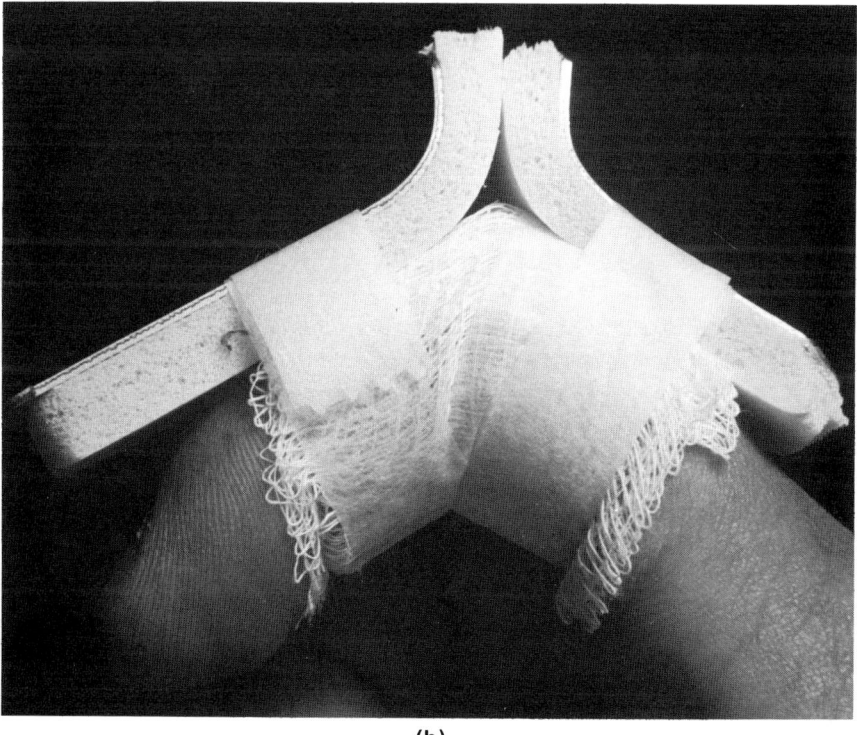

(b)

Fig. 14.49 A split metal splint can be worn following surgery to (**a**) prevent recurrent hyperextension at the PIP joint (**b**) yet allow flexion.

Table 14.7 Treatment programme for boutonnière deformity

Diagnosis	Characterized by	Non-operative/operative treatment
Boutonnière I (early)	1. Proliferative PIP synovitis or slowly progressive PIP joint contracture with dry synovitis	1. Splinting in extension of PIP 2. DIP free to flex to stretch ORL
Boutonnière II (mobile)	1. 30–50° of extensor lag of PIP with complete passive PIP extension	1. If no joint destruction, with proliferative synovitis, surgery may include synovectomy and extensor tendon reconstruction. 2. Conservative therapy would be static extension splinting of the PIP in neutral
Boutonnière III (intermediate)	1. Fixed flexion contracture of 30–40° 2. Loss of joint space on X-ray	1. Surgery: PIP arthroplasty 2. Therapy: Immobilized 3–3.5 weeks with PIP and DIP joints in neutral. If central slip only repaired, then begin movement of DIP only at 3–5 days to stretch ORL Gentle flexion of PIP at 3–3.5 weeks Active assistive motion at about 6 weeks Rest splinting always in extension for 8–10 weeks (longer if lag is present)
Boutonnière IV (late)	1. Fixed flexion contracture with subluxation and ankylosis	1. Treatment of choice is usually arthrodesis in a functional position

includes splinting, particularly at night to prevent increasing flexion contractures (Colditz 1984a). The splint or finger cast should provide extension of the PIP joint, but allow the DIP joint to be free so that the patient may flex the distal joint to stretch the oblique retinacular ligament. This treatment may be successful, but with flare-ups of the disease process, the contracture may increase despite splinting.

In the second or mobile stage of boutonnière deformity, a 30–50° extensor lag exists with nearly complete passive PIP joint extension. With the presence of proliferative synovitis and no joint destruction on X-ray, a synovectomy and extensor tendon reconstruction may be performed (Heywood 1969). Conservative treatment would be static extension splinting of the PIP joint in full extension (Colditz 1984a) (Fig. 14.50).

In the intermediate stage of boutonnière deformity, the patient has a fixed flexion contracture of 30–40°, loss of joint space on X-ray and is beyond the point of splinting. These patients are candidates for PIP implant arthroplasty with extensor reconstruction or distal tenotomy (Dolphin 1965).

After surgery, the finger is immobilized for 3–3.5 weeks with both the PIP and DIP joint in neutral. The treatment for a boutonnière reconstruction and an intermediate stage boutonnière arthroplasty are very similar. One difference in the programme includes early mobilization of the central slip.

The therapist may remove the splint in therapy at 3–5 d to begin movement of only the DIP joint to stretch the oblique retinacular ligament. The PIP joint is maintained in neutral while the DIP is moved. Gentle flexion of the PIP joint can begin after the period of immobilization. At approximately 6 weeks, more active motion can begin including active assistive exercise. Rest splinting in extension is applied between exercise and at night for 8–10 weeks. As with a primary boutonnière repair, if a lag persists, rest splinting in extension will have to continue for a prolonged period.

The late stage of boutonnière deformity has a fixed flexion contracture with subluxation and ankylosis. An arthroplasty attempt in a severely

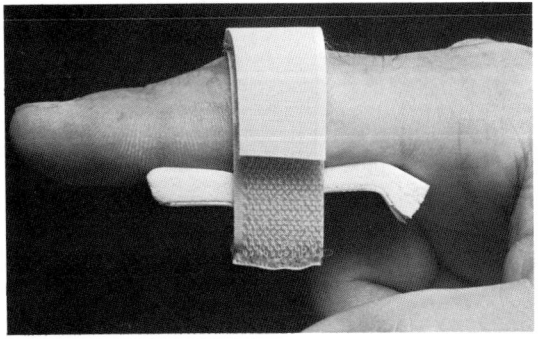

Fig. 14.50 Conservative treatment of the second stage boutonnière deformity is static splinting of the PIP joint in full extension.

contracted finger will require such extensive bone reconstruction for release that satisfactory seating of an implant plus tendon rebalancing may prove unsuccessful. Arthrodesis in a corrected position may be the surgery of choice in this case.

REMEDIAL STAGE TREATMENT: CHRONIC STIFF PIP JOINT

Evaluation procedures for a chronically stiff PIP joint are the same as for an acute injury. Problem areas that should be considered are the presence of 'brawny' oedema, skin or scar contracture, muscle (intrinsic or extrinsic) tightness, pain, instability and differences between active and passive range of motion. Many authors stress the importance of recognizing the 'end feel' of the stiff joint as a prognostic factor for treatment (Colditz 1984a, b, McEntee 1984). In performing a gentle passive range of motion, if there is a springy feel at the end of the joint's maximum range, the potential for improvement is more positive. However, if the joint moves to a certain point and stops in a solid, non-giving manner, it is said to have a 'hard end feel' (Colditz 1984a) Conservative management with this type of joint may be futile.

Ideally the goal of late treatment is to produce a pain-free, functional arc of motion. In some cases, the objective is to obtain maximum physiological homoeostasis of the joint and surrounding tissues prior to an operative procedure such as implant arthroplasty or capsulectomy. Contracture problems at the PIP joint are generally classified as chronic after 6–8 months whether treated primarily or not (Bowers 1983) and may involve all associated structures (Snow et al 1975, Tubiana 1985).

Specific treatment guidelines (Table 14.8)

Late, unresolved oedema is generally diffuse and requires vigorous management. Ice and retrograde massage, elevation, active exercise and compressive wraps or gloves are utilized to help reduce the swelling. An elastic glove or finger stalls often need to be worn for most of the day, even during activity, to produce a change in the condition (Fig. 14.51). Meticulous circumferential or volumetric measures are required to record the minute changes on a day-to-day basis.

Pain is often present with a chronic joint problem and is usually more difficult to control than in the acute phase (Redler 1967). Ice, massage, galvanic stimulation and TENS can help to produce local analgesia. Iontophoresis is not as successful with chronic problems as with acute inflammation unless the area can be specifically pinpointed.

Solving a longstanding problem requires a high level of patient motivation. Unfortunately after 6–

Table 14.8 Treatment programme for chronic stiff PIP joint

Diagnosis	Primary objectives	Timing factor to begin motion	Resistance
Chronic stiff PIP joint	1. To provide stable, pain-free, functional arc of motion 2. Or to obtain maximum physiological homoeostasis of digit prior to surgery	Usually considered chronic after 6–8 months from time of injury	Only limits are pain, instability or compression forces

Specific treatment procedures	Complications	Splinting
1. Oedema control—compression wraps, retrograde massage, active motion 2. Pain relief—TENS, ice massage, galvanic electrical stimulation, iontophoresis if pain is pin-pointed 3. Patient education—to accept slow process of recovery 4. Heat prior to passive stretching done with joint distraction 5. *No painful manipulation* 6. Directed exercises with blocking for FDP, FDS, long extensors and intrinsics 7. Resistive exercise 8. Joint mobilization	1. Increased inflammation and oedema 2. Reflex sympathetic dystrophy 3. PIP flexion contracture	1. Serial plaster cylindrical splinting and/or dynamic splinting with low intensity, prolonged traction 2. Alternate flexion and extension

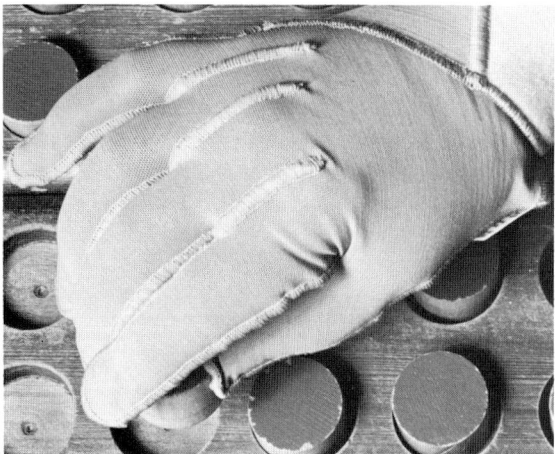

Fig. 14.51 An elastic glove or finger stalls may need to be worn for most of the day to help reduce chronic swelling.

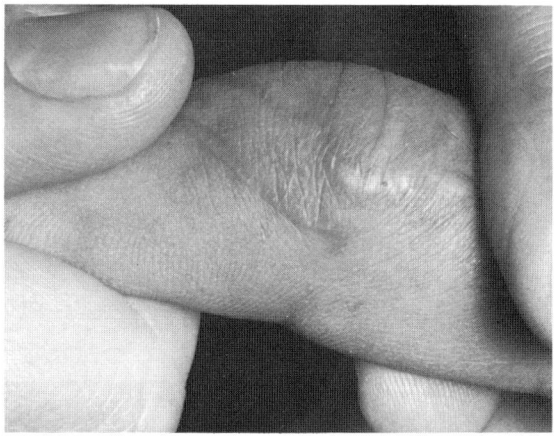

Fig. 14.52 In performing passive range of motion, the joints should be firmly supported and slightly distracted with motion performed in the comfort (stretch) range.

8 months of discomfort and poor function, most patients are justifiably discouraged. The therapist usually needs to provide realistic psychological support and patient education to help him accept the slow process to recovery and the need to adhere to a structured programme.

Joint mobilization techniques are often more appropriate with a small joint in this late stage than passive range of motion. Specific application of this technique is discussed in Chapter 16. If passive range of motion is performed, there must be no forceful motion that compresses and wedges the articular surfaces against each other (Enna & Zimny 1974, Bowers 1983). Rather, the joint should be firmly supported and slightly distracted with motion performed in the comfort 'stretch' range (Fig. 14.52). Intrinsic stretching is usually not possible at this stage due to the severe contracture of the joint. Both passive range of motion and joint mobilization with a chronically stiff, small joint require the skills of an experienced therapist (Bowers 1983).

Heat in elevation prior to or during stretching has been reported by Sapega et al (1981) as 'the best way to lengthen functional connective structures without compromising your structural integrity'. One suggested method of combining heat and stretch is through the use of Coban wrap applied to the involved joint in the direction requiring motion (Fig. 14.53). The bandage is either applied prior to dipping in paraffin or while under the hot pack (McEntee 1984). After 20–30 min of prolonged stretch in the heat, active exercise is immediately initiated.

As in the acute phase, the patient must perform specific exercises to encourage gliding of individual tendons, joint surfaces and surrounding soft tissues (Weeks et al 1978). A programme of active exercise should include blocking for isolated motions of FDP and FDS and abduction and adduction for individual intrinsic motion. For isolation of the long extensors, the fingers should attempt a claw position with the IPs flexed maximally while flexing and extending the MP joint. Finger extension in mass will help to include both extrinsic and intrinsic finger extensors. Care must be taken that the joints proximal to those being mobilized are stabilized to prevent incorrect balance of musculotendinous units. Positioning of both the MP joint and the wrist may have to be managed by splinting if the patient cannot actively maintain the desired position.

After 8 or more months, the only restriction in the use of resistance in exercise or activity is mandated by pain, instability or inappropriate compression force inherent in the task.

Philosophy concerning the splinting of the stiff PIP joint falls into two camps. The controversy concerns the use of static splints as opposed to dynamic splinting. One group feels that splinting corrections should be steady and inelastic (Watson et al 1979, Bowers 1983), while the other feels that low magnitude tension applied over a prolonged period of time through dynamic splinting is more appropriate (Colditz 1984b, McEntee 1984).

Serial splinting, which is advocated by many authors, is in actuality considered a dynamic splint because it is based on the same principle as dynamic splinting, 'in that the tissue is stressed to a new length each time' (Colditz 1984b).

The present author's choice is to use both serial and dynamic splinting for correction of small joint contractures. There is a wide variety of commercially available splints for PIP joint contractures and designs for custom PIP splinting are only limited by the imagination.

Stiff PIP joint implant arthroplasty

With degenerative or inflammatory arthritis, or chronic stiffness of the PIP joint, the patient may develop progressive loss of motion, pain with movement and deformity. One possible treatment that the surgeon may elect is an implant arthroplasty. When an implant arthroplasty has been performed for a stiff PIP joint, without tendon reconstruction, therapy can begin on the third to fifth day postsurgery (Swanson et al 1984).

Specific treatment guidelines (Table 14.9)

The finger is splinted in extension initially (Fig 14.54), but the distal strap of the splint is removed many times during the day to work on active flexion and extension (Fig. 14.55).

The resting position is always in extension to minimize extensor lag that can occur at the PIP joint. To achieve functional motion, a flexion cuff may be added at approximately 10–14 d postoperatively. Flexion begins with a loop over the middle phalanx providing a gentle dynamic force on the PIP joint (Fig. 14.56). The loop is worn 20 min out of each hour during the day with extension splinting at night. If a stronger dynamic pull is necessary for both DIP and PIP flexion, Velcro pile can be added to the fingernail providing a means of traction for both interphalangeal joints (Fig. 14.57). Even after flexion splinting is initiated, the finger is still rested in extension to prevent extensor lag.

Heat in elevation, prior to exercise helps to

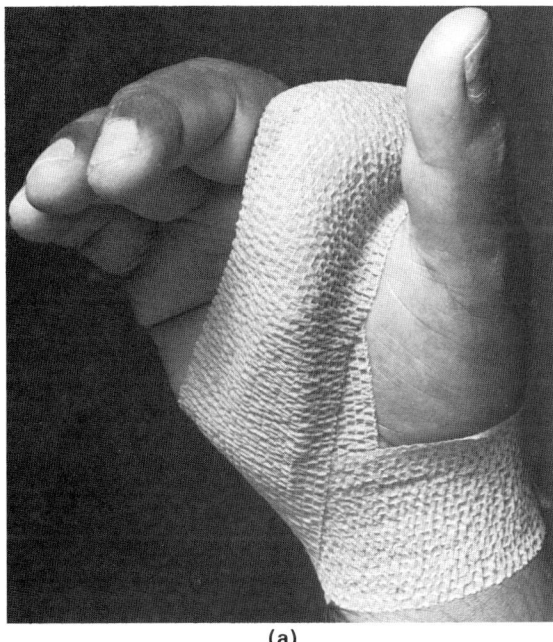

(a)

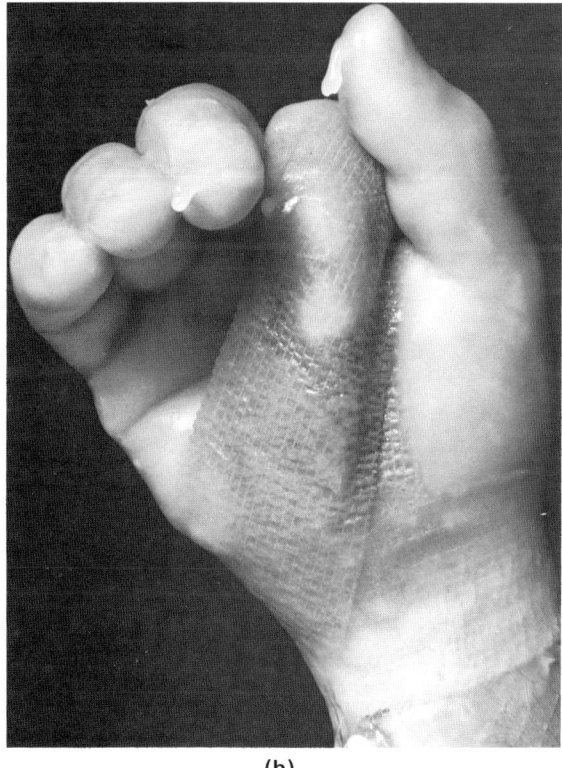

(b)

Fig. 14.53 One suggested method of combining heat and stretch is through the use of (**a**) Coban wrap applied to the involved joint followed by (**b**) paraffin or hot packs.

Table 14.9 Treatment programme for stiff PIP joint implant arthroplasty

Diagnosis	Primary objectives	Timing factor to begin motion	Resistance
Arthroplasty stiff PIP joint (e.g. osteoarthritis, or chronic PIP contracture from other cause)	To achieve active arc of 0–70° at the PIP joint	Begin therapy at 3–5 days	7–8 weeks (very gentle)

Specific treatment procedures	Complications	Splinting
1. Active blocking for individual flexors 2. Mass finger extension 3. MP flexion with IP extension 4. Hold MP in neutral, block DIP by splinting, direct flexion and extension at PIP	1. Extensor lag at PIP 2. Pain 3. Poor functional active range of movement	1. Initially a dorsal splint in extension with strap around proximal phalanx and another strap supporting IP joints. Remove distal strap frequently to allow active flexion and extension of PIP joint 2. Resting position—always in extension to prevent lag 3. Flexion cuff to alternate with extension at 10–14 days

reduce oedema and aid in comfortable active range of motion. After the sutures are removed, many patients prefer the circumferential application of paraffin as a therapeutic heating agent.

For active exercise, the patient is taught to block at each joint for individualized long flexor motion followed by mass finger extension. The goal is to achieve an active arc of approximately 0–70° at the PIP joint.

Specific active blocking exercises and dynamic splinting may be necessary for several months postsurgery if there is a tendency for recurrence of stiffness.

CAPSULECTOMY* (Table 14.10)

If non-operative management of the stiff joint fails to produce functional motion in either flexion or extension, a capsulectomy of the PIP joint may be necessary (Curtis 1954, 1964, Welsh & Hastings 1977).

Extension contracture

When a capsulectomy is performed for an extension contracture, the primary emphasis is on achieving maximum flexion while maintaining full extension (Curtis 1954, Laseter 1984). If therapy is started immediately postsurgery, ice packs in elevation

*Capsulectomy as descriptive of an operative procedure at the PIP joint may have historic value only. More specific terminology is desirable in order to convey what has, in fact, been done. Examples: for extensive contracture—extensor tenolysis, dorsal capsulotomy and collateral ligament release; for flexion contracture—release or resection of the volar plate etc. The therapist should request the information before beginning treatment.

followed by retrograde massage are used to control oedema and produce local analgesia for the first few days (Reynolds 1984) (Fig. 14.58). Light dressings are applied daily, but should not block motion.

Passive flexion and extension exercises are alternated with blocked assistive exercise. To help control oedema and pain, exercises are performed approximately five times every hour rather than in several long sessions (Laseter 1984, Reynold 1984). TENS is often helpful to control pain and produce local analgesia in the postoperative phase. Whether

Table 14.10 Treatment programme for capsulectomy

Capsulectomy	Postoperative management
Extension contracture	1. Therapy immediately following surgery or within 1–3 days 2. Ice packs in elevation to reduce oedema and produce local analgesia 3. TENS for pain 4. Passive/active range of movement 5. Active blocked flexion/extension 6. Intrinsic stretching 7. Short exercise sessions every hour 8. Continuous passive motion may be included 9. Alternate dynamic and static flexion, extension and intrinsic negative splinting
Flexion contracture	1. Therapy immediately, modalities and procedures same as for extension contracture with exception of: Emphasis on active extension. Hold MPs in flexion, actively extend PIP Individual active abduction/adduction for intrinsic pull through at PIP joint Stretch intrinsics and ORL Splinting—extension splinting may be needed long term to prevent recurrent flexion contracture

THERAPEUTIC MANAGEMENT OF THE PROXIMAL INTERPHALANGEAL JOINT 247

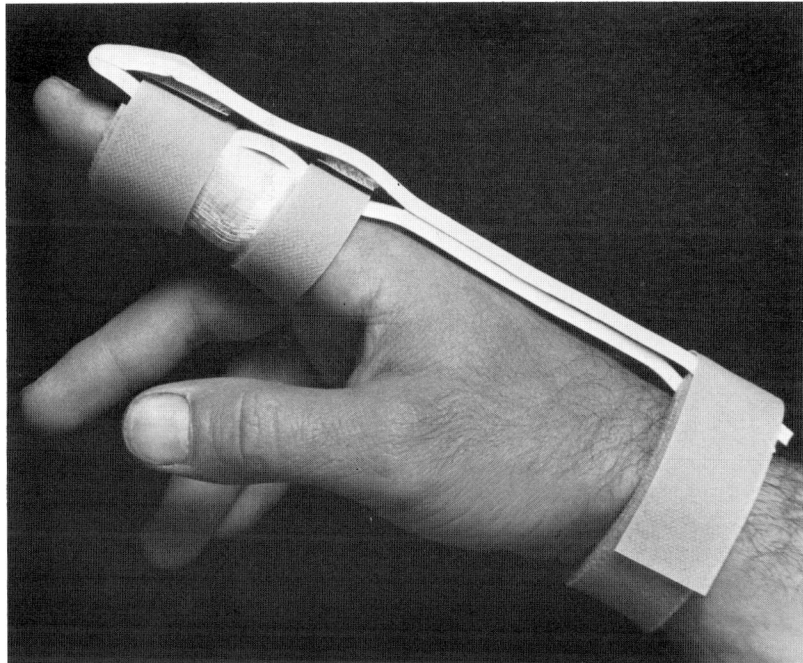

Fig. 14.54 Following an implant arthroplasty, the finger is splinted in extension initially.

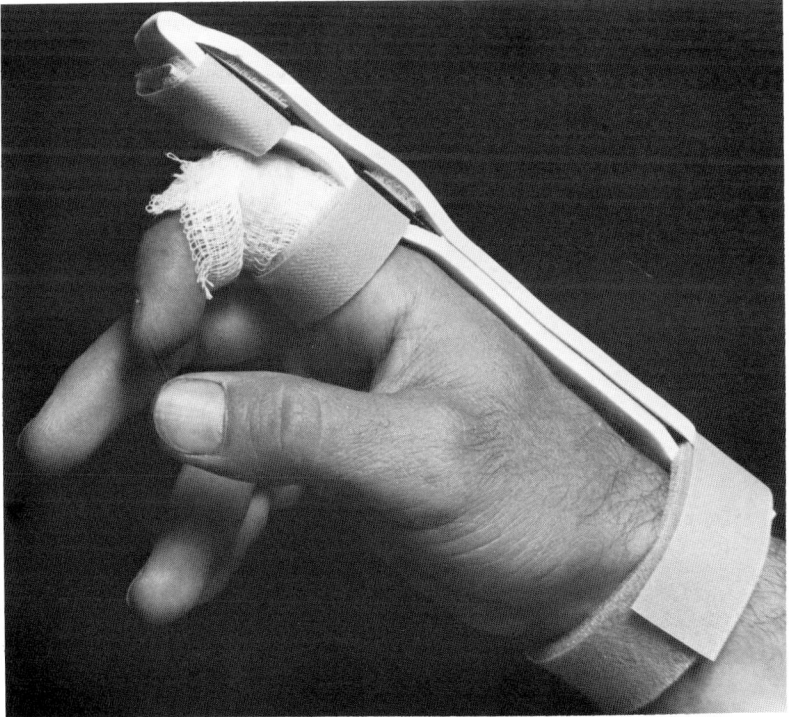

Fig. 14.55 The distal strap of the extension splint is removed many times during the day to work on active flexion and extension.

248 THE INTERPHALANGEAL JOINTS

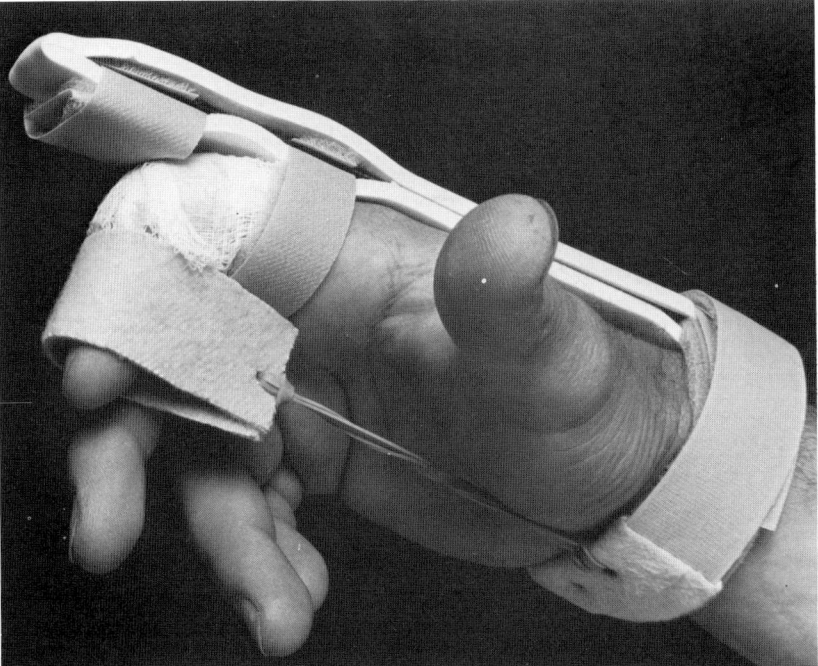

Fig. 14.56 Flexion begins with a loop over the middle phalanx providing a gentle dynamic force on the PIP joint.

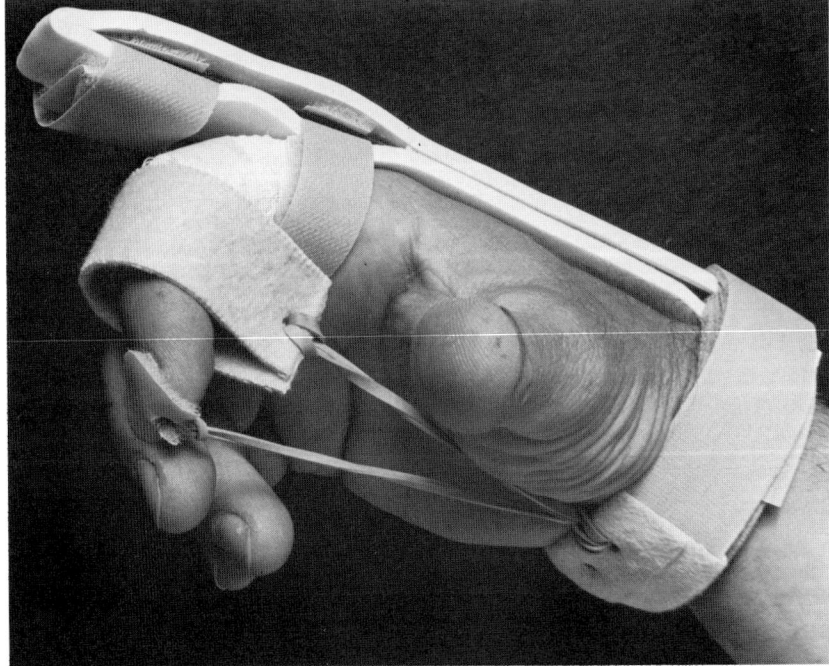

Fig. 14.57 If a stronger dynamic force is necessary for both DIP and PIP flexion, Velcro pile can be added to the fingernail to provide a means of traction for both IP joints.

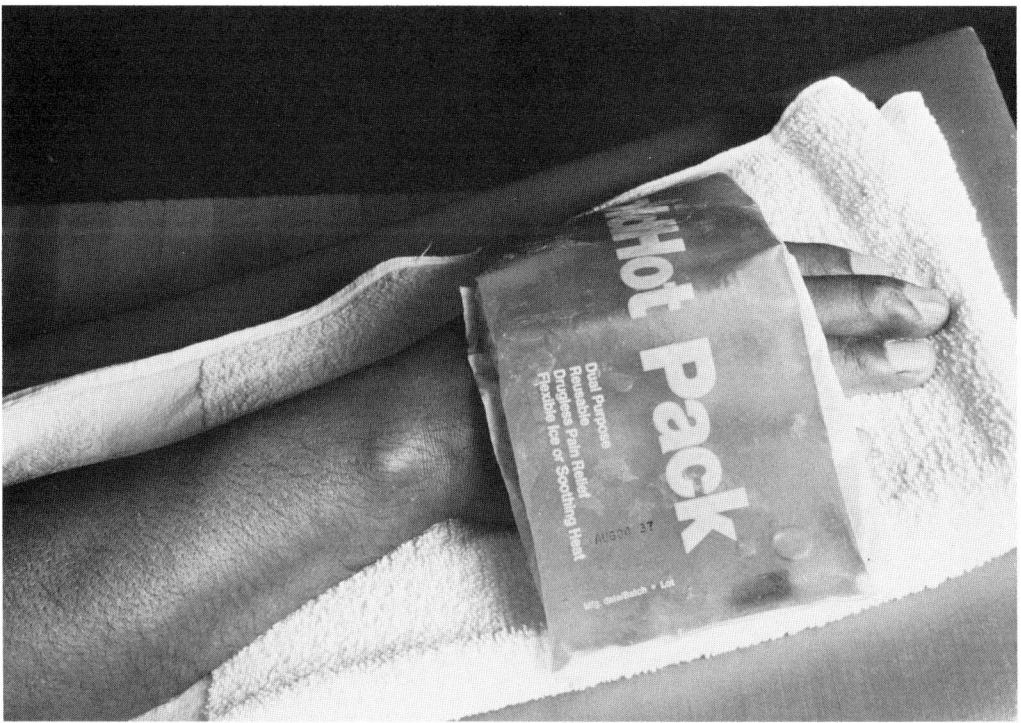

Fig. 14.58 Following a capsulectomy, ice packs in elevation help to control oedema and produce local analgesia for the first few days.

or not the intrinsic muscles have been released as part of the capsulectomy, they will need to be stretched to achieve maximum motion.

Alternate splinting in flexion, extension and an intrinsic negative position may be necessary (Curtis 1954, Laseter 1984, Tubiana 1985). Range of motion recordings, both active and passive must be taken frequently to help determine the most effective splinting position.

Recently in some centres, CPM has been used to prevent adhesions following capsulectomy. Since CPM has been used so little in the upper extremity at this time, its ultimate use in postoperative management of capsulectomy is hard to project. In current treatment protocol, 1–3 d after surgery the patient is fitted with a dorsal splint to allow motion of all three joints or specifically the PIP joints (Fig.14.59).

The CPM device is programmed to the passive flexion and extension limits comfortably tolerated by the patient. For the first week, the device should be worn in therapy for 1-h sessions to adjust limits as the patient can tolerate them. When maximum limits are achieved, the device can be rented for home use. Wearing time will vary depending on the discomfort and the patient's tolerance; 6–8-h a day during the first 3–4 weeks should be sufficient.

Flexion contracture

If a capsulectomy is performed for a flexion contracture of the PIP joint, active extension and prevention of recurrence of the deformity are the top priorities. While the exercise programme must include active and passive flexion and extension, active extension is emphasized (Curtis 1964). Holding the MP joint in flexion, the patient is taught to extend actively the PIP joint allowing the extrinsic extensors and the intrinsics to extend the joint. With the MP in extension, active abduction and adduction exercises of the involved digits help to isolate intrinsic pull through at the PIP level. The intrinsics and oblique retinacular ligament both need to be stretched to overcome the tightness produced from a prolonged contracture.

Extension splinting is often required for a long

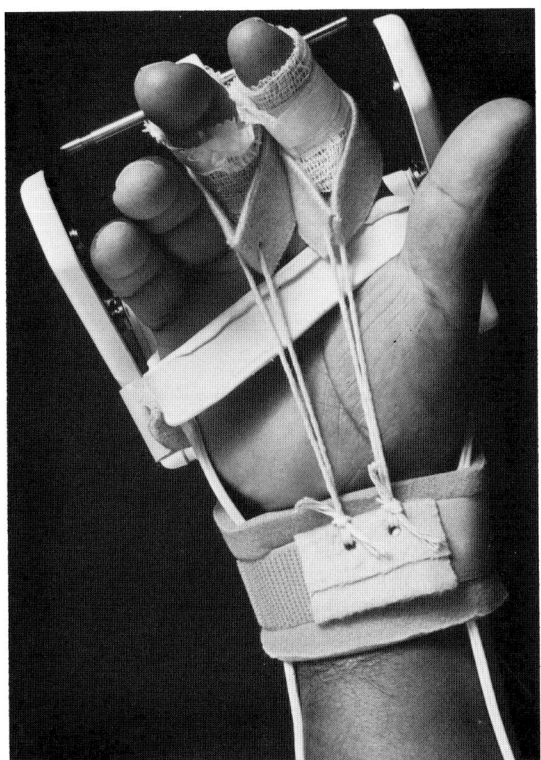

Fig. 14.59 Use of CPM following capsulectomy can allow motion of all three joints or specifically the PIP joints by blocking MP motion.

period postsurgically to prevent recurrence of the flexion contracture (Sprague 1976). Splinting is most effective if worn at all times except during exercise or bathing. Again, precise measurements are necessary to help determine the length of splinting necessary. While CPM may be used, the finger must be carefully observed to prevent repeated flexion contracture. If this occurs, CPM should be discontinued and static extension splinting instituted.

SUMMARY

Specific treatment guidelines for several of the more common acute and chronic conditions of the proximal interphalangeal joint have been presented to emphasize the need for a structured programme to achieve an optimum result following injury or surgery. The basis for any treatment programme must have its roots in the physiological principles of healing and then be validated through clinical experience. The reader must be aware that there is no cookbook or 'best' recipe for treating any disorder. As with all guidelines, there is leeway in most aspects of treatment since each presenting condition will be individual.

Two of the most important factors in planning the patient's treatment are continuous patient education and close communication between the therapist and the hand surgeon. This sharing of ideas and efforts among the three primary parties is the birthplace for guidelines of treatment.

REFERENCES

Adamson J E Treatment of the stiff hand. Orthopedic Clinics of North America 1: 467–480

Agee J M 1978 Unstable fracture dislocations of the proximal interphalangeal joint of the fingers. Journal of Hand Surgery 3: 386–389

American Academy of Orthopedic Surgeons 1965 Joint motion. Chicago

American Society for Surgery of the Hand 1978 The hand: examination and diagnosis. Colorado

Arem A J 1981 The stiff hand: an approach to prevention and treatment. Contemporary Orthopedics 3: 501–514

Bell J A 1984 Plaster cylinder casting of contractures of the interphalangeal joints. In: Hunter J, Schneider L, Mackin E, Callahan A (eds). Rehabilitation of the Hand. 2nd edn. C V Mosby, St Louis

Bowers W H 1983 Management of small joint injuries in the hand. Orthopedic Clinics of North America 14: 793–809

Bowers W H, Wolf J W Jr, Nehil J L et al 1980 The proximal interphalangeal joint volar plate. I. An anatomical and biomechanical study. Journal Hand Surgery 5: 79–88

Bowers W H 1981 The proximal interphalangeal joint plate. II: A clinical study of hyperextension injury. Journal of Surgery 6: 77–81

Brand P W, Wood H 1974 Hand volumeter instruction sheet. United States Public Health Service Hospital, Carville, La

Case R 1984 Iontophoresis as an alternative to trigger point injections. Eagle Medical Newsletter, December

Colditz J C 1984a Arthritis. In: Malick M H Kasch M H (eds) Manual on management of specific hand problems. Aren Publications, Pittsburgh

Colditz J C 1984b Dynamic splinting of the stiff hand. In: Hunter J, Schneider L, Mackin E, Callahan A (eds) Rehabilitation of the hand. C V Mosby, St Louis

Curtis R M 1984 Capsulectomy of the interphalangeal joints of the fingers. Journal of Bone and Joint Surgery 36A: 1219–1232

Curtis R M 1964 Treatment of injuries of proximal interphalangeal joints of fingers. Current Practice in Orthopedic Surgery 2: 125–139

Curtis R M 1984 Management of the stiff hand. In: Hunter J, Schneider L, Mackin E, Callahan A (eds) Rehabilitation of the hand C V Mosby, St Louis

Dolphin J A 1965 Extensor tenotomy for chronic boutonnière deformity of the finger. Report of two cases. Journal of Bone and Joint Surgery 47A: 161–164

Eaton R G, Dray G T 1982 Dislocations and ligament injuries in the digits. In: Green D P (ed) Operative hand surgery. Churchill Livingstone, New York

Enna E D, Zimny M 1974 A scanning electron microscopy study of articular cartilage obtained from joints of denervated hands. Hand 5: 65–68

Evans R B 1985 Extensor tendon injuries at PIP level, personal communication

Glass J M, Stephen R L, Jacobson S C The quantity and distribution of radiolabeled dexamethasone delivered to tissue by iontophoresis. International Journal of Dermatology 19: 519–525

Hamilton G F 1966 Mobilization of the proximal interphalangeal joint. Physical Therapy 47: 1111–1113

Heywood A W B 1969 Correction of the rheumatoid boutonnière deformity. Journal of Bone and Joint Surgery 51A: 1309–1314

Heywood A W B The pathogenesis of the rheumatoid swan-neck deformity. Hand, 11: 176–183

Kuczynski K The PIP joint: anatomy and causes of stiffness in the fingers. Journal of Bone and Joint Surgery 50B: 656–663

Kuczynski K Less known aspects of the proximal interphalangeal joint of the human hand. Hand 7: 31–33

Langley P L Iontophoresis to aid in releasing tendon adhesions. Physical Therapy 64: 1395

Laseter G A 1983 Management of the stiff hand. A practical approach. Orthopedic Clinics of North America 14: 749–765

Laseter G F 1984 Postoperative management of capsulectomies. In: Hunter J, Schneider L, Mackin E, Callahan A (eds) Rehabilitation of the hand. C V Mosby, St Louis

Lovett W L, McCalla M A 1983 Management and rehabilitation of extensor tendon injuries. Orthopedic Clinics of North America 14: 749–765

McCormack R M 1964 Stiffness of the injured hand: analysis, prevention and treatment. Journal of Trauma 4: 581–591

McElfresh E C, Dobyns J H, O'Brien E T 1972 Management of fracture-dislocation of the proximal interphalangeal joints by extension block splinting. Journal of Bone and Joint Surgery 54A: 1705–1710

McEntee P 1984 Therapist's management of the stiff hand, In: Hunter J, Schneider L, Mackin E, Callahan A (eds) Rehabilitation of the hand. C V Mosby, St Louis

Mullins-Taylor P, Cannon N M 1984 Modalities in upper extremity rehabilitation. In: Malick M H, Kasch M C (eds) Manual on management of specific hand problems. Aren Publications, Pittsburgh

Nalebuff E A, Millender L H 1975a Surgical treatment of the swan-neck deformity in rheumatoid arthritis. Orthopedic Clinics of North America 6: 733–752

Nalebuff E A, Millender L H 1975b Surgical treatment of the boutonnière deformity in rheumatoid arthritis. Orthopedic Clinics of North America 6: 753–763

Redler I 1967 Rupture of collateral ligaments of the PIP joint. Journal of Bone and Joint Surgery 49A: 323–326

Reynolds C C 1984 Stiff hand. In: Malick M H, Kasch M C (eds) Manual on management of specific hand problems. Aren Publications, Pittsburgh

Richards J S, Nepomueeno C, Riles M et al Assessing pain behavior: the UAB pain behavior scale. Pain 14: 393–398

Rosenthal E A 1978 The extensor tendons. In: Hunter J, Schneider L, Mackin E, Bell J (eds) Rehabilitation of the hand. C V Mosby, St Louis

Rosenthal E A 1985 Extensor tendon injuries at PIP level, personal communication

Salter R B, Harris O J 1979 The healing of intra-articular fractures with continuous passive motion. American Academy of Orthopedic Surgeons Lecture Series 6: 102–117

Sapega A A, Quedenfeld T C, Moyer R A et al 1981 Biophysical factors in range-of-motion exercise. Physical Sports Medicine 9: 57–65

Snow J W, Pohl R O, Obi L J 1975 Flexion contractures of the hand. Journal of the Florida Medical Association 62: 19–26

Sprague B L 1975 PIP injuries and their initial treatment Journal of Trauma 15: 380

Sprage B L 1975 Proximal interphalangeal joint contractures and their treatment. Journal of Trauma 16: 259–265

Swanson A B, Swanson G de G 1973 Pathogenesis and pathomechanics of rheumatoid deformities in the hand and wrist. Orthopedic Clinics of North America 4: 1039–1056

Swanson A B, Swanson G de G, Leonard J B 1984 Postoperative rehabilitation programs in flexible implant arthroplasty of the digits. In: Hunter J, Schneider L, Mackin E, Callahan A (eds) Rehabilitation of the hand. C V Mosby, St Louis

Tubiana R 1985 The treatment of stiffness of the fingers. In: Tubiana R (ed) The hand, vol II. W B Saunders, Philadelphia

Watson K H 1982 Stiff joints. In: Green D P (ed) Operative hand surgery. Churchill Livingstone, New York

Watson K H, Light T R, Johnson T R 1979 Checkrein resection for flexion contracture of the middle joint. Journal of Hand Surgery 4: 67–71

Weeks P M, Wray R C, Kuxhaus M 1978 The results of non-operative management of stiff joints in the hand. Journal of Plastic and Reconstructive Surgery 61: 58–63

Weeks P M, Wray C R (eds) 1978 Management of the stiff hand. In: Management of acute hand injuries, 2nd edn. C V Mosby, St Louis

Welsh R P, Hastings D E 1977 Swan-neck deformity in rheumatoid arthritis of the hand. Hand. 9: 109–116

Wilson R L 1981 RA: interphalangeal joints presentation, ASSH Annual Meeting, Las Vegas

Wilson R L, Carter M S 1984a Management of hand fractures. In: Hunter J, Schneider L, Mackin E, Callahan A (eds) Rehabilitation of the hand. C V Mosby, St Louis

Wilson R L, Carter M S 1984b Joint injuries in the hand: preservation of proximal interphalangeal joint function. In: Hunter J, Schneider L, Mackin E, Callahan A (eds) Rehabilitation of the hand C V Mosby, St Louis

S. Harkins Torkelson

15 Splinting the interphalangeal joints

Splinting the interphalangeal joints of the hand requires knowledge of the natural, untreated course of each diagnosed injury or disease process and the intervention necessary to prevent such an end. Splinting is a changeable, temporary management of many of these interphalangeal (IP) joint problems and must be used in conjunction with rest, hand therapy and exercise. Close continuous evaluation is required. Gone are the days of dispensing a commercial splint to the patient and releasing him for a month or more.

The case of the fixed, flexed proximal interphalangeal (PIP) joint is common and the history is usually related as: injury, self-treatment, medical consultation, immobilization, and perhaps some vigorous, passive and painful therapy. Ill-fitting commercial splints may have been used with a forced rehabilitation programme. The patient has become frustrated with his lack of progress and with his increasing disability due to pain and stiffness. If by referral or chance a hand team is asked to see this patient—a great opportunity awaits.

The patient's confidence is gained by the statement that therapy should not hurt. Joint range of motion is measured and the programme begins. Normal joint anatomy, the pathology present in the patient's hand, the game plan of the surgeon and therapist, and the natural expected course of the rehabilitation are all discussed. The pitfalls of non-compliance and the great weight of patient responsibility are emphasized. The patient should quickly become aware of the therapist's respect for the injured anatomy. He should leave the clinic more relaxed than when he arrived.

GENERAL PRINCIPLES

It is the therapist's responsibility to have reviewed thoroughly the patient's history with the surgeon. Operative notes, office notes, X-rays, and the patient's story are essential to the proper choice of treatment and splints. It is necessary to assess the patient's level of compliance, his understanding of the treatment and its goals, and the estimated time necessary to reach these goals. The therapist is sending the patient out to be his own therapist, splint monitor, hygienist, and protector until he returns. Precautions should be made clear and often written. The patient should be donning and removing his splints with confidence. If the therapist does not have a clear view of the rehabilitation course and its desired outcome, the patient cannot be expected to cooperate at the level required.

Koch & Mason (1939) described three purposes for splinting after hand injuries:

1. Securing rest for injured and inflamed tissues whether soft, tendon, muscle, joint capsule, or bone
2. Securing relaxation of muscles with divided tendons or an injured nerve supply
3. Bringing constant and prolonged tension to bear upon scar tissue, the gradual contraction of which interferes with the function of the hand

Immobilization and rest of injured tissues are very important but care should be taken that there is the least possible fixation of adjacent structures. This is especially important in the hand because of the closely articulating joints and their complex functional patterns (Peacock 1953). Kuczynski (1968) warned that the PIP joint should not be immobilized for too long and that extension contractures follow trauma to the extensors or longstanding immobilization. He also noted the dangers of immobilizing the PIP joints in greater than 15° of flexion. Bunnell (1944) described the efficacy of slow persistent, steady stretch just under that which would rupture the tissues when treating soft tissue contractures. He suggested semi-rigid splints to draw out the contracture and active dynamic splints to maintain the correction. Moberg (1964) preferred 'active' splinting at all times over static splints.

Static splints maintain a joint in a desired position and have no moving parts. Dynamic splints allow for or provide motion (Hopkins & Smith 1978). Therapists use static splints 'dynamically' as in serial casting, progressive splinting, or the patient-adjusted web straps. Clearly, there is controversy about the exact designation of these splint types. For clarity, the terms 'dynamic' and 'static' will be used in the strict sense—dynamic as splints with moving parts, static as splints with no moving parts.

DESIGN: FORM FOLLOWS FUNCTION

Consider the packaging of eggs for the market. Twelve fragile objects in a lightweight paper carton, protected only by the fit and design of the carton. The fit and design of splints for individual digits are no less important. With a poor design, one's treatment goals will not be met and with a poor fit, even the best design is harmful.

Splinting individual digits is a challenge to every therapist. One who has splinted the arm or hand of an infant can remember his frustration with the usual splint materials, seeming suddenly cumbersome and oversized. The scaling-down-to-size necessary for the infant splint must also be done for finger splints to avoid interference with other digits. These splints should be light, strong, thin, well-fitted, and firmly attached to the digit. Herein lies the challenge (Fig. 15.1).

Ready-made commercial splints are rarely used by hand therapists. Exceptions are the Stack mallet splint (Link America Inc., 10 Great Meadow Lane,

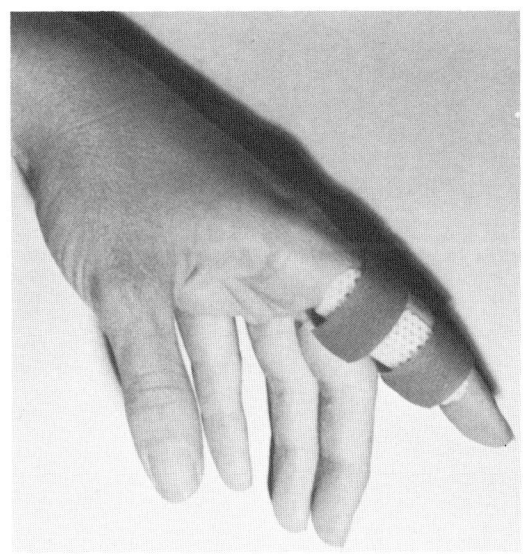

Fig. 15.1 Thin perforated thermoplastic material with 16 mm (⅝ inch) straps for immobilization of only the PIP joint.

East Hanover, NJ 07936, USA) (Fig. 15.2), the LMB wirefoam splints (LMB Hand Rehab Products, PO Box 1181, San Luis Obispo, CA 93406, USA) (Fig. 15.3), the LMB mallet splint (Fig. 15.4), and occasionally some uses are found for the aluminium-backed foam splints. The usual splinting requested by a hand surgeon is custom work. Today's requirements to build a splint around surgical hardware in the finger and to allow

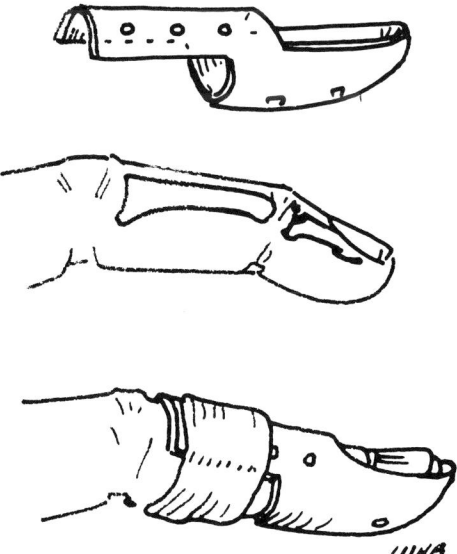

Fig. 15.2 Stack splint for mallet deformity.

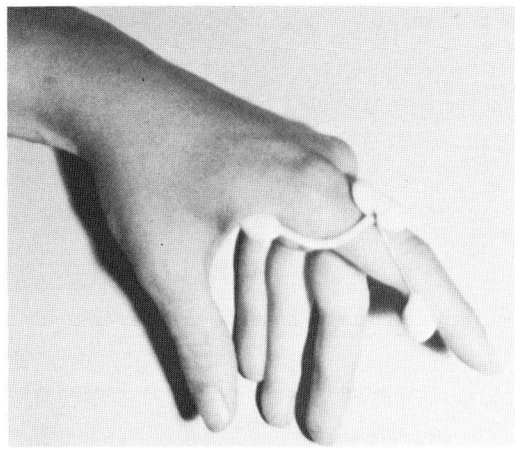

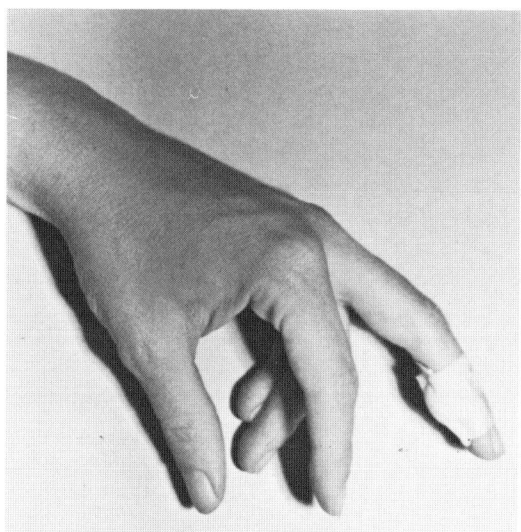

Fig. 15.4 LMB mallet splint for distal interphalangeal joint immobilization.

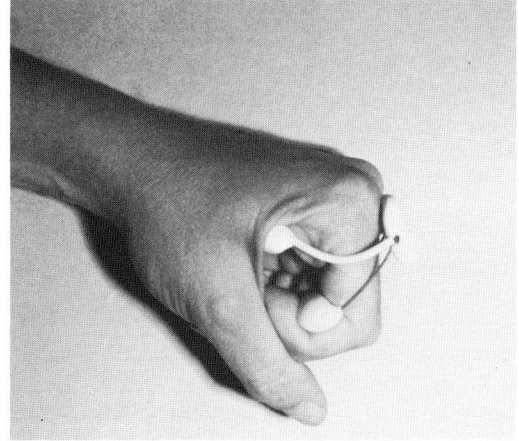

Fig. 15.3 LMB wirefoam splint—dynamic PIP joint extension—allows full active flexion.

only certain motion limits can best be accomplished with thermoplastic materials.

The attraction of the low temperature thermoplastics is that they are easily moulded to the hand. This allows the splint to fit the hand, not as historically, making the hand fit the splint (Colditz 1984a). The thinnest material available is 1.6 mm ($\frac{1}{16}$ inch) thick and is available in smooth or perforated form (WFR Corporation, PO Box 215, Ramsey, NJ 07446, USA). Changes in the splint can easily be made as healing occurs in the digit.

Thermoplastic finger splints are rarely padded because they are small and because *fit* is most important. Only if the padding is added in the 'plastic' phase of fabrication can the fit be preserved. A thin lining such as moleskin, gauze or perhaps a sock for the finger usually does not compromise the splint's fit if one thickness is used.

The gutter splint

The gutter is the most common design used in thermoplastic splinting of the fingers. The gutter may be dorsal (Fig. 15.5), volar (Fig. 15.6), or both (clamshell or bivalve splint). The splint type and the materials used are chosen depending on the diagnosis and objective. The form of the splint thus follows the function it must serve for the finger.

Serial cylinder casting

Serial casting was described by Brand (1952) and Bell (1984) as a painless and effective method of reducing flexion contractures of the PIP joints no matter how longstanding the deformity (Fig. 15.7). This method requires close follow-up and accurate assessment of joint range of motion with each cast change. The casts are changed every 2–5 d depending on the patient's situation. Removable casts are preferred so that active range of motion may be performed.

Easy removal of the plaster cast may not be possible until the contracture is less than 30° and the joint less swollen. A trap-door (Fig. 15.8) may be cut into the cast with scissors, but care must be taken that there are no tiny plaster particles loose under the cast. The casts then remove and replace

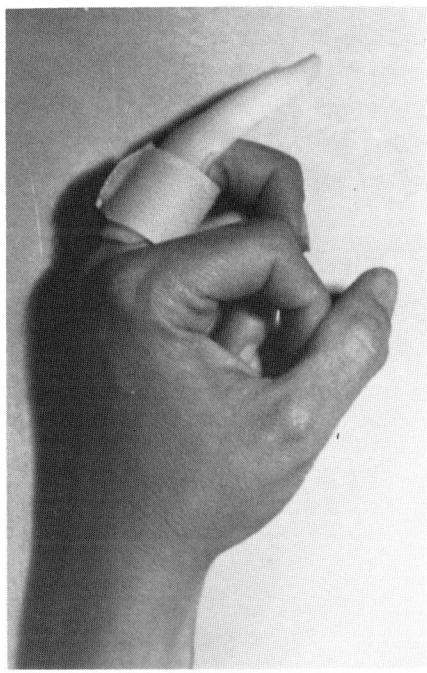
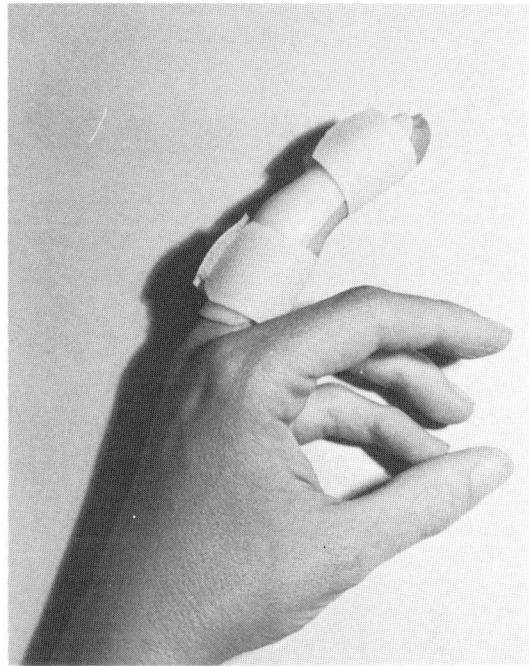

Fig. 15.5 Dorsal blocking splint—gutter type.

easily with Vaseline or lanolin. The finger should always be lubricated before the cast is replaced so that there is a minimum of scraping over the PIP joint with the cast. The course of casting usually begins with 24 h per day casting and removal only for brief exercise. This gradually tapers off to night casting or dynamic splinting. This progression may take several weeks to achieve the desired result.

An excellent step-by-step approach to the casting is described by Bell (1984) and will not be repeated here. The following are special points of emphasis:

1. No padding is placed under the cast. These are form-fitted casts and nothing but anhydrous lanolin should interface the plaster and skin during moulding

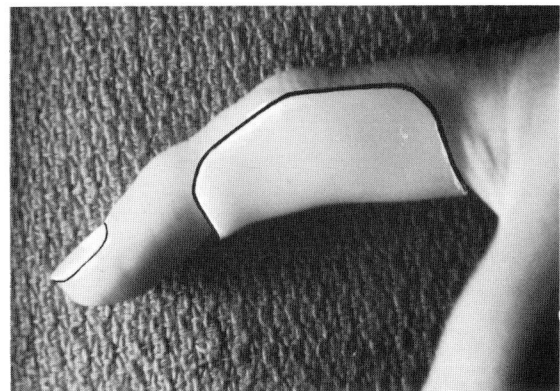

Fig. 15.6 Volar gutter splint.

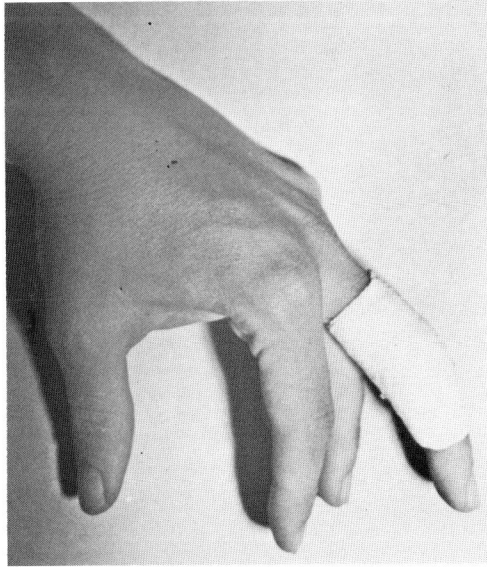

Fig. 15.7 Cylinder cast PIP joint.

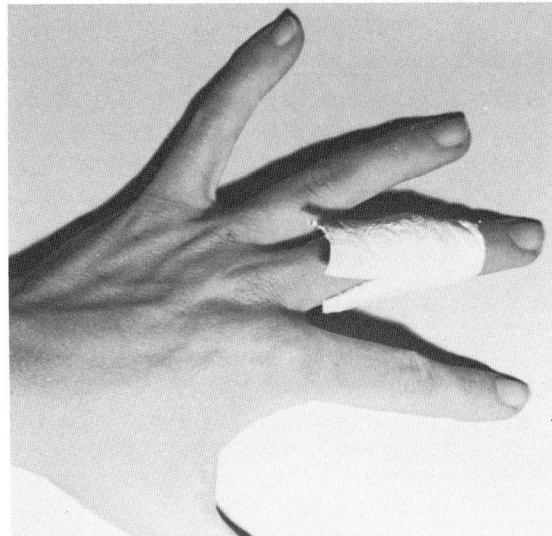

Fig. 15.8 Cylinder cast with trap door for easy removal.

2. Some traction and joint extension are performed during the plaster setting phase, after wrapping and during the smoothing. This force should be comfortable to the patient and not a painful stretch. The smoothing along with the joint manipulation is an acquired art

3. The metacarpophalangeal and distal interphalangeal joint creases should be visible after the cast is finished. This assures free motion at the joints which are not splinted (Fig. 15.9)

4. No pressure should be placed on the dorsum of the PIP joint during the setting of the cast. It is tempting to assist the extension force during setting but it is a sure way to cause an ischaemic ulcer of the skin beneath the cast indentation

5. Often the cast becomes loose the day after it is placed on the finger. This looseness is not desirable as motion can then occur in the cast and the rubbing may create a pressure area. It is best to replace the cast if the patient reports looseness. A well-fitting cast is essential.

Bell (1984) emphasized that this technique is not to be used in a flexion contracture that can be treated with a dynamic splint. Casting is best used with difficult contractures yielding to no other treatment. *Flexion* should be acceptable *before extension* casting is utilized.

Two-stage casting may be necessary for swan-neck or boutonnière deformity (Bell 1986). One joint is set in its desired position and the plaster is allowed to harden. The second joint is then positioned and casted.

Call it the 'inevitability of gradualness', or allowing tissues to 'grow longer' (Brand 1952), or plastic elongation when subjected to constant tension (Kottke et al 1966); the method works well

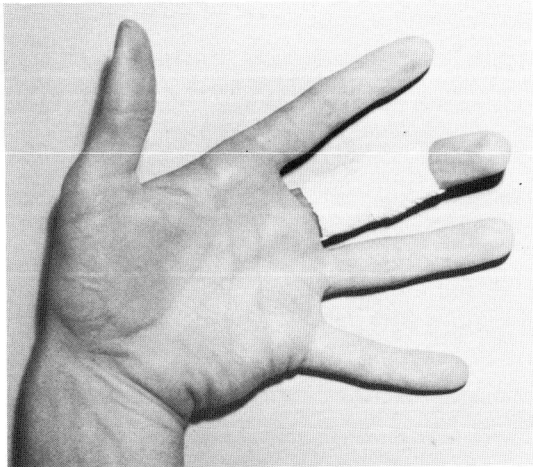

Fig. 15.9 PIP joint cylinder cast. MP and distal interphalangeal joint creases are visible to ensure full adjacent joint motion.

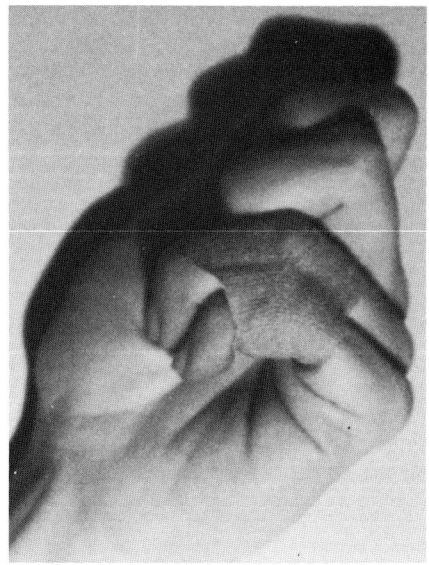

Fig. 15.10 Buddy taping using an elastic self-adhering material (Coban).

and painlessly through a prolonged stretch at moderate tension rather than a short duration, intense stretch. Patients are generally delighted with their quick progress and lack of discomfort.

BUDDY TAPING

This is a tried and true method of protection, prevention, assistance, and a free ride for adjacent digits (Fig. 15.10, 15.11). The buddy splint is usually made of 'velcro' (Aplix Co., Box 7505, Charlotte, NC 28217, USA) or Coban (3-M Corp., Medical Products Div., St Paul, MN 55101, USA) and carries one finger with another for any number of reasons. The buddy system is commonly used following collateral ligament injury to the PIP joint. The injured finger is taped to the adjacent finger on the injured side to prevent lateral stress to the injured joint. This taping can prevent shortening of the remaining collateral ligament complex in the absence of its partner. The buddy taping can act as an assist for the adjacent finger if it is unable to move passively through its range of motion. The taping can give a free ride to a digit lacking active motion such as in the Hunter stage I tendon reconstruction programme. Insensitive digits may be safer when carried with a sensate friend. Habitus or disuse tendencies will be curbed by buddy taping to an active finger. Carrying the little finger with the ring finger can be tricky as there is little, if any, common middle phalangeal area. One solution is to attach the buddy taping to the middle phalanx of the little finger and the proximal and middle phalangeal segments of the ring finger (see Fig. 15.11).

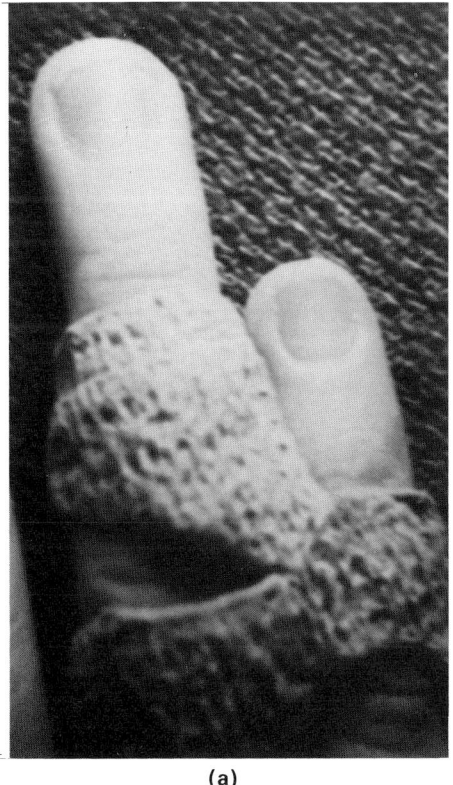
(a)

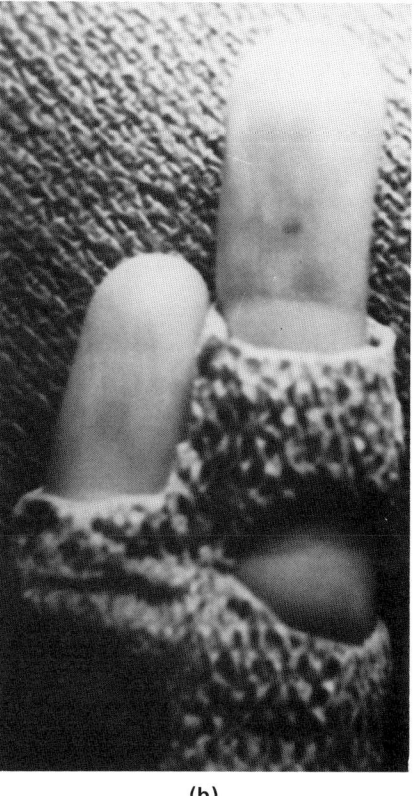
(b)

Fig. 15.11 (a) Dorsal and (b) volar views of Coban buddy taping for little and ring fingers.

DYNAMIC IP JOINT SPLINTS

There is general agreement among hand therapists that gentle exercise and long-term splinting to maintain gains accomplish more with stiff joints than vigorous passive exercises without splinting. The goal of dynamic splinting is to increase range of motion by the gradual lengthening of tissues. The splint tolerated well at low tension for a longer time is many times more useful than a high tension, painful, not-often-worn splint. Dynamic splinting takes advantage of the plastic properties of delicate anatomy and aims at long-term results. This is the soft therapy path, based on the belief that solid, gradual gains will last over time.

Wynn-Parry (1973) described the construction of the spring wire splint for correction of flexion or extension weakness in the fingers. The splint is more commonly known as the Capener splint, after its original designer.

Colditz (1983) described the step-by-step fabrication of the modified Wynn-Parry splint for correction of flexion deformities at the PIP joint and she exhorts its high patient tolerance and custom fit (Fig. 15.12). The spring wire coils are placed exactly at the PIP joint axis of motion so that the force is applied correctly. No finger is 'unfittable' with this splint which has a three-point-pressure design. It is best used with mild flexion contractures (45° or less). Colditz suggests that patients with full flexion of the PIP joint should use the splint while sleeping and remove it during daily activity. Should the deformity recur, the splint is worn all the time but removed for exercises. If almost the entire day passes without recurrence, then the splint is recommended for night wear only.

Other finger-based dynamic splints commonly used are:

1. LMB finger springs (LMB Hand Rehab Products, PO Box 1181, San Luis Obispo, CA 93406, USA). These splints are light, wirefoam constructions which come in a variety of sizes with variable tension. Two splints are for extension assist; one stronger than the other (see Fig. 15.3). One design is for flexion assist of the PIP joint

2. The Joint Jack (Joint Jack, 198 Millstone Road, Glastonbury, CT 06033, USA). This is a turnbuckle, wedge type of splint which has low tolerance by patients due to the pressure placed over the PIP joint dorsally and the DIP joint volarly. This is similar to the safety-pin splint (Bunnell 1924)

3. Bunnell knucklebender and reverse knuckle-

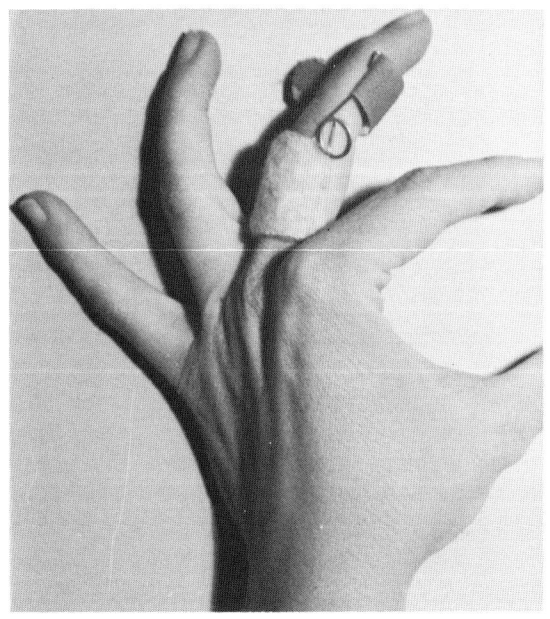

Fig. 15.12 Modified Wynn Parry PIP joint extension splint.

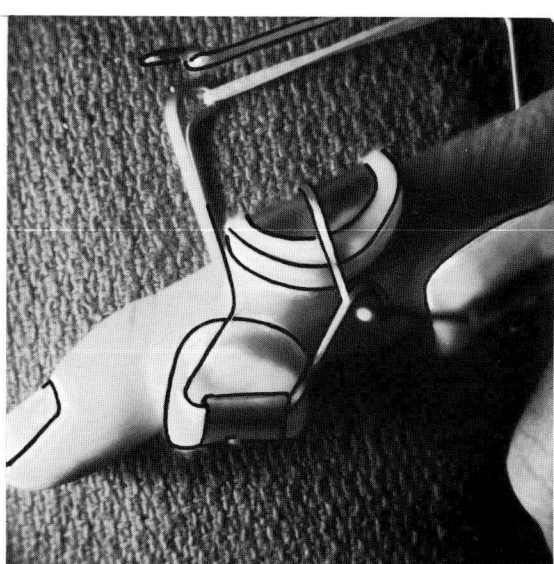

Fig. 15.13 Bunnell reverse knucklebender for PIP joint extension—rubber-band force.

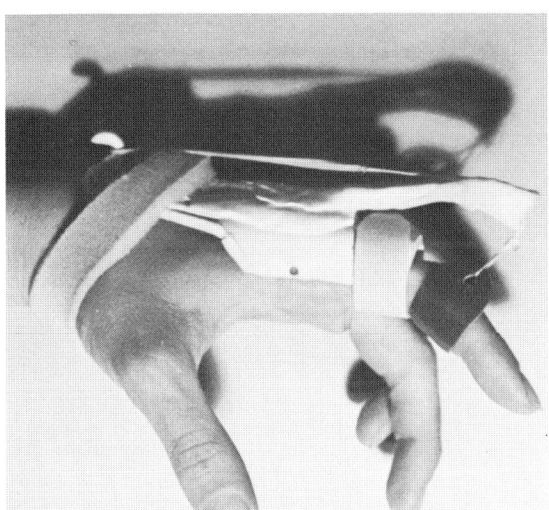

Fig. 15.14 Custom hand-based PIP joint extension splint with MP extension block.

bender (Bunnell & Howard 1950) splints. These splints are high-profile finger splints which use rubber-band force to flex or extend, respectively, the PIP joint. This is also a three-point-pressure splint. Pressure from the pads cause complaints from patients and fitting is sometimes difficult (Fig. 15.13)

4. Capener PIP extension splint and flexion splint for the PIP joints. This is similar to the modified Wynn-Parry splint for extension but delivers extension with less force (LMB Hand Rehab Products, PO Box 1181, San Luis Obispo, CA 93406, USA).

Hand-based dynamic splints usually provide metacarpophalangeal (MP) joint blocking for more effective work at the IP joints (Fig. 15.14). They are useful also when two or more digits on the same hand need splinting and digital splints would compromise hand usage. They offer the advantage of MP joint control (MP flexion with IP extension assist for flexion contracture, or MP extension with IP flexion assist for intrinsic tightness or dorsal scarring). Low profile dynamic splints as described by Colditz (1983) make this type of splint more attractive to the patient than the older more imposing designs.

Dynamic daytime splinting can be combined with progressive static night splinting to maintain daily gains in motion. Other types of splints acting 'dynamically' on the IP joints are the flexion gloves, rubber-band traction for flexion, small web straps flexing only the IP joints, and web straps which are usually made of Coban, 'velcro', or webbing with buckles wrapped in a figure-of-eight pattern for flexion of the fingers.

SPLINTING FOR CERTAIN PROBLEMS: SUGGESTIONS

Table 15.1 is a brief guideline to the current splinting used for IP joint problems. It is by no means the only way to manage these problems.

PERSPECTIVE

Splinting can assume many forms for many solutions to hand management problems. Close follow-up is essential with any splint to assure continued fit and need. Range of motion measurements and hand function are the ultimate yardstick for measuring successful splinting. Winning the battle but losing the war is not a valid strategy. Small joints gains at the expense of a person's livelihood and total hand function is not the goal of splinting the IP joints of the hand.

Table 15.1 Splinting for interphalangeal joint problems: suggestions

Problem	Goal	Splint description	Splint duration	Comments
Mallet finger (Stark et al 1962, Harris & Rutledge 1972, Stack 1969)	Maintain DIP joint extension	Stack mallet splint LMB mallet splint Dorsal alumnafoam	Maintain for 5–6 weeks	Allow *no* flexion of DIP joint Do not hyperextend the DIP joint in the splint
Swan neck deformity (Bell 1986)	Prevent PIP hyperextension	LMB 601 splint Dorsal block splint 2-stage casting		
Boutonnière deformity (Bell 1984, 1986, Souter 1974)	Decrease flexion contracture of PIP joint and increase DIP joint flexion	LMB 501, 502, 602 splints Volar gutter splint Cylinder casting PIP 2-stage casting		DIP joint must be left free for flexion

Problem	Goal	Splint description	Splint duration	Comments
Collateral ligament rupture (Redlar & Williams 1967, Bowers 1983)	Stability and healing following repair (immobilize)	Cylinder cast in full extension Volar gutter splint	3–4 weeks	Must provide good immobilization for adequate healing
	Allow protected motion of digit	Buddy taping	At 4 weeks full time	Watch out for inadvertent rotation of digit
Volar plate arthroplasty (Eaton & Malerich 1980)	Disallow full PIP joint extension	Dorsal block splint	3 weeks	Allow full flexion
	Regain extension	Dynamic PIP extension splint Buddy taping for protected motion	6 weeks	Only use if needed for extension by 6 weeks
PIP capsulectomy				
For extensor contracture PIP	Gain flexion of PIP joint	Alternate dynamic flexion and extension splints		Institute intrinsic stretch exercises
For flexion contracture PIP (Laseter 1984)	Gain extension of PIP joint	Volar extension splint (gutter type)	Full time	Remove splint for flexion exercises and replace
Collateral ligament sprains (Bowers 1983)	Prevent further injury to the joint	Buddy taping	1 month	
Dorsal dislocation of PIP joint (Bowers 1983, Eaton 1985)	Maintain reduction 30° PIP joint flexion	Dorsal gutter splint to block full extension	5–6 weeks	Do not allow full extension
	Protected motion	Buddy taping	At 6 weeks	
	Regain lost extension	Dynamic extension splint	After 6 weeks	Only if flexion deformity persists
PIP implant arthroplasty				
Stiff finger	Regain 0–70° active ROM	Volar or dorsal gutter with full PIP extension	Night wear	More time in splint if extension lag
Swan-neck	Regain 10–70° active ROM	Dorsal gutter 10–20° flexion at PIP joint		
	Obtain flexion contracture PIP joint			
	Extend DIP joint	K-wired or splinted in extension		
Boutonnière (Swanson et al 1984)	Maintain PIP extension Obtain 0–70° active ROM	Volar gutter PIP joint full extension, leave DIP joint free		
Extension contracture or dorsal skin tightness	Regain full flexion	LMB 601 Serial splinting Serial casting Hand-based dynamic IP flexion splint Flexion glove Web straps		Probably will require night and day splinting
Camptodactyly (Smith & Kaplan 1968)	Gain full PIP joint extension	Static volar gutter in progressive extension Serial casting	Night wear	
Lateral PIP dislocation (Bowers 1983, Eaton 1985)	Immobilize then protected motion	Dorsal gutter PIP 20–30° flexion	2–3 weeks	No motion
		Buddy taping to adjacent digit on injured side	Full time for 3–4 weeks	Careful active ROM
Pseudoboutonnière (Bowers 1983)	Regain PIP joint extension	Static extension splint for PIP joint with DIP joint left free		May need intrinsic stretch exercises
Joint fusions	Protect hardware and fusion	Volar gutter splints	Full time until solid	*No* motion or trauma

PIP: proximal interphalangeal
DIP: distal interphalangeal
ROM: range of motion
IP: interphalangeal

REFERENCES

Bell J A 1984 Plaster cylinder casting for contractures of the interphalangeal joints. In: Hunter J M, Schneider L H, Mackin E J, Callahan A D (eds) Rehabilitation of the hand, 2nd edn. C V Mosby, St Louis, ch 79, pp 875–880

Bell J A 1986 Cylinder casting. In: Fess E E, Philips C A (eds) Hand splinting principles and methods, 2nd edn. C V Mosby, St Louis (in press)

Bowers W H 1983 Management of small joint injuries in the hand. Orthopedic Clinics of North America 14: 793–810

Brand P W 1952 The reconstruction of the hand in leprosy. Annals of the Royal College of Surgeons of England 11: 350

Bunnell S 1924 Reconstructive surgery of the hand. Surgery, Gynecology and Obstetrics 39: 259–274

Bunnell S 1944 Surgery of the hand. J B Lippincott, Philadelphia, pp 200–202

Bunnell S, Howard L D 1950 Additional elastic hand splints. Journal of Bone and Joint Surgery 32A: 226–228

Colditz J C 1983 Low profile dynamic splinting of the injured hand. American Journal of Occupational Therapy 37: 182–188

Colditz J C 1984a Dynamic splinting of the stiff hand. In: Hunter J M, Schneider L H, Mackin E J, Callahan A D (eds) Rehabilitation of the hand, 2nd edn. C V Mosby, St Louis, ch 19, p 233

Colditz J C 1984b Spring-wire splinting of the proximal interphalangeal joint. In: Hunter J M, Schneider L H, Mackin E J, Callahan A D (eds) Rehabilitation of the hand, 2nd edn. C V Mosby, St Louis, ch 78, pp 862–874

Eaton R G 1985 Acute and chronic ligamentous injuries of the fingers and thumb. In: Tubiana R (ed) The hand Vol. II. W B Saunders, Philadelphia, ch 92, pp 880–887

Eaton R G, Malerich M M 1980 Volar plate arthroplasty of the PIP joint—a review of ten years experience. Journal of Hand Surgery 5: 260–268

Harris C, Rutledge G L 1972 The functional anatomy of the extensor mechanism of the finger. Journal of Bone and Joint Surgery 54A: 713–726

Hopkins H L, Smith H D (eds) 1978 Willard and Spackman's occupational therapy, 5th edn. J B Lippincott, Philadelphia, pp 731–738

Koch S L, Mason M L 1939 Purposeful splinting following injuries of the hand. Surgery, Gynecology and Obstetrics 68: 1–16

Kottke F J, Pauley D L, Ptak R A 1966 The rationale for prolonged stretching for correction of shortening of connective tissue. Archives of Physical Medicine and Rehabilitation 47: 345–352

Kuczynski K 1968 The proximal interphalangeal joint. Journal of Bone and Joint Surgery 50B: 656–663

Laseter G F 1984 Postoperative management of capsulectomies. In: Hunter J M, Schneider L H, Mackin E J, Callahan A D (eds) Rehabilitation of the hand, 2nd edn. C V Mosby, St Louis, ch 21, pp 246–252

LMB Hand Rehab Products 1984 Guidelines for use of LMB finger springs. Package insert.

Moberg E 1964 Dressings, splints and postoperative care in hand surgery. Surgery Clinics of North America 44: 941–949

Peacock E E 1953 Management of conditions of the hand requiring immobilization. Surgery Clinics of North America (Oct): 1297–1309

Redler I, Williams J T 1967 Rupture of a collateral ligament of the proximal interphalangeal joint of the fingers. Journal of Bone and Joint Surgery 49A: 322–326

Smith R J, Kaplan E B 1968 Camptodactyly and similar atraumatic flexion deformities of the PIP joints of the fingers. Journal of Bone and Joint Surgery 50A: 1187–1203

Souter W A 1974 The problem of boutonniere deformity. Clinical Orthopedics and Related Research 104: 116–133

Stack H G 1969 Mallet finger. Hand 1: 83–87

Stark H H, Boyes J H, Wilson J N 1962 Mallet finger. Journal of Bone and Joint Surgery 44A: 1061–1068

Swanson A B, Swanson G de G, Leonard J 1984 Postoperative rehabilitation programs in flexible implant arthroplasty of the digits. In: Hunter J M, Schneider L H, Mackin E J, Callahan A D (eds) Rehabilitation of the hand, 2nd edn. C V Mosby, St Louis, ch 61, pp 675–677

Wynn-Parry C B 1973 Rehabilitation of the hand, 3rd edn. Butterworths, Boston, pp 63–69

S. Bittinger

16 The art of joint mobilization: the restoration of joint play

INTRODUCTION

Hand rehabilitation, as a specialized field, utilizes a variety of treatment techniques including traditional massage and range of motion, biofeedback, transcutaneous nerve stimulation and joint mobilization—a specialized technique of obtaining range of motion.

This chapter defines and analyzes the specialized technique of joint mobilization (or more properly designated restoration of joint play) as it applies to the evaluation and treatment of the proximal interphalangeal (PIP) joint. It must be noted that this method is difficult to apply effectively to the distal interphalangeal joint because of its short skeletal levers.

A review of PIP joint anatomy is necessary in order to understand joint mobilization. This is well covered in Chapter 1 and should now be reviewed. Every therapist has on one occasion or another been awed, frustrated, perplexed or discouraged by the complexity of the PIP joint, and for good reasons. First, patients with PIP joint problems comprise the majority of the hand population that we evaluate and treat. Second, there are eight PIP joints per patient. Third, these joints are located at the end of the extremities where risk of injury is great. Lastly, the PIP joint is difficult to rehabilitate due to its anatomic composition.

Two anatomical points that are basic yet vitally significant to joint mobilization are (1) the PIP joint is small; the surface area is less than 100 mm^2. It is known that the smaller the surface the greater the effect of external forces (such as rubber-band tension, dynamic splinting, or passive range of motion). (2) The structural parts of this small joint fit together in a precise, compact design, providing stability, yet allowing mobility. Any alteration in the amount of space which these structures occupy is devastating to the function of this joint. Oedema is the major pathophysiological condition that alters the size of these joint elements. The collateral ligaments are lax in extension, but the joint remains stable due to the position of the volar plate. The volar plate is lax in flexion, but the joint remains stable due to the taut collateral ligaments (see Fig. 1.7). Due to the anatomical configuration of the distal end of the proximal phalanx (the condyles are flared) (see Fig. 1.8), the collateral ligaments ride over an asymmetric surface. Thus, although no change in ligament length occurs, the ligament tension does change. In the presence of oedema, the joint tends to take the midrange position, unable to flex or extend fully. The added space the oedema occupies does not allow the collateral ligaments to lengthen fully, hence, the inability of the joint to flex fully. The volar plate likewise with its unwelcome oedema cannot lengthen fully, hence, limiting full joint extension. Oedema must be attended to before full joint motion can be expected.

LITERATURE REVIEW

A review of the literature as recorded by Paris (1965) reveals none other than Hippocrates to be the first in recorded history to describe and illustrate joint mobilization (460–365 BC) in at least three works. In one entitled 'On setting joints by leverage', he describes the combination of extension (traction) and pressure (manipulation) exerted on a patient lying prone on a wooden bed. Considering these works are over 2000 years old, it makes one wonder how much we have accomplished both in practice and in acceptance of this modality. A further note extracted from Paris (1965) cites well-known contributors such as Galen (138–201) with his extensive teachings on fractures and dislocations. In 1543 Versalius described human anatomy through actual cadaver dissections which gave us a better understanding of the flexibility of tissue and the composition of joints. Thirty-six years later, Pare, a surgeon, utilized trunk supports and manipulation. Later in the 18th century, John Hunter (1728–1793) was teaching the value of movement of joints after injury in order to prevent stiffness and adhesions, and P. H. Ling (1776–1839) was perhaps the first authority to speak on the treatment of the sympathetic nervous system by manipulative therapy. In the 19th century Sir James Padgett (1814–1899) reported too long a rest as the most frequent cause of delayed recovery after the injury of joints, both those injured and those kept at rest because parts near them had been injured.

Contemporary authors who have contributed to this area are Cyriax (1975), Cyriax & Schiots (1975), Maigne (1965), Mennell (1964), Zohn & Mennell (1976), Paris (1965), Maitland (1977, 1978, 1980) and Kaltenborn (1980). Each employs his own school of thought and treatment emphasis.

THEORETICAL BASIS/DEFINITION

Terms synonymous with joint mobilization include manual therapy, manipulative therapy and restoration of joint play. It is a means to restore the functional range of motion sacrificed through prolonged immobilization, trauma or other pathological conditions. This technique requires only the clinician's hands and expertise. Although clinically simple to perform, it is imperative that the examiner has at least a basic understanding of joint anatomy, physiology and kinesiology, fundamental to quality hand rehabilitation.

The basis of Mennell's philosophy (Mennell 1964) is the pathological condition he calls 'joint dysfunction'. Joint dysfunction, as he uses the term, means the loss of joint movement that cannot be produced by the action of voluntary muscles, in contradistinction to the loss of a voluntary action of a joint. This non-voluntary movement of a joint is termed 'joint play'. To illustrate this motion, gently hold your left index finger in your right hand as if you were holding a golf club (Fig. 16.1 and see Fig. 16.4). Make sure your left hand is relaxed and gently distract your proximal phalanx in a longitudinal direction distally with your right golf grip. Notice the dimpling effect over the dorsum of your left metacarpophalangeal joint (Fig. 16.2). This movement cannot be reproduced by active contraction of any muscle group in the left hand. It is the laxity and flexibility of the normal ligamentous structures that allow this motion to occur. This motion can also occur in medial/lateral anterior/posterior and rotational directions. That joint play motions are small, often not more than 3.2 mm ($\frac{1}{8}$ inch) in any plane, does not mean that they are unimportant. In fact the performance of the gross voluntary movements of the synovial joints depend on the presence of these small involuntary movements. Their presence, not their range, is the basis of their importance.

Joint mobilization can and should be used in conjunction with other therapeutic modalities, such as active range of motion exercises, heat,

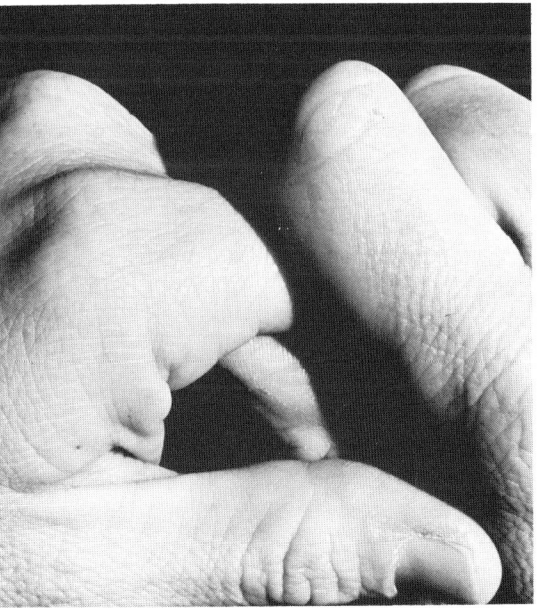

Fig. 16.1 Position of grip on digit if force is to be applied to metacarpophalangeal joint.

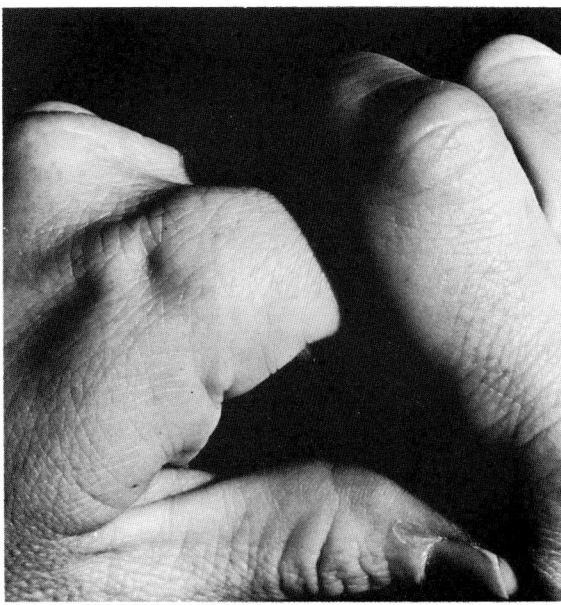

Fig. 16.2 'Dimpling' with long axis traction.

splinting, massage, and biofeedback. Mobilization of the PIP joint requires that the patient be relaxed as will be noted in the rules of manipulation which follow. Heat treatments as a relaxation modality are beneficial in preparation for mobilization. Joint mobilization is primarily employed when there is a loss of one or more movements in the normal range of joint play. This loss of motion may or may not be associated with pain, but definitely decreases functional ability. Although joint play movements are a prerequisite to joint motion, restoration of joint play does not mean necessarily that function will return; extra-articular tissue may need attention (skin contracture, extensor hood tightness, tendon contracture and dysfunction at or near adjacent joints which affect the involved PIP joint). Ligaments are living tissue that if short, will remain short but can be stimulated to become longer by adaptive lengthening. The key to overcoming elastic resistance or stiffness in a PIP joint is a slow, gentle stretching, accompanied by active exercise and serial splinting.

Example of joint mobilization programme

Step I Heat/relaxation techniques, biofeedback
Step II Mobilization
Step III Active range of motion (AROM) splinting

GOALS OF MOBILIZATION

The intermediate goals of mobilization are:

(1) To relieve pain

(2) To improve movement in a painless, stiff joint which does not have functional range

(3) To restore structures within a joint to their normal position

The ultimate goal is to allow the joint a full functional pain-free range of motion.

In order to determine whether mobilization can benefit a patient, the following must be obtained:

1. Discussion with referring physician regarding expectations and treatment
2. Complete patient history including age, hand dominance, occupation, and aetiology of joint stiffness, onset of injury, previous surgery affecting the involved joint, and current work status
3. Active and passive range of motion in all joints
4. Grip and pinch strengths if appropriate and bilateral
5. Intrinsic tightness is evaluated in affected as well as unaffected PIP joints
6. Tenodesis in affected as well as unaffected PIP joints
7. Sensory evaluation of affected extremity (not just affected digit)
8. Manual muscle test of affected and unaffected joints
9. Review of appropriate laboratory and radiographic results as they pertain to the joint problem
10. Patient goals
11. Family support
12. Assessment of pain, whether constant, at rest, during activity or a combination of factors, type, location, frequency, duration etc
13. Skin turgor, condition
14. Joint integrity: subluxed/dislocated, alignment, fusions, collateral ligament laxity, implants, volar plate laxity, surgical procedures, i.e. intrinsic releases etc
15. Prediction of residual function or potential: motivation, pending litigation, distance to therapy, other medical problems

Examination of joint play:

It is imperative that the patient be examined in a comfortable atmosphere—especially on the initial visit to the therapist. The examination should occur in a quiet area, not a busy clinic, otherwise the therapist may be easily distracted or the patient may not be able to relax fully. Joint play movements are small in range and their performance requires accuracy and precision. A distracted therapist and tense patient are wasting each other's time! The examiner's fingernails should be kept short so as not to pinch the patient's skin inadvertently during examination. Rings should be removed from the therapist and the patient to afford optimum sensory contact and no mechanical impingements. The position of the patient and therapist should be sitting adjacent to each other either on a mat or in chairs (Fig. 16.3).

MENNELL'S RULES OF MANIPULATION (1964)

1. Patient should be relaxed and the affected joint supported. Casual conversation and removal of tight fitting clothes may be helpful
2. The therapist must be relaxed. The examiner should not grab or tightly grip a joint or stretch the skin around it. The grasp must be firm, but not restrictive
3. Examine only one joint at a time. It is important to determine what entity is restricting joint motion. Is it a tight volar plate, tight collateral ligaments, restrictive dorsal capsule; bony impingement, skin contracture etc or any combination of the above?
4. Work on only one movement at each joint at a time. For instance, if there is an extension lag, restore extension primarily. Work on flexion with active motion rather than mobilization
5. There should always be a single mobilizing force and a single stabilizing force exerted on a joint. The therapist's hands should stabilize the joint to be mobilized proximally and the other hand should be the mobilizing force distal to that joint (Fig. 16.4)
6. To assess normal joint play, it is imperative to compare the 'feel' of the injured versus the uninjured joint on the unaffected hand. We are generally fortunate in our profession that most injuries we treat occur unilaterally; affording a 'control' side
7. No forceful or abnormal movements should be employed by the therapist mobilizing the injured joint
8. All manual techniques should be employed by the therapist mobilizing the injured joint
9. The collateral ligaments allow a certain amount of laxity around the joints and this laxity must be taken up before the manipulative movement can be performed

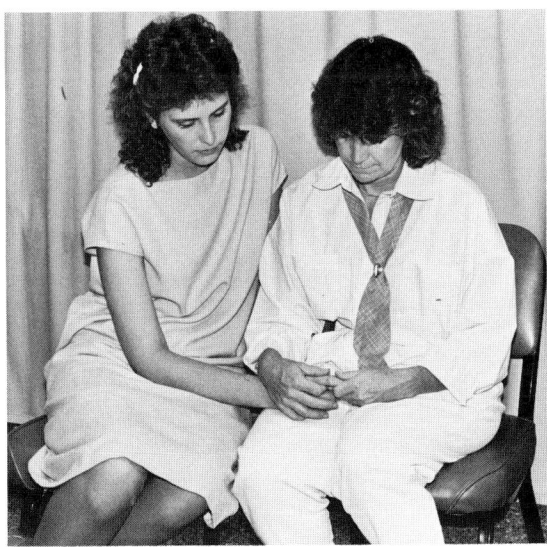

Fig. 16.3 Proper patient–therapist positioning.

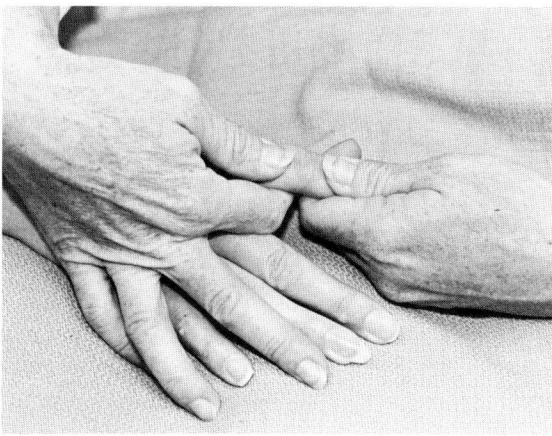

Fig. 16.4 Stabilizing hand (reader's left) and mobilizing hand (reader's right).

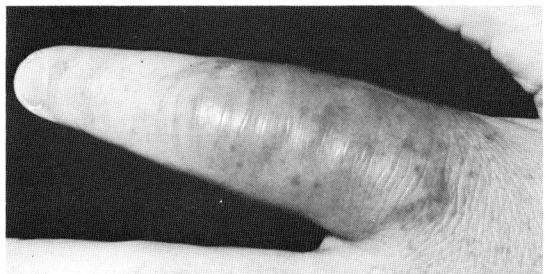

Fig. 16.5 Example of a digit which should not be mobilized.

10. No therapeutic movements need be or should be undertaken in the presence of clinical signs of joint or bone inflammation

INDICATIONS

Joint mobilization can be utilized with a variety of disorders. These include stiffness in joints secondary to prolonged casting, stiffness due to immobilization of the non-affected as well as affected joints, collateral ligaments, volar plate injuries, fractures in or about the interphalangeal joint and replants. Manipulative procedures can be utilized on other joints besides interphalangeal joints including the wrist, elbow, shoulder and other synovial joints. It is a treatment that is unique and specific for synovial joints. The clinician should be well aquainted with the 'feel' of joint play in normal joints in order to assess dysfunction in abnormal joints.

Contraindications for this modality are rheumatoid arthritis and osteoarthritis, implant, arthroplasty, infection, and acute injuries or inflammatory disorders (Fig. 16.5). The joint must be physiologically stable; that is at least 8 weeks' post injury. Time frames are not based on rules of thumb, but on an individual assessment of each patient.

TECHNIQUES

The joint must be distracted manually in order to perform the mobilization technique. Proper fixation of the joint is attained with the therapist's thumb touching over the joint to be mobilized (see Figs. 16.4 and 16.6).

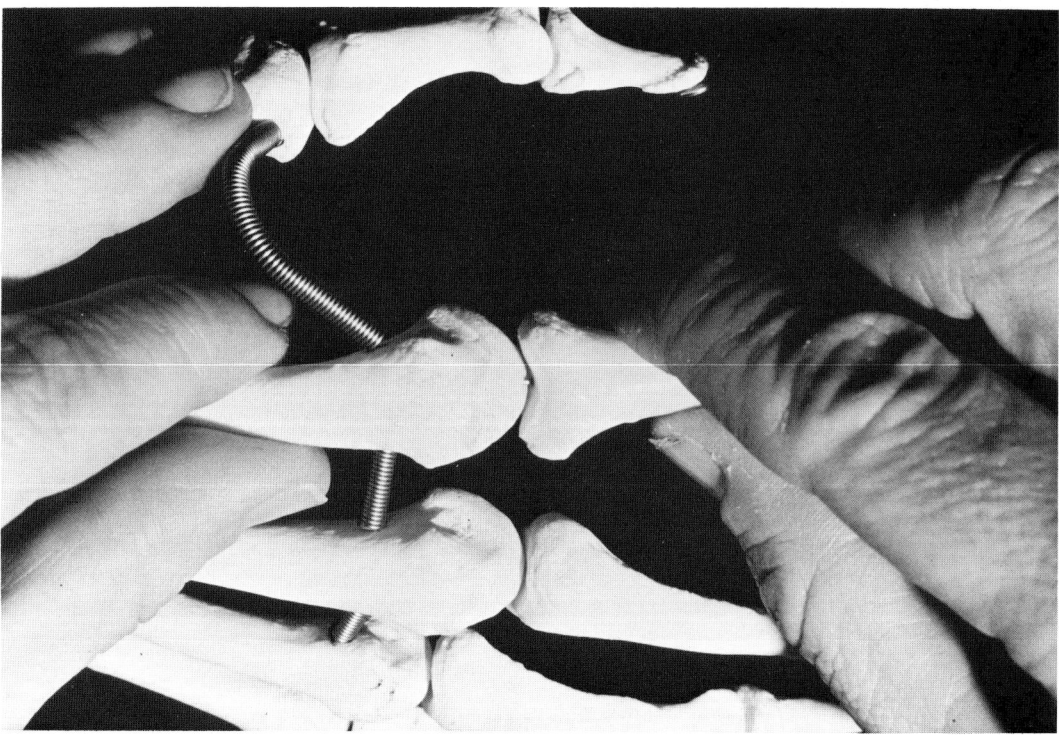

Fig. 16.6 Long axis traction.

1. Longitudinal traction

Long axis extension—the proximal phalanx is gently but firmly stabilized by one hand; the middle phalanx is slightly flexed (if possible). The skin is pushed together over the dorsum of the interphalangeal joint between the examiner's thumbs and the middle phalanx is gently, but firmly distracted in a straight line following the angle of the flexed phalanx until the laxity in the joint has been taken up. The middle phalanx is then further distracted only momentarily with a quick stretch and allowed immediately to spring back to its original state. This causes a slight stretch on the ligaments and volar plate.

2. Anterior/posterior glide

The examiner's thumbs are placed over dorsum of the proximal and middle phalanges in the same manner as long axis extension. The joint is gently, but firmly distracted in a straight line. While the joint is distracted, and the therapist's stabilizing hand is controlling the proximal phalanx; the therapist moves the middle phalanx in an anterior, then posterior plane (volar/dorsal). As the middle phalanx is moved in either direction, the slack is taken up; then a quick stretch is applied momentarily, allowing the middle phalanx to return to its resting position.

3. Rotation

The examiner's (therapist's) stabilizing hand is placed on the proximal phalanx in the same manner as the two previous techniques. However, the therapist places his/her mobilizing fingers laterally on the middle phalanx; distracts the phalanx and then rotates the phalanx in a clockwise then counter-clockwise direction (Fig. 16.7).

4. Medial/lateral tilt

The middle phalanx is gently distracted, then gently opened first in a radial and then in an ulnar direction (Fig. 16.8).

If assessment indicates a possible non-musculoskeletal problem and the patient is not responding, if the patient does not show progress after four to five treatments, or if the patient's condition is exacerbated, referral of the patient back to the physician is essential.

Joint mobilization is an art, and as with so many arts, not everyone can be expected to be able to learn to use it. Perhaps there are two main reasons why joint mobilization has not found the wide acceptance that it merits in the practice of medicine; first, the user has not learned the proper techniques, and second, the user is simply inept at the art. It is so much easier to blame a modality of treatment for failure than it is to blame someone

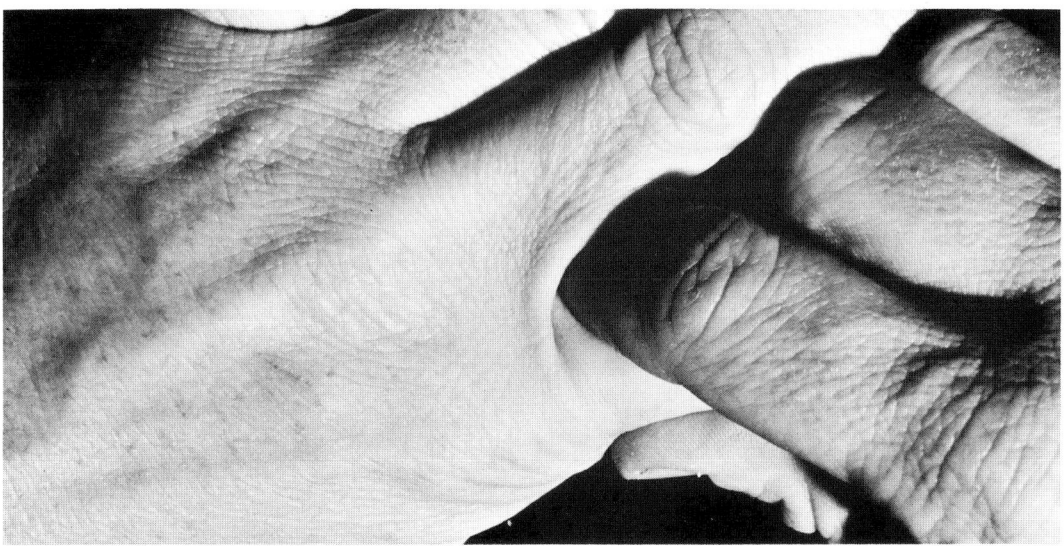

Fig. 16.7 Rotation.

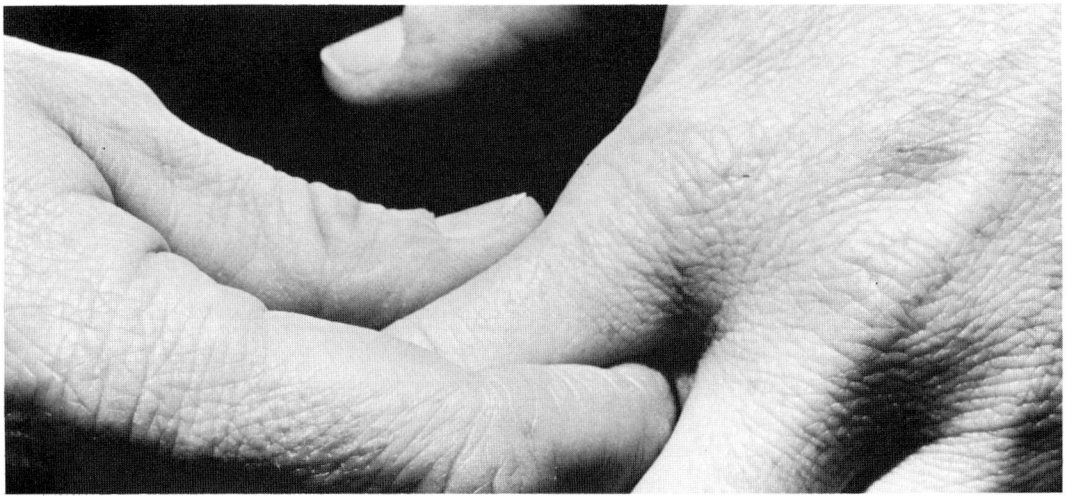

Fig. 16.8 Medial/lateral tilt.

who perhaps never should be using the modality in the first place. Mennell (1964) stresses there is one pitfall in teaching and learning these techniques. The therapist must learn to elicit the normal joint-play movements on the right and left extremities. It is essential to be ambidextrous in this field.

The present author's aim in this chapter has been to familiarize the treating registered or licensed therapist with the technique of joint mobilization as an adjunct to other therapeutic interventions. As with other treatment modalities, the clinician must obtain the proper schooling to utilize this valuable technique effectively to benefit the patient with a stiff or painful joint.

REFERENCES

Cyriax J 1975 Diagnosis of soft tissue lesions, textbook of orthopedic medicine: Vol I. Williams and Wilkins, Baltimore

Cyriax J, Schiotz E H 1975 Manipulation past and present. Heinemann, London

Kaltenborn F M 1980 Mobilization of extremity joints. Olaf Norlis Bokhandel, Oslo

Maigne R 1965 The concept of painlessness and opposite motion in spinal manipulation. American Journal of Physical Medicine 44: 55–59

Maitland G D 1977 Peripheral manipulation, 2nd edn. Butterworths, London

Maitland G D 1978 The hypothesis of adding compression when examining and treating synovial joints. Journal of Orthopedic and Sports Physical Therapy 2: 1–26

Maitland G D 1980 The development and possible future of manipulative therapy in Australia. Australian Journal of Physiotherapy 26: 63–66

Mennell J McM 1964 Joint pain: diagnosis and treatment using manipulative techniques. Little, Brown and Co, Boston

Paris S V 1965 The spinal lesion. Pegasus Press, Vashon Island, Washington, p 15–31

Zohn D A, Mennell J M 1976 Diagnosis and physical treatment, Muscloskeletal Pain. Little, Brown and Co, Boston

Index

Accessory collateral ligament, 4, 5, 12
  attachments, 5
  lateral stability and, 6, 7
Acetylsalicylic acid, 144
Active exercise programme, chronically stiff PIP joint, 236, 243, 244
Aminoglycosides, 147
Animal bites, 147
Apert's syndrome, 192
Arthrodesis, 16, 113, 116, 174–184
  bone graft, stability and, 181–182
  bone surface preparation, 175–177
  bone overgrowth, 167
  boutonnière deformity and, 128–129, 243
  complications, 183–184
  compression screws, 178–179
  external fixation, 182–183
  implant fracture, 167
  incisions, 175
  indications, 174
  infection and, 184
  intraosseous wiring, 179–180
  Kirschner wires, 177–178
  malunion, 184
  medullary peg, 180–181
  non-union, 183–184
  osteoarthritis and, 144, 145
  plate, 179
  position, 174–175
  psoriatic arthritis and, 135–136, 137
  splinting, 260
  scleroderma and, 139–140
  stabilization, 177–183
  swan-neck deformity and, 130, 131–132, 238
  systemic lupus erythematosus and, 138
  tension band wiring, 179
  thumb, 145
  vascular problems complicating, 184
Arthroplasty, 156–172
  active blocking exercises following, 246
  boutonnière deformity and, 242
  cemented-in prostheses, 144, 145, 157
  contraindications, 159
  DIP joint, 168
  dynamic splinting, 246
  heat in elevation, 245
  historical development, 157–158
  indications, 158–159
  metallic prosthetic replacements, 157
  microvascular transfer of joints, 170
  oedema control, 246
  osteoarthritis and, 144–145
  patient selection, 158–159
  perichondral arthroplasty of PIP joint, 172
  perioperative antibiotics, 167
  postoperative care/rehabilitation, 164–166, 245–246
  preoperative evaluation, 159
  psoriatic arthritis, 136
  resection arthroplasty, 157
  results, 166
  silastic implants, 157, 158
  silicone spacer arthroplasty, 144–145, 158
  silicone synovitis and, 167–168
  splinting, 260
  swan-neck deformity and, 132–133, 238
  systemic lupus erythematosus and, 138
  technique, 159, 160–164
  volar plate arthroplasty, 17, 168–170
Articular cartilage
  biochemistry, 142
  contusion, 188
  hydrodynamic lubrication and, 30
Atraumatic surgical technique, 14
Atypical mycobacteria, 146, 147
Avulsion injuries
  DIP joint, 112, 115, 116
  PIP joint, 77–78, 80–81, 100–104
    with central tendon rupture, 101
  pseudoboutonnière deformity, 98

Benign synovioma, see Pigmented villonodular synovitis
Biomechanics, 21–53
  balancing of moments between MP and PIP joints, 22–24
  balancing motion between IP joints, 24
  boundary lubrication, 29–30, 31
  boutonnière deformity, 53
  changing moment arms with flexion/extension of PIP joint, 45–50
  closely fitting synovial hinge joints, 29–31
  computer modelling, 26
  DIP joint
    extension moments, 43–44
    flexion strength, 42
  dorsal expansion reconstruction and, 32
  'drag', 29
  extension, 43–53
  flexion, 40–43
  flexion-extension moments, analysis of, 24–28
  flexor digitorum profundus (FDP), 40–41, 42
  free-body analysis of hand joints, 26–28
  hydrodynamic lubrication, 29–30
  hyperextension prevention, 50–51
  joint torque-angle measurements, see Torque-angle measurements
  kinematic chains, 21
  mathematical models and, 21
  MP joint, 44–45
  oedema fluid, 33–34
  PIP joint
    flexion strength, 43
    passive block to hyperextension, 51
  profundus tendon, estimate of tension, 27–28
  resistance to passive motion, 28–34
  sheets of tendon with relative motion, 32–33
  swan-neck deformity, 50, 52–53
  tendons with large bone interface, 31–32
  viscoelastic forces, 28
Blastomycosis, 146
Bone graft, arthrodesis and, 181–182
Bouchard's nodes, 143
Boundary lubrication, 29–30, 31

Boutonnière deformity, 32, 53, 95, 97, 98–99
  arthrodesis and, 128–129, 243
  arthroplasty and, 128, 129–130, 242
  attritional with intrinsic paralysis, 107
  biomechanics, 53
  burn boutonnière, 107
  central slip injury and, 233
  central slip reconstruction, 127, 128
  Dupuytren's contracture, 19
  extensor tendon tenotomy, 126, 127, 128, 242
  extrinsic tendon and, 95
  fixed, 107, 128–130, 242–243
  intermediate stage, 126–128, 242
  juvenile rheumatic arthritis and, 134, 135
  lateral band re-positioning, 127
  mobile, 104–107, 126, 240, 242
  post surgical exercise programme, 242
  retinacular fibres and, 95, 97
  rheumatic arthritis and, 121, 123, 126–130, 240–243
  serial cylinder casting, 256
  splinting, 242, 256, 259, 260
  stages of lesion, 97, 104–107, 126–130, 240, 242–243
  synovectomy, 126, 242
  systemic lupus erythematosus and, 137
  volar plate and, 17
Brachydactyly, 188
Buddy taping, 257–258
Bunnell knuckle bender, 259
Burn boutonnière deformity, 107

Calcium pyrophosphate deposition disease, 150
Campylodactyly, 200–201, 260
Capener PIP extension splint, 259
Capsule, 4–12
  dorsal elements, 4
  injuries, see Capsule injury
  innervation, 12
  lateral elements, 4–5
  lateral stability and, 5–8
  sheath relationships, 12
  volar, see Volar plate
  see also Collateral ligament system
Capsule injury, 56–75
  acute, 59–68
  classification, 59–60
  contracture following, 56, 58, 68–69
    extension, 69–71
    flexion, 71–73
  evaluation, 57–59
  instability following, see Capsule instability, post-traumatic
  management principles, 59
  natural history, 56, 57
  treatment 'insult' and, 56, 59

see also Collateral ligament injury; Volar plate injury
Capsule instability, post-traumatic, 56, 58, 73–75
  chronic lateral instability repair, 74–75
  ligament attenuation, 75
Capsulectomy, 246, 249–250
  continuous passive motion (CPM) following, 249, 250
  flexion contracture and, 249–250
  oedema management, 246
  pain control, 246
  post surgical exercises, 246, 249
  splinting, 249, 250, 260
Cemented prostheses, 144, 145, 157
Central slip, 94
  attachment, 4
  injuries, 101
  reconstruction, 101–104
  release, 116
  repair, 101
  rupture, 100
Central slip injury, 233–237
  active/active assistive exercise, 236
  boutonnière deformity and, 127, 128, 233
  dynamic splinting, 236
  mobilization, 233–234
  postoperative programme, 234–236
  rest splinting, 236, 237
Central tendon rupture, PIP joint, 100
Cephalosporins, 147
Check ligaments, hyperextension prevention and, 50
Chondrosarcoma, 209
Clinodactyly, 189–191, 192
  anatomical aspects, 189
  incidence, 189
  treatment, 190–191
Coccidioidomycosis, 146
Collagen
  articular cartilage, 142
  scar tissue, 32
Collateral ligament injury
  capsule instability following, see Capsule instability, post-traumatic
  classification, 59, 60
  evaluation, 58
  lateral dislocations, 218
  rehabilitation, 217–225
  rupture, 60–61, 64, 98, 100, 218, 260
  splinting, 260
  sprains, 60, 218, 260
  surgical intervention, 61, 64
  surgical technique, 62
  treatment, 60–61, 218–225
Collateral ligament system, 4–8
  accessory collateral ligament, 4, 5, 6, 7, 12
  attachments, 4
  hyperextension prevention and, 50
  lateral stability and, 5–8, 56
  proper collateral ligament (PCL), 4–5, 6, 7–8

Condylar fractures, 78–80
  open reduction, 78–79
  semi open technique, 79
  T-shaped fracture, 79
Cone epiphyses, 189
Congential conditions, 188–201
Continuous passive motion device, 231–232
Coordination testing, 216
Corticosteroids, 46, 63, 71, 77, 91, 135, 266, 279, 280
  iontophoretic administration, 218
Cortisone, local injection, 124
CREST syndrome, 138
Critical corner, 5, 6, 8
Crystalline deposition disease, 150
  see also Gout
Cysts, 203–206
  ganglion, 203
  mucous, 203–206

Decadron with xylocaine, 218
Delta phalanx
  anatomy, 191–192
  heredity, 193
  incidence, 193
  treatment, 193
Developmental conditions, 203–209
Dexamethasone, 218
Dexterity testing, 216
Digital joint transfers, 170, 172
Distal interphalangeal (DIP) joint
  acute extensor tendon injuries, 114–116
  acute flexor tendon injuries, 111–113
  arthroplasty, 168
  avulsion fracture, 112, 115, 116
  chronic extensor tendon injuries, 116
  chronic flexor tendon injuries, 113–114
  closed injuries of extensor tendon, 114
  condylar configuration, 3–4
  extension moments, 43–44
  flexion, 40, 41, 42
  flexion strength, 42
  flexion-extension arc and, 16
  flexor profundus closed rupture, 111–113
  fracture with simultaneous PIP fracture, 91
  fractures involving both sides of joint, 91
  head of middle phalanx fracture, 87–88
  mallet finger, 88, 89, 115
  open lacerations, 111, 114
  PIP movement and, 46–47
  stiffness, effect of, 77
  volar plate, 17
  see also Distal phalanx, fractures of base
Distal phalanx, fractures of base, 88–90
  dorsal lip, 88–90

Distal phalanx (*contd*)
  longitudinal fracture running into DIP joint, 90
  mallet finger fracture, 88, 89
  volar lip, 90
Dorsal dislocation, PIP joint, 260
  dorsal splint, 225–227
  exercise programme, 226, 227
  figure of eight (swan-neck) splint, 227, 229
  with fracture and volar plate advancement, 227–229
  oedema control, 226, 227
  pain control, 226, 227
  patient explanation, 226, 229
  post-traumatic arthritis and, 152
  splint removal, 227
Dorsal expansion
  tendon adherence, 32
  as 'torque tube', 33
Down's syndrome, 189
Drug addicts, 146
Dupuytren's contracture, 19
Dynamic splinting, 69, 227, 233, 236, 245–246
  splints, 258–259
Dynamometer, 215

Eikenella corrodens, 147
Elevation, 243
  see also Heat in elevation
Enchondroma, 209
'End feel' of stiff joint, 243
Erosive osteoarthritis, 145–146
Explanation/counselling, 59, 221, 252
Extension contracture
  splinting and, 260
  surgical release, 69–71
Extensor digitorum communis insertion, 4
Extensor plus phenomenon, 99
Extensor tendon injuries
  chronic, 116
  closed, 99–100, 114
  complex dislocations, 97–98
  DIP joint, 114–116
  free tendon grafting and, 102–104
  infected, 104
  open lacerations, 100–104, 114
  PIP joint, 97–108
  see also Central slip injury
  pseudoboutonnière deformity, 98
Extensor tenodesis, 99, 107–108
Extrinsic (extensor) tendon, PIP, 94
Extrinsic tendon tenotomy, 126, 127, 128

Figure of eight (swan-neck) splint, 227, 229, 237
Flexion contracture
  aetiology, 71

  capsulectomy, 249–250
  elevation, 71
  flexor digitorum superficialis (FDS) damage and, 17
  psoriatic arthritis and, 135
  scleroderma and, 139
  surgical release, 71–73
Flexion-extension arc
  anatomical aspects, 14–16
  final (total) encompassment, 14
  metacarpo–phalangeal (MP)-tip placement arc, 14
Flexion-extension moments, analysis of, 24–28
Flexor digitorum profundus (FDP)
  attachment points, 4
  biomechanics, 40–41, 42
  closed rupture, 111–113
  estimate of tension, 27–28
  flexion strength of DIP/PIP joints and, 42
  range of excursion, independent movement of fingers and, 42
  volar plate relationships, 8, 12
Flexor digitorum superficialis (FDS), 42
  flexion contracture following damage, 17
  flexion strength of PIP joints and, 43
  tenodesis, 130, 138
Flexor tendon graft, 113–114
  failed, 16
Flexor tendon injuries
  associated with open wounds, 111
  chronic, 113–114
  DIP, 111–114
Forces at IP joints, 22–28
Free tendon grafting, 102–104
Functional position splinting, 230
Functional testing, fingers, 28, 216
Fungal infection, 146, 147

Ganglion, 203
Giant cell tumour of tendon sheath, *see* Pigmented villonodular synovitis
Goniometer
  dynamic measurement of torque-angle relationships, 37–40
Gout, 148–150
  clinical presentation, 148–150
  surgical excision of tophaceous deposits, 149, 150
  tophaceous, untreated, 148, 149
Grip measurement, 215
Gutter splint, 254

Haemochromatosis, 150, 152
Heat in elevation, 219, 227, 244, 245, 263
  joint mobilization and, 264
Heberden's nodes, 143

High voltage electrical stimulation, 219, 221
Hinge joints, biomechanics
  close fit, 29–31
  hydrodynamic lubrication, 29–30
Human bites, 147
Hydrocortisone, local injection, 71
Hydrodynamic lubrication, 29–30
Hydroxyapatite deposition disease, 150
Hyperextension, 51–53
Hypermobile hands, 51–52
Hyperphalangy, 188

Ice massage, 219, 227, 243, 246
Infections, pyogenic, 146–148
  animal bites, 147
  antibiotics and, 147
  debridement/surgical drainage, 146–147
  in drug addicts, 146
  human bites, 147
Interaxial finger length, Fibonacci series and, 16
Intra-articular fractions, 231–233
  continuous passive motion device, 231–232
  dynamic splinting, 233
  exercise, 232
  pin care, 233
  splinting procedure of Agee, 231, 232
Intrinsic minus finger, 22
Intrinsic tendon, PIP, 94
Iontophoresis, 218–219, 243

Jebson Hand Function Test, 216
Joint jack, 258
Joint mobilization, 69, 244, 262–268
  anterior/posterior glide, 267
  contraindications, 266
  goals, 264
  heat treatment/relaxation and, 264
  historical aspects, 262–263
  indications, 266
  joint play and, 263, 265
  longitudinal traction, 267
  medial/lateral tilt, 267
  Mennell's rules of joint manipulation, 265–266
  rotation, 267
  technique, 266–268
  theoretical basis, 263–264
Joint play, 263
  examination, 265
Joint torque goniometer, 37
  mathematical model of joint, 37–40
Juvenile rheumatoid arthritis, 133–135
  boutonnière deformity, 134, 135
  longstanding fixed flexion deformity, 134, 135
  swan-neck deformity, 134
  treatment, 134–135

Kinematic chain, 21

Lateral bands, 94, 95
   repositioning, 127
Lateral PIP dislocation, splinting, 260
Lateral stability, 5
   accessory collateral ligament and, 6, 7
   collateral ligament system and, 5–8, 56
   dynamic, 5
   passive, 5–6
   proper collateral ligament and, 6, 7–8
   volar plate system and, 7, 8
LMB finger springs, 258
LMB mallet splint, 253
LMB wirefoam splints, 253

Macrodactyly, 189
Mallet finger, 88, 89–115
   splinting, 289
Mennell's rules of joint manipulation, 265–266
Metacarpal bone length, Fibonacci series and, 16
Metacarpo-interphalangeal flexion-extension curve, 14
Metacarpo–phalangeal (MP) joint
   balancing of moments with PIP joints, 22–24
   biomechanics of extension, 44–45
   blocking, splints and, 259
   independent movement of fingers and, 41, 42
   passive hyperextension, 51
   structures limiting hyperextension, 45
Microvascular joint transfer, 170, 172
Middle phalanx, fractures of base, 80–86
   avulsion fracture of dorsal lip, 80–81
   avulsion fracture of volar lip, 81
   dorsal subluxation with volar fracture, 81–84
   lateral compression fractures, 86
   longitudinal middle phalanx fracture running into PIP joint, 86
   volar subluxation with dorsal fracture, 84–85
Motions, analysis at IP joints, 22–28
Mucous cyst, 154, 203–206
   clinical presentation, 204–205
   origin, 203–204
   osteoarthritis and, 204, 205, 206
   treatment, 205–206
Musculotendinous tightness, tests for, 214–215
Mycobacteria, 147
Mycobacterium marinum, 146

Non-steroidal anti-inflammatory agents (NSAIDs), 135, 144, 150

Oblique retinacular ligament, 18–19
   DIP flexion/extension and, 18
   hyperextension prevention and, 50–51
Oedema, 243, 246, 262
   biomechanical considerations, 33–34
   control, 218, 219, 230
   evaluation of viscous tissue factors, 37
   measurement, 212–213, 230, 243
Oligosyndactyly, 192
Osseous anatomy, 2–4
   asymmetry of articulation, 2–3
   central slip attachment, 4
   collateral ligament attachment, 4
   extensor digitorum communis insertion, 4
   flexor digitorum profundus (FDP) attachment, 4
   relative motion of articulating phalanges, 2
   rotation and, 2
   translation and, 2
   volar plate attachment points, 4
Osteoarthritis
   aetiology, 143
   articular cartilage biochemistry and, 142
   clinical presentation, 143
   DIP arthrodesis and, 144
   management, 143–145
   mucous cyst and, 204, 205, 206
   PIP arthrodesis and, 144, 145
   PIP arthroplasty and, 144–145, 245–246
   thumb arthrodesis, 145
Osteochondroma, 209
Osteosarcoma, 209

Pain, joint stiffness and, 243
   evaluation, 213–214
   relief, 218–221
Pain scale records, 214
Palmar plate, 51
Paratendon, 31
Pasteurella multocida, 147
Pedicle flaps, tendon repair and, 101–102
Penicillin, 147
Percutaneous Kirschner wiring, 83, 115
Perichondral arthroplasty, 172
Phalangeal bone length, Fibonacci series and, 16
Phenylbutazone, 150
Pigmented villonodular synovitis, 206–208
   aetiology, 206
   clinical presentation, 206–207
   pathological appearance, 207
   treatment, 207–208
   X-ray appearance, 207
Pin care programme, 230, 233
Pinch meter, 215

Polydactyly, bifid joints with, 197–199
   anatomical aspects, 197–198
   treatment, 198–199
   with triphalangeal thumb, 195
Polymethylmethacrylate-stabilized implants, 144, 145
Polysyndactyly, 192
Post-traumatic arthritis, 143, 152–154
   follow-up, 152–153
Power grip, osseous anatomy and, 2, 3
Proper collateral ligament (PCL), 4
   attachment, 4–5
   lateral stability and, 6, 7–8
Proteoglycans, 142
Proximal interphalangeal (PIP) joint
   adhesion prevention, exercise programme, 221, 223
   arthroplasty, 168–170, 245–246
   balancing of moments with MP joint, 22–24
   capsular innervation, 12
   changing moment arms with flexion/extension, 45–50
   condylar configuration, 3
   differential loading of fibres during movement, 45–46
   DIP movement and, 46–47
   extensor surface
      anatomy, 94–95
      injuries, 94–108
   extrinsic extensor common tendon and, 147
   flexion, 41
   flexion strength, 43
   flexion-extension arc, 16
   fractures
      base of middle phalanx, 80–86
      head of proximal phalanx, 77–80
      involving both sides of joint, 86–87
      necessitating amputation, 87
      with simultaneous DIP fracture, 91
   mathematical relationships, 16
   passive block to hyperextension, 51
   perichondral arthroplasty, 172
   retrocondylar space, 17–18
   stiffness, *see* Stiffness, joint
   volar plate, 17
Proximal phalanx fracture, 77–80, 229–233
   avulsion fractures of head, 77–78
   condylar fractures, 78–80
   delayed presentation, 79–80
   elevation programme, 230
   exercise, 230
   functional position splinting, 230
   light activities, 230
   oedema control, 230
   oedema evaluation, 230
   protected motion, 230
   treatment aims, 229, 230
Pseudoboutonnière deformity, 98
   splinting, 260
Psoriatic arthritis, 135–137
   arthrodesis, 135–136, 137
   medical treatment, 135

Psoriatic arthritis (contd)
  PIP arthroplasty, 136
  PIP flexion contracture, 135
  X-ray findings, 135

Radian, 22
Rehabilitation, stiff joints
  coordination/dexterity testing, 216
  elevation, 212–216
  functional testing, 216
  goniometric measurements, 214
  grip/pinch measurements, 215
  intrinsic/extrinsic tests for musculo-tendinous tightness, 214–215
  lateral stress, avoidance of, 221
  manipulative activities, 224
  oedema control, 218, 219
  oedema evaluation, 212–213
  pain evaluation, 213–214
  pain relief, 218–221
  palpation, 215
  patient counselling, 221, 252
  prevention of protective posturing, 218
  progressive resistive programme, 223
  range of motion evaluation, active/passive, 214
  remedial stage treatment, see Remedial stage treatment, PIP stiffness
  sensibility evaluation, 216
  splinting, 224–225
  treatment principles, 216–217
  visual inspection, 215
Remedial stage treatment, PIP stiffness
  active exercise programme, 244
  'end feel', prognosis and, 243
  evaluation procedure, 243
  heat in elevation, 244
  joint mobilization, 244
  oedema and, 243
  pain and, 243
  passive range of motion and, 244
  patient motivation and, 243–244
  splinting, 244–245
Renal arthropathy, 152
Resection arthroplasty, 157
Retinacular ligaments, 94–95, 96
  boutonnière deformity and, 95, 97
Retrocondylar space, PIP joint, 17–18
Retrograde massage, 226, 243, 246
Rheumatoid arthritis, 120–133
  arthrodesis and, 120
  arthroplasty and, 120
  boutonnière deformity
    pathogesesis, 121, 123
    treatment, 126–130, 240–243
  DIP joint, 120, 121
  extrinsic factors affecting PIP joint motion, 120–121
  flexor tenosynovitis and, 121
  intrinsic tightness secondary to MCP joint involvement, 121

  MCP joint, 120, 121
  rehabilitation of joints, 237–243
  rupture of terminal extensor tendon at DIP, 121
  sinovitis treatment, 124–126
  swan-neck deformity, 121–123, 130–133, 159, 237–239
  synovectomy, 123–126
Rotational movements, anatomical aspects, 2, 7
Rubenstein-Taybi syndrome, 192

Sarcoma, 209
Scar tissue
  biomechanical aspects, 32
  viscoelastic forces and, 29
Scleroderma, 138–140
  arthrodesis, 139–140
  distal ulcerations, 139
  MCP arthroplasty, 139
  MCP extension contracture, 139
  PIP flexion contracture, 139
  subcutaneous calcification, 139
Sensibility evaluation, 216
Serial cylinder casting, 69, 245, 254–259
  moulding, 255–256
Silastic implants, 157, 158
  joint replacement technique, 159, 160–164
Silicone spacer arthroplasty, 158
  osteoarthritis in PIP, 144–145
Silicone synovitis, 167–168
Splinting, 252–260
  boutonnière deformity, 242, 256, 259, 260
  buddy taping, 257–258
  design, 253–257
  dynamic IP joint splints, 258–259
  functional position, 230
  gutter splint, 254
  immobilization, 252–253
  purposes, 252
  ready-made commercial splints, 253
  rehabilitation, 224–225
  remedial stage treatment, 244–245
  serial cylinder casting, 254–257
  thermoplastic materials, 254
Sporotrichosis, 146
Spring wire (Capener) splint, 258, 259
Stack splint, 89, 92, 253
Staphylococcus aureus infection, 146
Stiffness, joint, 77, 212
  biomechanical aspects, 29, 31
  capsulectomy, 246, 249–250
  evaluation of viscoelastic constraints, 36
  oedema and, 33–34
  therapeutic management, see Rehabilitation, stiff joints
Stiles-Bunnel operation for intrinsic palsy, 52
Streptococcus infection, 146

Swan-neck deformity, 32
  arthrodesis, 130, 131–132, 238
  arthroplasty, 132–133, 238
  biomechanical aspects, 50, 52–53
  classification, 122
  figure of eight splint, 237
  flexor superficialis tenodesis, 130
  juvenile rheumatoid arthritis, 134
  mild, 130, 237, 238–239
  moderate, 130–131, 237–238
  pathogenesis, 121–123
  PIP rehabilitation, 237–239
  post-surgical exercise programme, 238, 239
  rheumatoid arthritis, 121–123, 130–133, 159, 237–239
  serial cylinder casting, 256
  severe, 131–133, 238–239
  splinting, 237, 259, 260
  systemic lupus erythematosus, 137–138
  tendon resection, 130, 238
  volar plate and, 17
Swanson burrs, 162
Symbrachydactyly, 188
Symphalangism, 199–200
  anatomical aspects, 199
  inheritance, 199
  treatment, 199–200
Syndactyly, 188
  with triphalangeal thumb, 195
  see also Polysyndactyly
Synovectomy
  boutonnière deformity and, 126, 242
  evaluation of results, 126
  indications, 124
  juvenile rheumatoid arthritis and, 134, 135
Synovial fluid, 30–31
Synovial sheath lubrication, 31
Synovitis in rheumatoid arthritis, 124–126
Systemic lupus erythematosus, 137–138
  arthrodesis, 138
  boutonnière deformity, 137
  causes of PIP joint deformity, 138
  MCP flexion deformities, 137–138
  MCP silicone arthroplasties, 138
  superficialis tenodesis, 138
  swan-neck deformity, 137–138

Tenodermadesis, 116
Tenosynovitis, 31
Thumb
  osteoarthritis, arthrodesis and, 145
  duplication/hypoplasia, 189
  joint fractures, 91–93
    bone of distal phalanx, 92–93
    head of proximal phalanx, 92
  see also Triphalangeal thumb
Torque, 22
  analysis at IP joints, 22–28
Torque-angle measurements, 34, 36–40
  dynamic measurements, 37–40

Torque-angle measurements (*contd*)
  evaluation of viscoelastic constraints, 36
  evaluation of viscous tissue factors, 37
  static measurements, 36
Transcutaneous electrical nerve stimulation (TENS), 71, 291, 227, 243, 246
Translational movement, 2, 7
Triamcinolone, 135
Triphalangeal thumb
  anatomical aspects, 194–195
  brachymesophalangeal, 194, 196
  dolichophalangeal, 194–195, 196
  incidence, 195
  intermediate type, 195, 197
  with polydactyly, 195
  with syndactyly, 195
  treatment, 196–197
Tuberculosis, IP joint involvement, 146
Tumours, developmental, 209

Volar capsule, *see* Volar plate
Volar lip fracture, 152
Volar metal splint, 115
Volar plate, 8–12
  arthroplasty, *see* Volar plate arthroplasty
  attachment points, 4, 8
  boutonnière deformity and, 17
  DIP, 17
  injury, *see* Volar plate injury
  hyperextension prevention and, 17, 50, 51
  lateral stability and, 6, 7, 8, 56
  'suspended sheaths' concept and, 12
Volar plate arthroplasty, 17, 168–170
  for dorsal fracture dislocation, 168
  splinting, 260
Volar plate injury
  capsular instability and, *see* Capsular instability, post-traumatic
  classification, 159, 160
  dorsal dislocation, 63–64
    with chip fracture, 64, 81
  evaluation, 58, 64
  management, 62–66
  patterns of, 62–64
  volar dislocation management, 66–68
    with central slip injury, 66, 67
    with collateral ligament injury, 66

Webs, finger skin, 17
Wedge osteotomy, 190–191, 193, 196
Wynn-Parry splint, 258

Xanthoma, 17